Injury & Trauma Sourcebook

Learning Disabilities Sourcebook, 2nd Edition

Leukemia Sourcebook

Liver Disorders Sourcebook

Lung Disorders Sourcebook

Medical Tests Sourcebook, 3rd Edition

Men's Health Concerns Sourcebook, 2nd Edition

Mental Health Disorders Sourcebook, 3rd Edition

Mental Retardation Sourcebook

Movement Disorders Sourcebook

Multiple Sclerosis Sourcebook

Muscular Dystrophy Sourcebook

Obesity Sourcebook

Osteoporosis Sourcebook

Pain Sourcebook, 3rd Edition

Pediatric Cancer Sourcebook

Physical & Mental Issues in Aging Sourcebook

Podiatry Sourcebook, 2nd Edition

Pregnancy & Birth Sourcebook, 2nd Edition

Prostate Cancer Sourcebook

Prostate & Urological Disorders Sourcebook

Reconstructive & Cosmetic Surgery Sourcebook

Rehabilitation Sourcebook

Respiratory Disorders Sourcebook, 2nd Edition

Sexually Transmitted Diseases Sourcebook, 3rd Edition

Sleep Disorders Sourcebook, 2nd Edition

Smoking Concerns Sourcebook

Sports Injuries Sourcebook, 3rd Edition

Stress-Related Disorders Sourcebook, 2nd Edition

Stroke Sourcebook, 2nd Edition

Surgery Sourcebook, 2nd Edition

Thyroid Disorders Sourcebook

Transplantation Sourcebook

Traveler's Health Sourcebook

Urinary Tract & Kidney Diseases & Disorders Sourcebook, 2nd Edition

Vegetarian Sourcebook

Women's Health Concerns Sourcebook, 2nd Edition

Workplace Health & Safety Sourcebook

Worldwide Health Sourcebook

Teen Health Series

Abuse and Violence Information for Teens

Alcohol Information for Teens

Allergy Information for Teens

Asthma Information for Teens

Body Information for Teens

Cancer Information for Teens

Complementary & Alternative Medicine Information for Teens

Diabetes Information for Teens

Diet Information for Teens, 2nd Edition

Drug Information for Teens, 2nd Edition

Eating Disorders Information for Teens

Fitness Information for Teens, 2nd Edition

Learning Disabilities Information for Teens

Mental Health Information for Teens, 2nd Edition

Pregnancy Information for Teens

Sexual Health Information for Teens, 2nd Edition

Skin Health Information for Teens

Sleep Information for Teens

Sports Injuries Information for Teens, 2nd Edition

Stress Information for Teens

Suicide Information for Teens

Tobacco Information for Teens

Medical Tests
SOURCEBOOK
Third Edition

Health Reference Series

Third Edition

Medical Tests
SOURCEBOOK

Basic Consumer Health Information about X-Rays, Blood Tests, Stool and Urine Tests, Biopsies, Mammography, Endoscopic Procedures, Ultrasound Exams, Computed Tomography, Magnetic Resonance Imaging (MRI), Nuclear Medicine, Genetic Testing, Home-Use Tests, and More

Along with Facts about Preventive Care and Screening Test Guidelines, Screening and Assessment Tests Associated with Such Specific Concerns as Cancer, Heart Disease, Allergies, Diabetes, Thyroid Disfunction, and Infertility, a Glossary of Related Terms, and a Directory of Resources for Additional Help and Information

Edited by
Karen Bellenir

Omnigraphics

P.O. Box 31-1640, Detroit, MI 48231

Bibliographic Note

Because this page cannot legibly accommodate all the copyright notices, the Bibliographic Note portion of the Preface constitutes an extension of the copyright notice.

Edited by Karen Bellenir

Health Reference Series

Karen Bellenir, *Managing Editor*
David A. Cooke, M.D., *Medical Consultant*
Elizabeth Collins, *Research and Permissions Coordinator*
Cherry Stockdale, *Permissions Assistant*
EdIndex, Services for Publishers, *Indexers*

* * *

Omnigraphics, Inc.

Matthew P. Barbour, *Senior Vice President*
Kevin M. Hayes, *Operations Manager*

* * *

Peter E. Ruffner, *Publisher*

Copyright © 2008 Omnigraphics, Inc.

ISBN 978-0-7808-1040-2

Library of Congress Cataloging-in-Publication Data

Medical tests sourcebook : basic consumer health information about x-rays, blood tests, stool and urine tests, biopsies, mammography, endoscopic procedures, ultrasound exams, computed tomography, magnetic resonance imaging (mri), nuclear medicine, genetic testing, home-use tests, and more; along with facts about preventive care and screening test guidelines, screening and assessment tests associated with such specific concerns as cancer, heart disease, allergies, diabetes, thyroid disfunction, and infertility, a glossary of related terms, and a directory of resources for additional help and information / edited by Karen Bellenir. -- 3rd ed.
    p. cm.
Includes bibliographical references and index.
Summary: "Provides basic consumer health information about medical testing for disease diagnosis, screening, and monitoring in children and adults. Includes index, glossary of related terms, and other resources"--Provided by publisher.
ISBN 978-0-7808-1040-2 (hard cover : alk. paper) 1. Diagnosis--Popular works. 2. Diagnosis, Laboratory--Popular works. 3. Medicine, Popular. I. Bellenir, Karen.
RC71.3.M45 2008
616.07'5--dc22

2008031326

Table of Contents

Visit www.healthreferenceseries.com to view *A Contents Guide to the Health Reference Series*, a listing of more than 14,000 topics and the volumes in which they are covered.

Part III: Laboratory Tests of Body Fluids and Specimens

Part IV: Imaging Tests

Part V: Electrical, Endoscopic, and Functionality Exams

Part VI: In-Home and Self-Ordered Medical Tests

Part VII: Additional Help and Information

Preface

About This Book

Medical testing processes can be found at every stage of the lifespan. Screening tests serve as tools to identify people at risk for certain disorders. Diagnostic tests can help pinpoint specific markers of disease or rule out alternate possibilities. Medical tests can also be used to monitor the course of disease progression, to make crucial decisions about initiating or withdrawing therapies, and to evaluate the effects of treatment. Despite their widespread use, however, medical testing technologies may seem confusing to many people, and the process of deciphering test reports can be bewildering.

Medical Tests Sourcebook, Third Edition provides updated information about the vast and ever-growing arena of screening, diagnostic, and disease-monitoring exams. It provides an overview of tests for preventive care in infants, children, and adults. It discusses screening and assessment tests associated with such specific concerns as cancer, heart disease, diabetes, kidney disease, thyroid dysfunction, infertility, osteoporosis, sexually transmitted diseases, allergies, hearing loss, and vision problems. It offers details about blood testing, biopsy procedures, imaging tests—including x-rays, ultrasounds, computed tomography, magnetic resonance imaging, and nuclear medicine—electrical and endoscopic procedures, and tests designed for home use. The book concludes with a glossary of related terms, information about on-line health screening tools, and resources for more information about medical tests.

How to Use This Book

This book is divided into parts and chapters. Parts focus on broad areas of interest. Chapters are devoted to single topics within a part.

Part I: Routine Screening Tests provides information about procedures used to detect genetic, metabolic, hormonal, and functional disorders in newborns. It also describes assessments used to evaluate children's growth and development, and it explains guidelines for preventive healthcare services for adults.

Part II: Screening and Assessment Tests Associated with Specific Concerns provides facts about the types of tests that are commonly used to identify and monitor such conditions as cancer, heart disease, diabetes, kidney disease, and infectious diseases. The part concludes with information about tests used to assess hearing loss and vision-related concerns.

Part III: Laboratory Tests of Body Fluids and Specimens describes processes that are used to evaluate samples of blood, urine, stool, or other tissues or substances of the body. It explains how test results can be used to identify or rule out specific health problems or to evaluate the results of a particular course of treatment. A separate chapter on genetic testing discusses the benefits, limitations, and risks of tests that are used to identify chromosome, gene, or protein changes that are associated with inherited disorders.

Part IV: Imaging Tests explains how x-rays, ultrasounds, and other imaging technologies are used to allow physicians to see inside the body in order to detect health concerns or guide treatments. Individual chapters describe how the various procedures work and explain patient safety precautions.

Part V: Electrical, Endoscopic, and Functionality Exams includes information about procedures that monitor and evaluate the performance of the body's organs and systems. These include electrocardiograms (EKGs) and other tests used to evaluate how well the heart is functioning, electroencephalograms (EEGs), electromyography, and endoscopic tests.

Part VI: In-Home and Self-Ordered Medical Tests discusses the advantages and disadvantages of using kits to perform certain medical tests at home. It offers suggestions for ensuring that purchased at-home tests are approved by the U.S. Food and Drug Administration, and it explains when test results should be evaluated by a healthcare professional.

Part VII: Additional Help and Information includes a glossary of terms related to medical tests, a list of online health screening tools, and a directory of resources for more information about medical tests.

Bibliographic Note

This volume contains documents and excerpts from publications issued by the following U.S. government agencies: Agency for Healthcare Research and Quality; National Cancer Institute; National Center for Biotechnology Information; National Center on Birth Defects and Developmental Disabilities; National Digestive Diseases Information Clearinghouse; National Eye Institute; National, Heart, Lung, and Blood Institute; National HIV Testing Resources; National Human Genome Research Institute; National Institute for Allergies and Infectious Diseases; National Institute of Diabetes and Digestive and Kidney Diseases; National Kidney and Urologic Diseases Information Clearinghouse; National Library of Medicine; National Women's Health Information Center; NIH Clinical Center; and the U.S. Food and Drug Administration.

In addition, this volume contains copyrighted documents from the following organizations and individuals: A.D.A.M. Inc.; AIDS Treatment Data Network – The Network; American Academy of Family Physicians; American Academy of Orthopaedic Surgeons; American Academy of Pediatrics; American Association for Clinical Chemistry; American Cancer Society, Inc.; American Heart Association, Inc.; American Optometric Association; American Pregnancy Association; American Rhinologic Society; American Society for Clinical Laboratory Science; American Society for Gastrointestinal Endoscopy; American Society for Reproductive Medicine; American Society of Echocardiography; American Society of Radiologic Technologists; American Speech-Language-Hearing Association; American Thyroid Association; David E. Bernstein, M.D.; Cleveland Clinic Foundation; Cystic Fibrosis Foundation; Dartmouth-Hitchcock Medical Center; Frederick Memorial Healthcare System; Glaucoma Research Foundation; Hepatitis B Foundation; Imaginis Corporation; March of Dimes Birth Defects Foundation; Medical College of Wisconsin, *HealthLink*; Muscular Dystrophy Association of the United States; MyThyroid.com; Nemours Foundation; New Zealand Dermatological Society; James Norman, MD,

FACS, FACE; Society for Vascular Ultrasound; Society of American Gastrointestinal Endoscopic Surgeons; Sue Stiles Program in Integrative Oncology at the UCLA Jonsson Cancer Center; University of California, Los Angeles (UCLA) Medical Center; University of Michigan Health System; University of Washington Medical Center; and the University of Washington, Seattle.

Full citation information is provided on the first page of each chapter or section. Every effort has been made to secure all necessary rights to reprint the copyrighted material. If any omissions have been made, please contact Omnigraphics to make corrections for future editions.

Acknowledgements

In addition to the organizations who have contributed to this *Sourcebook*, special thanks go to editorial assistants Nicole Salerno and Elizabeth Bellenir, research and permissions coordinator Liz Collins, and permissions assistant Cherry Stockdale.

About the Health Reference Series

The *Health Reference Series* is designed to provide basic medical information for patients, families, caregivers, and the general public. Each volume takes a particular topic and provides comprehensive coverage. This is especially important for people who may be dealing with a newly diagnosed disease or a chronic disorder in themselves or in a family member. People looking for preventive guidance, information about disease warning signs, medical statistics, and risk factors for health problems will also find answers to their questions in the *Health Reference Series*. The *Series*, however, is not intended to serve as a tool for diagnosing illness, in prescribing treatments, or as a substitute for the physician/patient relationship. All people concerned about medical symptoms or the possibility of disease are encouraged to seek professional care from an appropriate health care provider.

A Note about Spelling and Style

Health Reference Series editors use *Stedman's Medical Dictionary* as an authority for questions related to the spelling of medical terms and the *Chicago Manual of Style* for questions related to grammatical structures, punctuation, and other editorial concerns. Consistent adherence is not always possible, however, because the individual volumes within the *Series* include many documents from a wide variety of different producers and copyright holders, and the editor's primary goal is to present material from each source as accurately as is possible following the terms specified by each document's producer. This sometimes means that information in different chapters or sections may follow other guidelines and alternate spelling authorities. For example, occasionally a copyright holder may require that eponymous terms be shown in possessive forms (Crohn's disease *vs.* Crohn disease) or that British spelling norms be retained (leukaemia *vs.* leukemia).

Locating Information within the Health Reference Series

The *Health Reference Series* contains a wealth of information about a wide variety of medical topics. Ensuring easy access to all the fact sheets, research reports, in-depth discussions, and other material contained within the individual books of the *Series* remains one of our highest priorities. As the *Series* continues to grow in size and scope, however, locating the precise information needed by a reader may become more challenging.

A Contents Guide to the Health Reference Series was developed to direct readers to the specific volumes that address their concerns. It presents an extensive list of diseases, treatments, and other topics of general interest compiled from the Tables of Contents and major index headings. To access *A Contents Guide to the Health Reference Series*, visit www.healthreferenceseries.com.

Medical Consultant

Medical consultation services are provided to the *Health Reference Series* editors by David A. Cooke, M.D. Dr. Cooke is a graduate of Brandeis University, and he received his M.D. degree from the University of Michigan. He completed residency training at the University of Wisconsin Hospital and Clinics. He is board-certified in Internal Medicine. Dr. Cooke currently works as part of the University of Michigan Health System and practices in Ann Arbor, MI. In his free time, he enjoys writing, science fiction, and spending time with his family.

Our Advisory Board

We would like to thank the following board members for providing guidance to the development of this *Series*:

- Dr. Lynda Baker,
  Associate Professor of Library and Information Science,
  Wayne State University, Detroit, MI

- Nancy Bulgarelli,
  William Beaumont Hospital Library, Royal Oak, MI

- Karen Imarisio,
  Bloomfield Township Public Library, Bloomfield Township, MI

- Karen Morgan,
  Mardigian Library, University of Michigan-Dearborn,
  Dearborn, MI

- Rosemary Orlando,
  St. Clair Shores Public Library, St. Clair Shores, MI

Health Reference Series *Update Policy*

The inaugural book in the *Health Reference Series* was the first edition of *Cancer Sourcebook* published in 1989. Since then, the *Series* has been enthusiastically received by librarians and in the medical community. In order to maintain the standard of providing high-quality health information for the layperson the editorial staff at Omnigraphics felt it was necessary to implement a policy of updating volumes when warranted.

Medical researchers have been making tremendous strides, and it is the purpose of the *Health Reference Series* to stay current with the most recent advances. Each decision to update a volume is made on an individual basis. Some of the considerations include how much new information is available and the feedback we receive from people who use the books. If there is a topic you would like to see added to the update list, or an area of medical concern you feel has not been adequately addressed, please write to:

Editor
Health Reference Series
Omnigraphics, Inc.
P.O. Box 31-1640
Detroit, MI 48231-1640
E-mail: editorial@omnigraphics.com

Part One

Routine Screening Tests

Chapter 1

Newborn Screening Tests

Every state and U.S. territory routinely screens newborns for certain genetic, metabolic, hormonal, and functional disorders. Most of these birth defects have no immediate visible effects on a baby but, unless detected and treated early, can cause physical problems, mental retardation, and, in some cases, death.

Except for hearing screening, all newborn screening tests are done using a few drops of blood from the newborn's heel. Fortunately, most babies are given a clean bill of health when tested. However, in 2002, about 3,300 babies were found to have metabolic disorders and another 12,000 to 16,000 to have hearing impairment.[1, 2] In these cases, early diagnosis and proper treatment can make the difference between healthy development and lifelong impairment.

Which newborn screening tests are most likely to be given to my baby?

This depends on where your baby is born. Currently each state or region operates by law its own newborn screening program. Individual programs vary widely in the number and types of conditions for which they test. Some states test for as few as four disorders, while others test for 30 or more.[3]

You can find out which tests are routinely done in your state by asking your health care provider or state health department. You can also visit the National Newborn Screening and Genetics Resource Center website available online at http://genes-r-us.uthscsa.edu. This site also lists commercial and nonprofit laboratories that provide comprehensive newborn screening for parents considering having their baby tested for more disorders than those screened for by their state.

All states and U.S. territories screen newborns for phenylketonuria (PKU), hypothyroidism, and galactosemia.[3] The test for PKU was the nation's first newborn screening test. Developed with the help of the March of Dimes, it has been routinely administered since the 1960s. PKU affects about one baby in 25,000.[4] Babies with the disorder cannot process a part of protein called phenylalanine, which is found in nearly all foods. Without treatment, phenylalanine builds up in the blood stream and causes brain damage and mental retardation.

When PKU is detected early, mental retardation can be prevented by feeding the baby a special formula that is low in phenylalanine. This low-phenylalanine diet will need to be followed throughout childhood, adolescence, and generally, for life.

Women of childbearing age with PKU need to remain on this special diet before and during pregnancy. This will often prevent mental retardation in their children by avoiding fetal exposure to high maternal phenylalanine levels.[5]

Congenital hypothyroidism is the most common disorder identified by routine screening. It affects at least one baby in 5,000.[4] Congenital hypothyroidism is a thyroid hormone deficiency that retards growth and brain development. If it is detected in time, a baby can be treated with oral doses of thyroid hormone to permit normal development.

Galactosemia, which affects about one baby in 50,000, can cause death in infancy, or blindness and mental retardation.[4] A baby with galactosemia is unable to convert galactose, a sugar in milk, into glucose, a sugar the body uses as an energy source. The treatment for galactosemia is to eliminate milk and all other dairy products from the baby's diet; this dietary restriction is lifelong.[5]

Almost all states also screen for sickle cell anemia, congenital adrenal hyperplasia (CAH), and hearing loss. Sickle cell anemia is an inherited blood disease that can cause bouts of pain, damage to vital organs, and, sometimes, death in childhood. Young children with sickle cell anemia are especially prone to dangerous bacterial infections such as pneumonia and meningitis. Vigilant medical care and early treatment with penicillin, beginning in infancy, can dramatically reduce these serious complications and the deaths that can result from them. Sickle cell anemia affects about one in 400 African-American babies[1] and at least one in 5,000 of all babies in the United States.[4]

CAH is a group of disorders in which there is a deficiency of certain hormones, sometimes affecting genital development. In severe cases, CAH also can cause life-threatening salt loss from the body. Lifelong treatment with the missing hormones suppresses this disease, which occurs in about one in 25,000 babies.[4]

Up to three to four in 1,000 newborns have significant hearing impairment.[2] Without testing, most babies with hearing loss are not diagnosed until two or three years of age.[2] By this time, they often have delayed speech and language development. Detection of hearing loss in the neonatal period allows the baby to be fitted with hearing aids before six months of age, helping prevent serious speech and language problems.

The National Center for Hearing Assessment and Management provides resources for both health care providers and families. The center has produced a 6-minute educational video for parents "Giving Your Baby a Sound Beginning," which is available in English and Spanish. The video may be viewed online at no charge (http://www .infant hearing.org/videos/index.html), or a VHS copy may be purchased for $15.

What other disorders can newborn screening detect?

Recent advances in technology, such as tandem mass spectrometry, now make it possible to screen for about 55 disorders. The March of Dimes would like to see all babies in all states screened for at least 29 specific disorders for which effective treatment is available. This March of Dimes recommendation is based on endorsement of a report by the American College of Medical Genetics (commissioned by the Health Resources and Services Administration) urging screening for the 29 disorders,[4] and will be updated when appropriate. (In addition to these 29 disorders, the March of Dimes recommends that states report screening results of 25 "secondary target" conditions. However, treatment for these additional disorders is generally not yet available.)

Treatment for the 29 disorders is likely to improve the health of children who are affected by them. The disorders are grouped into five categories:

Organic acid metabolism disorders: Each disease in this group of inherited disorders results from the loss of activity of an enzyme

5

involved in the breakdown of amino acids, the building blocks of proteins, and other substances (lipids, sugars, steroids). When any of these chemicals is not properly broken down, toxic acids build up in the body. Without treatment, these disorders can result in coma and death during the first month of life.

- IVA (isovaleric acidemia)
- GA I (glutaric acidemia)
- HMG (3-OH 3-CH3 glutaric aciduria)
- MCD (multiple carboxylase deficiency)
- MUT (methylmalonic acidemia due to mutase deficiency)
- Cbl A,B (methylmalonic acidemia)
- 3MCC (3-methylcrotonyl-CoA carboxylase deficiency)
- PROP (propionic acidemia)
- BKT (beta-ketothiolase deficiency)

Fatty acid oxidation disorders: This group of disorders is characterized by inherited defects of enzymes needed to convert fat into energy. When the body runs out of glucose (sugar), it normally breaks down fat to support production of alternate fuels (ketones) in the liver. Because individuals with these disorders have a block in this pathway, their cells suffer an energy crisis when they run out of glucose. This is most likely to occur when an individual is ill or skips meals. Without treatment, the brain and many organs can be affected, sometimes progressing to coma and death.

- MCAD (medium-chain acyl-CoA dehydrogenase deficiency)
- VLCAD (very long-chain acyl-CoA dehydrogenase deficiency)
- LCHAD (long-chain L-3-OH acyl-CoA dehydrogenase deficiency)
- TFP (trifunctional protein deficiency)
- CUD (carnitine uptake defect)

Amino acid metabolism disorders: This is a diverse group of disorders with varying degrees of severity. Some individuals lack enzymes that are needed to break down the building blocks of protein called amino acids. Others have deficiencies in enzymes that help the body rid itself of the nitrogen incorporated in amino acid molecules. Toxic levels of amino acids or ammonia can build up in the body causing a variety of signs and symptoms, and even death.

- PKU (phenylketonuria)
- MSUD (maple syrup urine disease)
- HCY (homocystinuria due to CBS deficiency)
- CIT (citrullinemia)
- ASA (argininosuccinic acidemia)
- TYR I (tyrosinemia type I)

Hemoglobinopathies: These inherited diseases of red blood cells result in varying degrees of anemia (shortage of red blood cells) and other health problems. The severity of these disorders varies greatly from one person to the next.

- Hb SS (sickle cell anemia)
- Hb S/Th (hemoglobin S/beta-thalassemia)
- Hb S/C (hemoglobin S/C disease)

Others: This mixed group of disorders includes some diseases that are inherited and others that are not. This group of disorders varies greatly in severity, from mild to life threatening.

- CH (congenital hypothyroidism)
- BIOT (biotinidase deficiency)
- CAH (congenital adrenal hyperplasia due to 21-hydroxylase deficiency)
- GALT (classical galactosemia)
- HEAR (hearing loss)
- CF (cystic fibrosis)

How are screening tests done?

All of these disorders, except for hearing loss, are detected by a blood test. The baby's heel is pricked to obtain a few drops of blood for laboratory analysis. The same blood sample can be used to screen for 55 or more disorders. Usually, the baby's blood specimen is sent to a state public health laboratory for testing, and findings are sent to the health care professional responsible for the infant's care. Babies are screened for hearing loss with one of two tests that measure how the baby responds to sounds. These tests are done in the newborn hospital nursery, using either a tiny soft earphone or microphone that is placed in the baby's ear. If either of these tests shows abnormal results, the baby needs more extensive hearing testing to see if he does have hearing loss.

How soon after birth should screening tests be done?

A blood specimen should be taken from every newborn before hospital release, usually at 24 to 48 hours of life. Some of the tests (such as the one for PKU) may not give accurate results, however, if they are done too soon after birth. Because of early hospital discharge, some babies are tested within the first 24 hours of life. Because some cases of PKU can be missed when the test is performed this early, the American Academy of Pediatrics recommends that a repeat specimen be taken one to two weeks later from infants whose initial test was taken within the first 24 hours of life.[6] Some states routinely screen twice in the newborn nursery and again approximately two weeks later. Hearing tests are usually performed before the baby is discharged from the hospital. Babies born outside the hospital should have newborn screening tests done before the seventh day of life.[6]

What does an abnormal test result mean?

Parents should not be overly alarmed by abnormal test results, as the initial screening tests give only preliminary information that must be immediately followed by more precise testing. Most babies with abnormal thyroid screening test results, for example, prove normal in further testing, as do most with abnormal hearing test results.[6, 7]

What should I do if my child is diagnosed with one of the conditions for which he was tested?

Your child may need follow-up treatment at a pediatric center that specializes in children with metabolic or genetic conditions. It is essential for your child's healthy development that you follow the health care provider's treatment recommendations. As your child grows, he or she may need careful, continued evaluations and monitoring.

If one of my children has a disorder, will my other children have it?

For most of the disorders detected by newborn screening, when one child in a family is affected, the chance of the same birth defect occurring in a sibling is one in four. The chances remain the same with each pregnancy. Parents who have a baby with one of these disorders can discuss their risk of having another affected child with their health care provider or a genetic counselor. These disorders are inherited when both parents have the same abnormal gene and pass it on to their baby. A parent who has the abnormal gene, but not the disease, is called a carrier. The health of a carrier is rarely affected.

Congenital hypothyroidism usually is not inherited from parents.[6] The siblings of those who have this disorder are seldom affected.

Hearing loss can be passed on through parents' genes. However, other causes of hearing loss, such as infections that are passed on to the baby during pregnancy or birth, are unlikely to recur in another pregnancy.

Does the March of Dimes fund research on newborn screening?

The March of Dimes has long supported research related to newborn screening. In the 1960s, a March of Dimes grantee developed the first PKU screening test. Other grantees developed screening tests for biotinidase deficiency and congenital adrenal hyperplasia and contributed to the development of testing for hypothyroidism. The March of Dimes also funds research aimed at improving the treatment of children with a number of the screened disorders, and for many years, has worked to expand and improve newborn screening programs.

References

1. General Accounting Office. *Newborn Screening: Characteristics of State Programs*. Washington, DC: U.S. General Accounting Office, 2003. Publication GAO-03-449. Data from the National Newborn Screening and Genetics Resource Center.

2. National Center for Hearing Assessment and Management, Utah State University. http://www.infanthearing.org/index.html. Accessed 9/28/04.

3. National Newborn Screening and Genetics Resources Center. U.S. National Screening Status Report. Updated 9/8/04.

4. American College of Medical Genetics. Newborn Screening: Toward a Uniform Screening Panel and System. Final Report, March 8, 2005. http://mchb.hrsa.gov/screening.

5. Tuerck, J., et al. *The Northwest Regional Newborn Screening Program Oregon Practitioner's Manual, 7th edition.* Oregon Health & Science University and Oregon Department of Human Services, 2004.

6. American Academy of Pediatrics Committee on Genetics. Newborn Screening Fact Sheets. *Pediatrics*, volume 98, number 3, September 1996.

7. American Academy of Pediatrics. Hearing: Understanding Screening Results. http://www.medem.com/medlb/article _detaillb.cfm?article_ID=ZZZ88BR175D&sub_cat=108. Accessed 9/30/04.

Chapter 2

Checkups for Children

Chapter Contents

Section 2.1

Routine Checkups and Tests

"Checkups, Tests, and Immunizations," Chapter 2 in
The Pocket Guide to Good Health for Children, Agency for
Healthcare Research and Quality (www.ahrq.gov).

Checkups allow your doctor to review your child's growth and development, perform tests, or give shots.

Checkups also are a good time for parents to ask questions. Make a list of your questions and concerns and bring it with you. The doctor will have answers to many questions about your child, such as whether your child is eating too much or too little, whether he or she seems uncoordinated, or what to do if your child isn't sleeping well.

Some authorities recommend checkups at ages 2–4 weeks; 2, 4, 6, 9, 12, 15, and 18 months; and 2, 3, 4, 5, 6, 8, 10, 12, 14, 16, and 18 years.

Some children may need to be seen more often, others less.

Newborn Screening

Required newborn screening tests vary depending on which state you live in. With new scientific discoveries, state newborn screening programs are growing rapidly. A few states screen for more than 30 disorders.

Some common tests check for phenylketonuria (PKU), thyroid disease, and sickle cell disease. If you are pregnant, check with your doctor or local health department about tests required by your state.

Immunizations

Immunizations (shots) protect your child from many serious diseases. Below is a list of immunizations and when most children should receive them. Some children, for example those with chronic illnesses or those in certain areas of the country, may need to follow a different schedule. Your child's doctor can help you decide which immunizations your child needs and when. Be sure to talk with the doctor or nurse about possible reactions and what you should do if your child has one.

12

- **Hepatitis B:** At birth, 1–4 months, and 6–18 months.

- **Diphtheria, tetanus, pertussis:** At 2 months, 4 months, 6 months, 15–18 months, and 4 to 6 years.

- **Tetanus-diphtheria:** At 11–12 years.

- **Haemophilus influenzae type B:** At 2 months, 4 months, 6 months, and 12–15 months. Depending on the type of vaccine your doctor uses, the 6-month dose may not be needed.

- **Inactivated poliovirus:** At 2 months, 4 months, 6–18 months, and 4–6 years.

- **Measles, mumps, rubella:** At 12–15 months and 4–6 years. Children who have not previously received the second dose should receive it by 11–12 years.

- **Chickenpox (varicella):** At 12–18 months if your child lacks a reliable history of chickenpox.

- **Pneumococcal disease (PCV vaccine):** At 2 months, 4 months, 6 months, and 12–15 months.

- **Pneumococcal disease (PPV vaccine):** Recommended in addition to PCV for certain high-risk groups. Ask your doctor.

- **Hepatitis A:** For children in selected areas or in certain high risk groups. At two years or older, two doses at least six months apart. Ask your doctor.

- **Influenza:** Yearly for children six months or older with risk factors such as asthma, cardiac disease, sickle cell disease, HIV, and diabetes; and household members of persons in groups at high risk. Government experts recently recommended that all children aged 6–23 months receive annual influenza vaccine starting in the fall of 2004. Immunization schedules for influenza may change. For the latest information, check with your doctor or go to: www .cdc.gov/flu.

From time to time, other immunization schedules may change, too. Check with your doctor or go to: www.cdc.gov/nip.

Vision and Hearing

Your children's vision should be tested before age five. Some experts recommend vision testing in infancy. Your children also may need vision tests as they grow.

Many states require newborn hearing screening.

If at any age your child has any of the vision or hearing warning signs listed below, be sure to talk with your child's doctor.

Vision Warning Signs

- Eyes turning inward (crossing) or outward
- Squinting
- Headaches
- Not doing as well in school work as before
- Blurred or double vision

Hearing Warning Signs

- Poor response to noise or voice
- Slow language and speech development
- Abnormal-sounding speech

Warning: Listening to very loud music, especially with earphones, can permanently damage your child's hearing.

Lead

Lead can harm your child, slowing physical and mental growth and damaging many parts of the body. The most common way children get lead poisoning is by being around old house paint that is chipping or peeling. Some authorities recommend lead tests at one and two years of age.

Look at the questions below. If you answer "yes" to any of them, it may mean that your child needs lead tests earlier and more often than other children.

- Has your child lived in or regularly visited a house built before 1950? (This could include a day care center, a preschool, or the home of a babysitter or relative)

- Has your child lived in or regularly visited a house built before 1978 (the year lead-based paint was banned for residential use) with recent, ongoing, or planned renovation or remodeling?

- Has your child had a brother or sister, housemate, or playmate been followed or treated for lead poisoning?

Tuberculosis

Children may need a tuberculosis skin test if they have had close contact with a person who has tuberculosis (TB), live in an area where TB is more common than average (such as a Native American reservation, a homeless shelter, or an institution), or have recently moved from Asia, Africa, Central America, South America, the Caribbean, or the Pacific Islands.

Section 2.2

Developmental Screening

From "Child Development," 2005, and "Learn the Signs. Act Early: Developmental Screening," 2007, Centers for Disease Control and Prevention (www.cdc.gov).

What is child development?

A child's growth is more than just physical. Children grow, develop, and learn throughout their lives, starting at birth. A child's development can be followed by how they play, learn, speak, and behave.

What is a developmental delay? Will my child just grow out of it?

Skills such as taking a first step, smiling for the first time, and waving "bye bye" are called developmental milestones. Children reach milestones in playing, learning, speaking, behaving, and moving (crawling, walking). A developmental delay is when your child does not reach these milestones at the same time as other children the same age. If your child is not developing properly, there are things you can do that may help. Most of the time, a developmental problem is not something your child will "grow out of" on his or her own. But with help, your child could reach his or her full potential.

What is developmental screening?

Doctors and nurses use developmental screening to tell if children are learning basic skills when they should, or if they might have problems. Your child's doctor may ask you questions or talk and play with your child during an exam to see how he or she learns, speaks, behaves, and moves. Since there is no lab or blood test to tell if your child may have a delay, the developmental screening will help tell if your child needs to see a specialist.

Why is developmental screening important?

Many children with behavioral or developmental disabilities are missing vital opportunities for early detection and intervention.

Many children with developmental delays are not being identified early. In the United States, 17% of children have a developmental or behavioral disability such as autism, mental retardation, and attention-deficit/hyperactivity disorder. In addition, many children have delays in language or other areas, which also impact school readiness. However, less than 50% of these children are identified as having a problem before starting school, by which time significant delays may have already occurred and opportunities for treatment have been missed.

Early identification and intervention for children with developmental delays is mandated. The Individuals with Disabilities Education Act (IDEA) Amendments of 1990 to 1997 require states to provide early identification and provision of services to infants and toddlers with 1) developmental delays, 2) established conditions that are associated with developmental delays, and, 3) at the state's option, children at risk for developmental delays. States that do not serve the at-risk population are encouraged to track and monitor these children's development, so that they may be referred in the future if needed. IDEA also mandates that states refer children, free of charge, for a comprehensive, multi-disciplinary evaluation by a team who, with the family, decides on which services are needed for the child (via the Individualized Family Service Plan). Furthermore, it mandates states to implement coordinated, family-centered, and culturally competent community-based systems of care, to provide early intervention services for children identified with developmental problems. The National Early Childhood Technical Assistance Center, lists early intervention programs by state and provides their contact information for interested parents and professionals.

Parents are interested in knowing more about their child's development and pediatric practitioners need to be better prepared for this.

Recent surveys indicate that parents want information and guidance from their health care provider about their child's development. However, studies sponsored by the American Academy of Pediatrics show that about 65% of pediatricians feel inadequately trained in assessing children's developmental status.

Who provides developmental screening services?

Developmental screening can be done by various professionals in healthcare, community, or school settings. The role of health professionals has become particularly important, because of the greater emphasis placed on early identification of children with delays. Through well-child visits, health professionals have regular contact with children zero to three years of age, allowing them an opportunity to monitor development through periodic developmental screening. This has led healthcare professional organizations, such as the American Academy of Pediatrics (AAP) and the American Academy of Neurology, to recommend that all infants and young children be screened for developmental delays periodically in the context of office-based primary care.

I have concerns that my child could have a developmental delay. Who can I contact in my state to get my child a developmental assessment?

Talk to your child's doctor or nurse if you have concerns about how your child is developing. If you or your doctor think there could be a problem, you can take your child to see a developmental pediatrician or other specialist, and you can contact your local early intervention agency (for children under three) or public school (for children three and older) for help. To find out who to speak to in your area, you can contact the National Dissemination Center for Children with Disabilities by logging on to http://www.nichcy.org or calling 800-695-0285. In addition, the Centers for Disease Control and Prevention (CDC) has links to information for families at www.cdc.gov/ncbddd/dd/aic/resources. If there is a problem, it is very important to get your child help as soon as possible.

How can I help my child's development?

Proper nutrition, exercise, and rest are very important for children's health and development. Providing a safe and loving home and spending time with your child—playing, singing, reading, and even just talking—can also make a big difference in his or her development.

Chapter 3

Preventive Care and Screening Test Guidelines for Adults

Adult Care Timeline: Screening and Counseling

The most important things you can do to prevent disease and be healthy are these: Be tobacco free, be physically active, eat a healthy diet, and get the right kinds of preventive health services—screenings, counseling, and preventive medicines—at the right times.

Heart Health

- **Blood pressure checked:** Men and women at least every two years: 18 years and older

- **Cholesterol checked:** Men and women, based on age and risk:
  - Men: 35–65 years; Men at risk, also 18–35 years; 65 years and older
  - Women: 45–65 years; Women at risk, also 18–45 years; 65 years and older

- **Dietary counseling:** Men and women with high cholesterol and those at risk for heart disease and diabetes: 18 years and older

This chapter includes excerpts from "Adult Preventive Care Timeline," AHRQ Publication No. APPIP06-IP001, June 2006. Agency for Healthcare Research and Quality (AHRQ), and from "Chapter 3: Checkups, Tests, and Shots," *The Pocket Guide to Good Health for Children*, AHRQ, May 2003.

- **Diabetes screening:** Men and women at risk for heart disease: 18 years and older
- **Aspirin:** To prevent heart attack
  - Men at risk: 18–40 years; Men: 40 years and older
  - Women at risk: 18–50 years; Women: 50 years and older
- **Abdominal aortic aneurysm screening:** Once for men who have ever smoked: 65–75 years

Health Risks

- **Tobacco use counseling:** All adults: 18 years and older
- **Obesity screening and counseling:** All adults: 18 years and older
- **Alcohol misuse counseling:** All adults: 18 years and older

Sexual Health

- **Chlamydia and gonorrhea screening:** Women, based on age and risk:
  - Women: 18–25 years
  - Women at risk: 25 years and older
- **HIV screening:** All adults at risk: 18 years and older
- **Syphilis screening:** All adults at risk: 18 years and older

Bone Health

- **Osteoporosis screening:** Women, based on age and risk:
  - Women at risk: 60–65 years
  - Women: 65 years and older

Mental Health

- **Depression screening:** All adults: 18 years and older

Checkups, Tests, and Shots

Checkups and tests, such as vision tests or cholesterol tests, help find diseases or conditions early, when they are easier to treat. Shots (immunizations) protect you from different diseases.

Dental, Hearing, and Vision Care

Teeth and gums: Here are some simple tips to follow for dental health:

- Visit your dentist once or twice a year for checkups.
- Brush after meals with a toothbrush that has soft or medium bristles.
- Use toothpaste with fluoride.
- Use dental floss every day.
- Eat fewer sweets, especially between meals.
- Do not smoke or chew tobacco products.

Hearing: Hearing loss is one of the most common health problems. Your risk for hearing loss increases after age 50. How can you tell if you have a hearing problem? Here are some signs:

- You may have to strain to hear a normal conversation.
- You may find yourself turning up the volume of the TV and radio so loud that others complain.

If you are worried about your hearing, talk to your doctor or nurse. They may suggest a hearing test. Hearing aids can help you hear well.

Vision: People 45 and older have more vision problems than younger people, and the problems are more likely to result in accidental injuries. By age 65, you should have regular eye exams.

Glaucoma can lead to vision problems and even cause blindness. Glaucoma is more common in people older than 45 than it is earlier in life. You are more likely to get glaucoma, and you should see an eye doctor for a glaucoma test, if these conditions apply to you:

- you are severely near-sighted
- you have diabetes
- you have a family history of glaucoma
- you are older than 65 or older than 40 and black

If you have vision problems, eyeglasses or contact lenses can improve your vision. Doctors also have other ways to improve your vision and

21

prevent you from losing your sight. Be sure to tell your doctor if you are having trouble with your vision.

Tests to Find Other Diseases or Conditions Early

Tuberculosis: Tuberculosis (TB) is an infection that affects the lungs and eventually other parts of the body. This infection can be passed from one person to the next. It is treated more easily if caught early.

You are at greater risk for TB and may need a TB test if any of the following conditions apply to you:

- You have been in close contact with someone who has TB.

- You have recently moved from Asia, Africa, Central or South America, or the Pacific Islands.

- You have kidney failure, diabetes, HIV, or alcoholism.

- You have injected or now inject street drugs.

Colorectal cancer: Colorectal cancer is second only to lung cancer as a cause of death from cancer. But if colorectal cancer is caught early, it can be treated.

Older men and women are more likely to get colorectal cancer than those who are younger. Starting at age 50, you should be tested for colorectal cancer. Tell your doctor if you have had polyps or if you have family members who have had colorectal cancer, breast cancer, or cancer of the ovaries or uterus. If so, you may need to be tested more often and at an earlier age.

There are a number of effective tests, used separately or in combination, for colorectal cancer. Each has advantages and disadvantages.

Breast cancer: Breast cancer is the most common cancer among women in the United States.

If you are at high risk for breast cancer, talk with your doctor about whether you should take medicine to reduce your risk. While medicines can reduce some women's risk for breast cancer, they also may cause blood clots and cancer of the uterus.

From age 40 on, your risk for breast cancer increases. If you have a sister or mother who has had breast cancer, your risk is even higher. A mammogram every one to two years beginning at age 40 can help find this disease early when it is easier to treat.

Mammograms have a few risks. They may not find all breast cancers. Also, they may show that you have cancer when you really do not. These false-positive results could lead to unnecessary biopsies.

Cervical cancer: All women who are or have been sexually active are at risk for cancer of the cervix unless their uterus has been completely removed. Most deaths from cancer of the cervix can be prevented if the cancer is found and treated early. A Pap test is used to find cervical cancer.

Women need to have a Pap test at least every three years, and women at increased risk for cervical cancer may need the test more often.

You are at increased risk for cervical cancer if you have had a sexually transmitted disease, you have had more than one sex partner, or you have had previous abnormal Pap tests.

Your doctor may suggest stopping Pap tests if you are older than 65, have had regular, normal Pap tests, and are not at increased risk for other reasons, or you have had a hysterectomy.

Prostate cancer: Prostate cancer is most common in men older than 50. You also may be at increased risk for prostate cancer if you are black or your father or brother has had prostate cancer.

Tests such as a PSA (prostate-specific antigen) blood test or a digital rectal exam can help detect prostate cancer, but these tests also have risks. They sometimes have false positive results, which may lead to avoidable anxiety and unnecessary biopsies and treatment. It is not yet clear whether these tests save lives.

Oral cancer: Oral cancer includes cancers of the lip, tongue, pharynx, and mouth. Most oral cancers occur in people older than 40 who use tobacco or alcohol. People who are in the sun a lot are at risk for cancer of the lip.

You can help prevent oral cancer by not smoking or abusing alcohol. If you are outdoors a lot, use a sun block on your lips.

If you chew or smoke tobacco or abuse alcohol, you may want your dentist to examine your mouth for signs of oral cancer during your regular dental checkup. You also may need to see your dentist more often.

Shots to Prevent Diseases

You can prevent some serious diseases by getting shots (immunizations). This section tells you which shots you need and when. Make sure to keep track of the shots you receive.

Measles-mumps-rubella shot: If you have never had a measles-mumps-rubella shot or never had measles, mumps, and rubella, you should receive at least one dose of this vaccine if you are a woman and able to become pregnant or you were born after 1956.

This shot is especially important for women. If a pregnant woman gets rubella, she could have a miscarriage, or her baby could have birth defects.

Tetanus-diphtheria shot: Most people need this shot every 10 years.

Flu shots: Most people 50 or older need a flu shot every year. You may need flu shots before age 50 if any of these situations apply to you:

- You have lung, heart, or kidney disease, diabetes, or cancer.

- You are a health care worker.

- You are infected with HIV or have AIDS.

Pneumonia shot: Everyone needs a pneumonia shot once around age 65. If you have lung, heart, or kidney disease; HIV; diabetes; or cancer, you may need this shot sooner.

Hepatitis B shots: You should receive hepatitis B shots if any of these situations apply to you:

- You have had sex with more than one partner or with someone infected with hepatitis B.

- You are a man and have had sex with a man.

- You have had any other sexually transmitted disease within the last six months.

- You have injected street drugs.

- You have a job that involves contact with human blood or blood products.

- You travel to areas where hepatitis B is common.

Part Two

Screening and Assessment Tests Associated with Specific Concerns

Chapter 4

Common Cancer Screening Tests

Chapter Contents

Section 4.1

Bladder and Other Urothelial Cancers Screening

Excerpted from PDQ® Cancer Information Summary. National Cancer Institute; Bethesda, MD. Bladder and Other Urothelial Cancers Screening (PDQ®): Patient Version. Updated 09/07/2007. Available at: http://cancer.gov. Accessed December 28, 2007.

There is no standard or routine screening test for bladder cancer. Screening for bladder cancer is under study and there are screening clinical trials taking place in many parts of the country. Information about ongoing clinical trials is available from the National Cancer Institute's (NCI) website (available online at http://www.cancer.gov/clinicaltrials).

Two tests may be used to screen for bladder cancer in patients who have had bladder cancer in the past:

- **Cystoscopy:** Cystoscopy is a procedure to look inside the bladder and urethra to check for abnormal areas. A cystoscope (a thin, lighted tube) is inserted through the urethra into the bladder. Tissue samples may be taken for biopsy.

- **Urine cytology:** Urine cytology is the examination of urine under a microscope to check for abnormal cells.

Hematuria tests may also be used to screen for bladder cancer. Hematuria (red blood cells in the urine) may be caused by cancer or by other conditions. A hematuria test is used to check for blood in a sample of urine by viewing it under a microscope or using a special test strip. The test may be repeated over time.

Risks of Screening for Bladder and Other Urothelial Cancers

Screening tests have risks. Decisions about screening tests can be difficult. Not all screening tests are helpful and most have risks. Before having any screening test, you may want to discuss the test with your doctor. It is important to know the risks of the test and whether it has been proven to reduce the risk of dying from cancer.

False-positive test results can occur: Screening test results may appear to be abnormal even though no cancer is present. A false-positive test result (one that shows there is cancer when there really isn't) can cause anxiety and is usually followed by more tests (such as cystoscopy or other invasive procedures), which also have risks. False-positive results often occur with hematuria testing; blood in the urine is usually caused by conditions other than cancer.

False-negative test results can occur: Screening test results may appear to be normal even though bladder cancer is present. A person who receives a false-negative test result (one that shows there is no cancer when there really is) may delay seeking medical care even if there are symptoms.

Your doctor can advise you about your risk for bladder cancer and your need for screening tests.

Section 4.2

Breast Cancer Screening

Excerpted from PDQ® Cancer Information Summary. National Cancer Institute; Bethesda, MD. Breast Cancer Screening (PDQ®): Screening - Patient. Updated 06/14/2007. Available at: http://cancer.gov. Accessed December 28, 2007.

Three tests are commonly used to screen for breast cancer:

- **Mammogram:** A mammogram is an x-ray of the breast. This test may find tumors that are too small to feel. A mammogram may also find ductal carcinoma in situ, abnormal cells in the lining of a breast duct, which may become invasive cancer in some women. The ability of a mammogram to find breast cancer may depend on the size of the tumor, the density of the breast tissue, and the skill of the radiologist.

- **Clinical breast exam (CBE):** A clinical breast exam is an exam of the breast by a doctor or other health professional. The doctor will carefully feel the breasts and under the arms for lumps or anything else that seems unusual.

- **Breast self-exam (BSE):** Breast self-exam is an exam to check your own breasts for lumps or anything else that seems unusual.

If a lump or other abnormality is found using one of these three tests, ultrasound may be used to learn more. It is not used by itself as a screening test for breast cancer. Ultrasound is a procedure in which high-energy sound waves (ultrasound) are bounced off internal tissues or organs and make echoes. The echoes form a picture of body tissues called a sonogram.

New screening tests are being studied in clinical trials.

MRI (magnetic resonance imaging): MRI is a procedure that uses a magnet, radio waves, and a computer to make a series of detailed pictures of areas inside the body. This procedure is also called nuclear magnetic resonance imaging (NMRI). Screening trials of MRI in women with a high genetic risk of breast cancer have shown that MRI is more sensitive than mammography for finding breast tumors.

MRI scans are used to make decisions about breast masses that have been found by a clinical breast exam or a breast self-exam. MRIs also help show the difference between cancer and scar tissue. MRI does not use any x-rays.

Tissue sampling: Breast tissue sampling is taking cells from breast tissue to examine under a microscope. Abnormal cells in breast fluid have been linked to an increased risk of breast cancer in some studies. Scientists are studying whether breast tissue sampling can be used to find breast cancer at an early stage or predict the risk of developing breast cancer. Three methods of tissue sampling are under study:

- *Fine-needle aspiration:* A thin needle is inserted into the breast tissue around the areola (darkened area around the nipple) to withdraw cells and fluid.

- *Nipple aspiration:* The use of gentle suction to collect fluid through the nipple. This is done with a device similar to the breast pumps used by nursing women.

- *Ductal lavage:* A hair-size catheter (tube) is inserted into the nipple and a small amount of salt water is released into the duct. The water picks up breast cells and is removed.

Risks of Breast Cancer Screening

The risks of breast cancer screening tests include the following:

- Finding breast cancer may not improve health or help a woman live longer
- False-negative test results can occur
- False-positive test results can occur
- Mammograms expose the breast to radiation

The risks and benefits of screening for breast cancer may be different for different groups of people. The benefits of breast cancer screening may vary among age groups:

- In women who have a life expectancy of five years or less, finding and treating early stage breast cancer may reduce their quality of life without helping them live longer.

- In women older than 65 years, the results of a screening test may lead to more diagnostic tests and anxiety while waiting for the test results. Also, the breast cancers found are usually not life-threatening.

- In women 35 years or younger who go to the doctor for breast symptoms, mammogram results may not be helpful in managing their care.

Routine breast cancer screening is advised for women who have had radiation treatment to the chest, especially at a young age. The benefits and risks of mammograms and MRIs for these women are not known. There is no information on the benefits or risks of breast cancer screening in men.

No matter how old you are, if you have risk factors for breast cancer you should ask for medical advice about when to begin having mammograms and how often to be screened.

Section 4.3

Cervical Cancer Screening

Excerpted from "Pap Tests: Things to Know,"
National Cancer Institute (www.cancer.gov), November 6, 2007.

The Pap test (or Pap smear) looks for abnormal changes in the cells of the cervix, the narrow, lowest part of the uterus. It forms an opening between the uterus (where the baby grows when a woman is pregnant) and the vagina. Almost all cervical cancer is caused by an infection from a virus called HPV or human papillomavirus.

The Pap test is a simple and routine way to find cell changes. During a Pap test the doctor or nurse will collect a few cells from your cervix to send to a medical lab for testing. You can get the Pap test at your doctor's office, clinic, or community health center.

Why should I have a Pap test?

Sometimes cells in a woman's cervix begin to change and look abnormal. These abnormal cells may not be cancer yet. But if you don't have the cell changes treated, the changes may become cancer. Having Pap tests regularly gives you the best chance of finding cell changes or cervical cancer early, when they are easy to treat.

When should I have a Pap test?

- Have your first Pap test about three years after the first time you have sex, or when you reach age 21 (whichever comes first).

- Keep getting Pap tests every one to three years. If you are 30 or older, an HPV test may be done along with the Pap test.

- Talk with your doctor or nurse about whether and when you should get a Pap test if you are 65 or older.

What should I expect with a Pap test?

Before the Pap test: For two days before your Pap test, do not douche or use any vaginal medicines, spermicidal foams, creams, or jellies unless directed by your doctor. If you have heavy bleeding from your period the day of the test, call your doctor or nurse to change the appointment to another day.

During the Pap test: A female staff member will be with you during the test. Your hips and legs will be covered. Your doctor or nurse will use an instrument called a "speculum" to open the vagina and see your cervix. Your doctor or nurse will then collect some cells from the cervix using a swab or a small brush. You may feel some discomfort.

After the Pap test: Your doctor or nurse will send the cells to a medical lab. The results will come back to your doctor or nurse in one or two weeks.

- If the test results are normal (or "negative"), your doctor's office may not notify you at all. If you do not hear from your doctor's office, you should call to be sure that the results are normal.

- If there is something abnormal on the test (or "positive"), your doctor should tell you. It is very important that you see your doctor for follow-up as soon as possible. Most times, an abnormal (or "positive") test does not mean that you have cancer. It only means that your doctor needs to do more tests.

When can I stop getting a Pap test?

- If you are 65 or older, talk to your doctor or nurse about whether or not you should keep having Pap tests. Your doctor or nurse will tell you how often you should get one. This will depend on the results of your previous tests, and whether you are sexually active.

- A total hysterectomy is when both the uterus and cervix have been taken out. If you had a hysterectomy to treat pre-cancer or cancer, you should continue to have Pap tests. If you had a total hysterectomy that was not done to treat pre-cancer or cancer, you do not need a Pap test. Talk with your doctor or nurse if you are not certain.

Section 4.4

Colorectal Cancer Screening

Excerpted from PDQ® Cancer Information Summary. National Cancer Institute; Bethesda, MD. Colorectal Cancer Screening (PDQ®): Screening - Patient. Updated 07/12/2007. Available at: http://cancer.gov. Accessed December 28, 2007.

Five tests are commonly used to screen for correctable cancer:

- **Fecal occult blood test:** A fecal occult blood test is a test to check stool (solid waste) for blood that can only be seen with a microscope. Small samples of stool are placed on special cards and returned to the doctor or laboratory for testing. Blood in the stool may be a sign of polyps or cancer.

- **Sigmoidoscopy:** Sigmoidoscopy is a procedure to look inside the rectum and sigmoid (lower) colon for polyps, abnormal areas, or cancer. A sigmoidoscope is inserted through the rectum into the sigmoid colon. A sigmoidoscope is a thin, tube-like instrument with a light and a lens for viewing. It may also have a tool to remove polyps or tissue samples, which are checked under a microscope for signs of cancer. A sigmoidoscopy and a digital rectal exam (DRE) may be used together to screen for colorectal cancer.

- **Barium enema:** A barium enema is a series of x-rays of the lower gastrointestinal tract. A liquid that contains barium (a silver-white metallic compound) is put into the rectum. The barium coats the lower gastrointestinal tract and x-rays are taken. This procedure is also called a lower GI series.

- **Colonoscopy:** Colonoscopy is a procedure to look inside the rectum and colon for polyps, abnormal areas, or cancer. A colonoscope is inserted through the rectum into the colon. A colonoscope is a thin, tube-like instrument with a light and a lens for viewing. It may also have a tool to remove polyps or tissue samples, which are checked under a microscope for signs of cancer.

- **Digital rectal exam:** A digital rectal exam (DRE) is an exam of the rectum. The doctor or nurse inserts a lubricated, gloved finger into the lower part of the rectum to feel for lumps or anything else that seems unusual.

New screening tests are being studied in clinical trials.

Virtual colonoscopy: Virtual colonoscopy is a procedure that uses a series of x-rays called computed tomography to make a series of pictures of the colon. A computer puts the pictures together to create detailed images that may show polyps and anything else that seems unusual on the inside surface of the colon. This test is also called colonography or CT colonography. Clinical trials are comparing virtual colonoscopy with commonly used colorectal cancer screening tests. Other clinical trials are testing whether drinking a contrast material that coats the stool, instead of using laxatives to clear the colon, shows polyps clearly.

DNA stool test: This test checks DNA in stool cells for genetic changes that may be a sign of colorectal cancer.

Table 4.1. American Cancer Society Guidelines on Screening and Surveillance for the Early Detection of Colorectal Adenomas and Cancer—Women and Men at Increased Risk or at High Risk (*continued on next page*)

Risk Category	Age to Begin	Recommendation	Comments
Increased Risk			
People with a single, small (< 1 cm) adenomas	3–6 years after the initial polypectomy	Colonoscopy[1]	If the exam is normal, the patient can thereafter be screened as per average risk guidelines.
People with a large (1 cm +) adenoma, multiple adenomas, or adenomas with high-grade dysplasia or villous change.	Within 3 years after the initial polypectomy	Colonoscopy[1]	If normal, repeat examination in 5 years; If normal then, the patient can thereafter be screened as per average risk guidelines.

Table 4.1. (*continued*) American Cancer Society Guidelines, on Screening and Surveillance for the Early Detection of Colorectal Adenomas and Cancer—Women and Men at Increased Risk or at High Risk (*continued on next page*)

Risk Category	Age to Begin	Recommendation	Comments
Increased Risk (*continued*)			
Personal history of curative-intent resection of colorectal cancer	Within 1 year after cancer resection	Colonoscopy[1]	If normal, repeat examination in 3 years; If normal then, repeat examination every 5 years.
Either colorectal cancer or adenomatous polyps, in any first-degree relative before age 60, or in two or more first-degree relatives at any age (if not a hereditary syndrome).	Age 40, or 10 years before the youngest case in the immediate family, whichever is earlier	Colonoscopy[1]	Every 5–10 years. Colorectal cancer in relatives more distant than first-degree does not increase risk substantially above the average risk group.
High Risk			
Family history of familial adenomatous polyposis (FAP)	Puberty	Early surveillance with endoscopy, and counseling to consider genetic testing	If the genetic test is positive, colectomy is indicated. These patients are best referred to a center with experience in the management of FAP.
Family history of hereditary non-polyposis colon cancer (HNPCC)	Age 21	Colonoscopy and counseling to consider genetic testing	If the genetic test is positive or if the patient has not had genetic testing, every 1–2 years until age 40, then annually. These patients are best referred to a center with experience in the management of HNPCC.

Table 4.1. (*continued*) American Cancer Society Guidelines, on Screening and Surveillance for the Early Detection of Colorectal Adenomas and Cancer—Women and Men at Increased Risk or at High Risk

Risk Category	Age to Begin	Recommendation	Comments
High Risk (continued)			
Inflammatory bowel disease Chronic ulcerative colitis Crohn's disease	Cancer risk begins to be significant 8 years after the onset of pancolitis, or 12–15 years after the onset of left-sided colitis	Colonoscopy with biopsies for dysplasia	Every 1–2 years. These patients are best referred to a center with experience in the surveillance and management of inflammatory bowel disease.

[1] If colonoscopy is unavailable, not feasible, or not desired by the patient, double contrast barium enema alone, or the combination of flexible sigmoidoscopy and double contrast barium enema are acceptable alternatives. Adding flexible sigmoidoscopy to double contrast barium enema (DCBE) may provide a more comprehensive diagnostic evaluation than DCBE alone in finding significant lesions. A supplementary DCBE may be needed if a colonoscopic exam fails to reach the cecum, and a supplementary colonoscopy may be needed if a DCBE identifies a possible lesion, or does not adequately visualize the entire colorectum.

Source: "American Cancer Society Guidelines on Screening and Surveillance for the Early Detection of Colorectal Adenomas and Cancer in People at Increased Risk or at High Risk, " is reprinted by permission of the American Cancer Society, Inc. from www.cancer.org. All rights reserved. © 2008.

Risks of Colorectal Cancer Screening

The risks of colorectal cancer screening tests include the following:

- Damage to the colon can occur
- False-negative test results can occur
- False-positive test results can occur

Your doctor can advise you about your risk for colorectal cancer and your need for screening tests.

Section 4.5

Lung Cancer Screening

Excerpted from PDQ® Cancer Information Summary. National Cancer Institute; Bethesda, MD. Lung Cancer Screening (PDQ®): Screening - Patient. Updated 02/17/2006. Available at: http://cancer.gov. Accessed December 28, 2007.

Two tests have commonly been used to screen for lung cancer. It has not yet been shown that screening for lung cancer with either of the following tests decreases the chance of dying from lung cancer:

- **Chest x-ray:** A chest x-ray is an x-ray of the organs and bones inside the chest. An x-ray is a type of energy beam that can go through the body and onto film, making a picture of areas inside the body.

- **Sputum cytology:** Sputum cytology is a procedure in which a sample of sputum (mucus that is brought up from the lungs by coughing) is viewed under a microscope to check for cancer cells.

New tests are being studied in clinical trials. Screening clinical trials are taking place in many parts of the country. Information about NCI's lung screening trial can be found at the National Lung Screening Trial (NLST) website (available online at http://www.cancer.gov/nlst). Information about other clinical trials is available from the NCI Cancer.gov website (http://www.cancer.gov/clinicaltrials).

Risks of Lung Cancer Screening

The risks of lung cancer screening tests include the following:

- Finding lung cancer may not improve health or help you live longer
- False-negative test results can occur
- False-positive test results can occur
- Chest x-rays expose the chest to radiation

Your doctor can advise you about your risk for lung cancer and your need for screening tests.

Section 4.6

Oral Cancer Screening

Excerpted from PDQ® Cancer Information Summary. National Cancer Institute; Bethesda, MD. Oral Cancer Screening (PDQ®): Screening - Patient. Updated 07/23/2007. Available at: http://cancer.gov. Accessed December 28, 2007.

Oral cancer may develop in any of the following areas:

- Lips

- Oral cavity, which includes the front two thirds of the tongue, the gingiva (gums), the buccal mucosa (the lining of the inside of the cheeks), the floor (bottom) of the mouth under the tongue, the hard palate (the roof of the mouth), and the retromolar trigone (the small area behind the wisdom teeth)

- Oropharynx, which includes the middle part of the pharynx (throat) behind the mouth, the back one-third of the tongue, the soft palate, the side and back walls of the throat, and the tonsils

Salivary glands are located throughout the oral cavity and oropharynx.

Risk of Oral Cancer

The number of new cases of oral cancer, as well as the number of deaths from oral cancer, has been decreasing. Anything that increases a person's chance of developing a disease is called a risk factor. Some of these risk factors for oral cancer are as follows:

- **Sex:** Men have a slightly higher risk of developing oral cancer than women.

- **Race:** The risk of developing oral cancer is higher in blacks than in whites.

- **Age:** The risk of developing oral cancer increases after age 45 years.

- **Tobacco and alcohol use:** The use of tobacco (including smokeless tobacco) and alcohol increases the risk of developing oral cancer.

- **HPV infection:** Infection with human papillomavirus (HPV) increases the risk of developing cancer of the oropharynx.

Screening Tests for Oral Cancer

Screening for oral cancer may be done during a physical examination by the dentist or doctor. High-risk areas of the mouth that can be checked for early detection are the floor of the mouth, the front and sides of the tongue, and the soft palate. The exam will include looking for lesions on the mucous membranes, including leukoplakia (white patches) and erythroplakia (red patches). Oral cancer sometimes develops in areas with these lesions. It is not known, however, if screening decreases the risk of dying from oral cancer. Early-stage oral cancer can be cured, but most oral cancers have spread by the time they are found.

Section 4.7

Prostate Cancer Screening

Excerpted from "The Prostate-Specific Antigen (PSA) Test:
Questions and Answers," National Cancer Institute (www.cancer.gov),
August 21, 2007.

Prostate-specific antigen (PSA) is a protein produced by the cells of the prostate gland. The PSA test measures the level of PSA in the blood. The doctor takes a blood sample, and the amount of PSA is measured in a laboratory. Because PSA is produced by the body and can be used to detect disease, it is sometimes called a biological marker or tumor marker.

It is normal for men to have low levels of PSA in their blood; however, prostate cancer or benign (not cancerous) conditions can increase PSA levels. As men age, both benign prostate conditions and prostate cancer become more frequent. The most common benign prostate conditions are prostatitis (inflammation of the prostate) and benign prostatic hyperplasia (BPH) (enlargement of the prostate). There is no evidence that prostatitis or BPH causes cancer, but it is possible for a man to have one or both of these conditions and to develop prostate cancer as well.

PSA levels alone do not give doctors enough information to distinguish between benign prostate conditions and cancer. However, the doctor will take the result of the PSA test into account when deciding whether to check further for signs of prostate cancer.

For whom might a PSA screening test be recommended?

Doctors' recommendations for screening vary. Some encourage yearly screening for men over age 50, and some advise men who are at a higher risk for prostate cancer to begin screening at age 40 or 45. Others caution against routine screening, while still others counsel men about the risks and benefits on an individual basis and encourage men to make personal decisions about screening. Currently, Medicare provides coverage for an annual PSA test for all men age 50 and older.

How are PSA test results reported?

PSA test results report the level of PSA detected in the blood. The test results are usually reported as nanograms of PSA per milliliter (ng/mL) of blood. In the past, most doctors considered PSA values below 4.0 ng/mL as normal. However, recent research found prostate cancer in men with PSA levels below 4.0 ng/mL. Many doctors are now using the following ranges with some variation:

- 0 to 2.5 ng/mL is low
- 2.6 to 10 ng/mL is slightly to moderately elevated
- 10 to 19.9 ng/mL is moderately elevated
- 20 ng/mL or more is significantly elevated

There is no specific normal or abnormal PSA level. The higher a man's PSA level, the more likely it is that cancer is present. But because various factors (such as age) can cause PSA levels to fluctuate, one abnormal PSA test does not necessarily indicate a need for other diagnostic tests. When PSA levels continue to rise over time, other tests may be needed.

It should be noted that it is common for normal PSA ranges to vary somewhat from laboratory to laboratory.

What if the screening test results show an elevated PSA level?

A man should discuss elevated PSA test results with his doctor. There can be different reasons for an elevated PSA level, including prostate cancer, benign prostate enlargement, inflammation, infection, age, and race. If cancer is suspected, a biopsy is needed to determine if cancer is present in the prostate.

What if the test results show a rising PSA level after treatment for prostate cancer?

A man should discuss rising PSA test levels with his doctor. Doctors consider a number of factors before recommending further treatment. Additional treatment based on a single PSA test result is often not recommended. Rather, a rising trend in PSA test results over a period of time combined with other findings, such as an abnormal DRE, positive prostate biopsy results, or abnormal CT (computed tomography) scan results, may lead to a recommendation for further treatment.

What are some of the limitations of the PSA test?

- Detection does not always mean saving lives
- False positive tests
- False negative tests

Why is the PSA test controversial in screening?

Using the PSA test to screen men for prostate cancer is controversial because it is not yet known if this test actually saves lives. Moreover, it is not clear if the benefits of PSA screening outweigh the risks of follow-up diagnostic tests and cancer treatments. For example, the PSA test may detect small cancers that would never become life threatening. This situation puts men at risk for complications from unnecessary treatment such as surgery or radiation.

The procedure used to diagnose prostate cancer (prostate biopsy) may cause side effects, including bleeding and infection. Prostate cancer treatment may cause incontinence (inability to control urine flow) and erectile dysfunction (erections inadequate for intercourse). For these reasons, it is important that the benefits and risks of diagnostic procedures and treatment be taken into account when considering whether to undertake prostate cancer screening.

Section 4.8

Skin Cancer Screening

Excerpted from PDQ® Cancer Information Summary. National Cancer Institute; Bethesda, MD. Skin Cancer Screening (PDQ®): Screening - Patient. Updated 10/20/2004. Available at: http://cancer.gov Accessed December 28, 2007.

Regular examination of the skin by both you and your doctor increases the chance of finding melanoma early. Most melanomas that appear in the skin can be seen by the naked eye. Usually, there is a long period of time when the tumor grows beneath the top layer of skin but does not grow into the deeper skin layers. This period of slow growth allows time for skin cancer to be found early. Skin cancer may be cured if the tumor is found before it spreads deeper. Monthly self-examination of the skin may help find changes that should be reported to a doctor. Regular skin checks by a doctor are important for people who have already had skin cancer.

If an area on the skin looks abnormal, a biopsy is usually done. The doctor will remove as much of the suspicious tissue as possible with a local excision. A pathologist then looks at the tissue under a microscope to check for cancer cells. Because it is sometimes difficult to tell if a skin growth is benign (not cancer) or malignant (cancer), you may want to have the biopsy sample checked by a second pathologist.

Other screening tests are being studied in clinical trials. Screening clinical trials are taking place in many parts of the country. Information about ongoing clinical trials is available from the NCI Cancer.gov website (http://www.cancer.gov/clinicaltrials).

Risks of Skin Cancer Screening

The risks of melanoma screening tests include the following:

- Finding melanoma may not improve health or help a person live longer
- False-negative test results can occur
- False-positive test results can occur
- A biopsy may cause scarring

Your doctor can advise you about your risk for skin cancer and your need for screening tests.

Section 4.9

Testicular Cancer Screening

Excerpted from PDQ® Cancer Information Summary. National Cancer Institute; Bethesda, MD. Testicular Cancer Screening (PDQ®): Screening - Patient. Updated 02/28/2008. Available at: http://cancer.gov Accessed December 28, 2007.

The testicles are male sex glands involved in the production of sperm. They are located behind the penis in a pouch of skin called the scrotum. The testicles are the body's main source of male hormones.

Risk of Testicular Cancer

Testicular cancer is rare. Despite a slow increase in the number of new cases, the number of deaths due to testicular cancer has decreased dramatically since the 1960s as a result of treatment improvements.

Anything that increases a person's chance of developing a disease is called a risk factor. Some risk factors for testicular cancer are as follows:

- **Age:** Young men have a higher risk of testicular cancer. In men, testicular cancer is the most common cancer between the ages of

20 to 34, the second most common cancer between the ages of 35 to 39, and the third most common cancer between the ages of 15 to 19.

- **Family history:** Men with a family history of testicular cancer may have an increased risk of developing testicular cancer.

- **Hereditary conditions:** Men born with gonadal dysgenesis or Klinefelter syndrome have a greater risk of developing testicular cancer.

- **Personal history:** Men with undescended testicles have a higher-than-average risk of developing testicular cancer. Men who have already had testicular cancer have a higher risk of developing a tumor in the other testicle. There is an increased risk of second cancers for at least 35 years after treatment for testicular cancer.

- **Race:** Testicular cancer is more common among white men than black men. Hispanic, American Indian, and Asian men develop testicular cancer at a higher rate than black men, but less than white men.

Screening Tests for Testicular Cancer

Most testicular cancers are first detected by the patient, either unintentionally or by self-examination. Some are discovered by routine physical examination. However, no studies have been done to determine whether self-examination or examination during routine physicals can help reduce the number of deaths caused by testicular cancer.

Harms of screening for testicular cancer may include unnecessary diagnostic tests which could cause rare but serious complications.

Section 4.10

Tumor Markers: Questions and Answers

Excerpted from "Tumor Markers: Questions and Answers,"
National Cancer Institute (www.cancer.gov), February 3, 2006.

What are tumor markers?

Tumor markers are substances produced by tumor cells or by other cells of the body in response to cancer or certain benign (noncancerous) conditions. These substances can be found in the blood, in the urine, in the tumor tissue, or in other tissues. Different tumor markers are found in different types of cancer, and levels of the same tumor marker can be altered in more than one type of cancer. In addition, tumor marker levels are not altered in all people with cancer, especially if the cancer is early stage. Some tumor marker levels can also be altered in patients with noncancerous conditions.

To date, researchers have identified more than a dozen substances that seem to be expressed abnormally when some types of cancer are present. Some of these substances are also found in other conditions and diseases. Scientists have not found markers for every type of cancer.

What are risk markers?

Some people have a greater chance of developing certain types of cancer because of a change, known as a mutation or alteration, in specific genes. The presence of such a change is sometimes called a risk marker. Tests for risk markers can help the doctor to estimate a person's chance of developing a certain cancer. Risk markers can indicate that cancer is more likely to occur, whereas tumor markers can indicate the presence of cancer.

How are tumor markers used in cancer care?

Tumor markers are used in the detection, diagnosis, and management of some types of cancer. Although an abnormal tumor marker level may suggest cancer, this alone is usually not enough to diagnose cancer. Therefore, measurements of tumor markers are usually combined with other tests, such as a biopsy, to diagnose cancer.

Tumor marker levels may be measured before treatment to help doctors plan appropriate therapy. In some types of cancer, tumor marker levels reflect the stage (extent) of the disease. (More information about staging is available in the National Cancer Institute (NCI) fact sheet Staging: Questions and Answers, which can be found at http://www.cancer.gov/cancertopics/factsheet/Detection/staging on the internet.)

Tumor marker levels also may be used to check how a patient is responding to treatment. A decrease or return to a normal level may indicate that the cancer is responding to therapy, whereas an increase may indicate that the cancer is not responding. After treatment has ended, tumor marker levels may be used to check for recurrence (cancer that has returned).

How and when are tumor markers measured?

The doctor takes a blood, urine, or tissue sample and sends it to the laboratory, where various methods are used to measure the level of the tumor marker.

If the tumor marker is being used to determine whether a treatment is working or if there is recurrence, the tumor marker levels are often measured over a period of time to see if the levels are increasing or decreasing. Usually these "serial measurements" are more meaningful than a single measurement. Tumor marker levels may be checked at the time of diagnosis; before, during, and after therapy; and then periodically to monitor for recurrence.

Can tumor markers be used as a screening test for cancer?

Screening tests are a way of detecting cancer early, before there are any symptoms. For a screening test to be helpful, it should have high sensitivity and specificity. Sensitivity refers to the test's ability to identify people who have the disease. Specificity refers to the test's ability to identify people who do not have the disease. Most tumor markers are not sensitive or specific enough to be used for cancer screening.

Even commonly used tests may not be completely sensitive or specific. For example, prostate-specific antigen (PSA) levels are often used to screen men for prostate cancer, but this is controversial. It is not yet known if early detection using PSA screening actually saves lives. Elevated PSA levels can be caused by prostate cancer or benign conditions, and most men with elevated PSA levels turn out not to have prostate cancer. Moreover, it is not clear if the benefits of PSA screening outweigh the risks of follow-up diagnostic tests and cancer treatments.

Another tumor marker, CA 125, is sometimes used to screen women who have an increased risk for ovarian cancer. Scientists are studying whether measurement of CA 125, along with other tests and exams, is useful to find ovarian cancer before symptoms develop. So far, CA 125 measurement is not sensitive or specific enough to be used to screen all women for ovarian cancer. Mostly, CA 125 is used to monitor response to treatment and check for recurrence in women with ovarian cancer.

Chapter 5

Cardiovascular Screening Tests

Chapter Contents

Section 5.1

Recommended Schedule for Cardiovascular Screening Tests

"Recommended Schedule for Screening Tests," reprinted with permission www.americanheart.org © 2008, American Heart Association, Inc.

To stay heart healthy, it's important to keep track of your numbers by getting screened regularly.

If you're an adult age 20 or older, use this information (approved by the American Heart Association) to keep track of which tests you should have done and how often:

Recommended Screening: Blood pressure

How often?

Each regular healthcare visit or at least once every two years if blood pressure is less than 120/80 mm Hg.

Starting when?

Age 20.

Recommended Screening: Cholesterol ("Fasting Lipoprotein Profile" to Measure Total, HDL and LDL Cholesterol, and Triglycerides)

How often?

Every five years for normal-risk people; more often if any of the following apply to you:

- Total cholesterol above 200 mg/dL
- You are a man over age 45 or a woman over age 50
- Your HDL (good) cholesterol is less than 40 mg/dL (if you're a man) or less than 50 mg/dL (if you're a woman)

- You have other risk factors for heart disease and stroke

Starting when?

Age 20.

Recommended Screening: Weight (Body Mass Index)

How often?

Each regular healthcare visit.

Starting when?

Age 20.

Recommended Screening: Waist Circumference

How often?

As needed to help evaluate cardiovascular risk.

Starting when?

Age 20.

Recommended Screening: Blood Glucose Test

How often?

Every three years.

Starting when?

Age 45.

After your screenings, talk to your doctor about your numbers. To find out the optimum levels for blood pressure, cholesterol, and other risk factors, visit the American Heart Association's page on "numbers that count" (available online at http://www.americanheart.org/presenter .jhtml?identifier=3038638).

Section 5.2

Cholesterol Screening for Adults and Children

AHA Scientific Position

Public screenings have the potential to detect large numbers of people with high blood cholesterol levels besides those detected in the physician's office. Public screenings can also raise awareness of high blood cholesterol as a risk factor for coronary heart disease, the first step toward modifying lifestyle to reduce risk. However, public screenings must meet acceptable criteria for recruitment, reliability of measurement of cholesterol levels, appropriate educational information, properly trained staff, and referral.

High-density lipoprotein (HDL) cholesterol as well as total cholesterol should be measured. However, if HDL cholesterol measurements aren't available in the screening setting, measuring total cholesterol levels still gives valuable information that can be used to manage cholesterol.

The American Heart Association doesn't recommend mass screenings of blood cholesterol for all children and adolescents.

The American Heart Association shares the concern expressed by federal agencies and congressional committees about the potential dangers of poorly conducted community cholesterol screening programs. Our association recommends focusing on smaller-scale screenings with potential for higher return. There are many such possibilities.

- American Heart Association Heart At Work locales and other business and industry worksites provide major opportunities to reach a high-risk population of middle-aged men and women and especially younger males not yet identified as being at risk. Essential follow-up and referral can be carried out more readily at a job locale. Worksite screenings held cooperatively with a third party such as a hospital, health club, university, or medical school are an example. National Heart At Work companies now have access to a national screening referral service. Vendors providing this service conduct screenings that follow American Heart Association guidelines and specifications.

- Screenings targeting low-income, low-education level groups are another way to reach a population that's often under-represented in other voluntary screenings. These programs have great potential for identifying high-risk people who are often from minority communities and not connected to traditional healthcare and information systems. Such screenings may be held in schools, churches, community centers, or neighborhood clinics. Again it's preferable that qualified groups conduct the testing.

Wherever public screenings are held, they should be at reasonable cost and at convenient sites that efficiently accommodate the numbers of screenees, and ensure quality-control procedures and privacy. Screenings should include reliable verbal and printed information about cholesterol levels from knowledgeable staff who can provide referrals or follow up.

The American Heart Association urges all Americans to have their physicians determine their total and HDL blood cholesterol levels. This is very important for those people with a family history of heart disease, high blood pressure, or stroke.

Getting blood cholesterol and blood pressure measurements should be part of an overall plan of medical care. Physicians or para-professionals working at the direction of the physician should order the cholesterol tests and interpret the result for the patient. The physician should then direct any follow-up care if needed, such as prescribing a diet, exercise program, or drug therapy.

Repeat cholesterol tests, specifically those to determine LDL cholesterol and triglycerides, should be completed before therapy is begun, according to the detailed directions and guidelines of the National Cholesterol Education Program and the American Heart Association.

The American Heart Association recommends integrating community health risk assessment programs into the medical care system. These systems should ensure that test results are interpreted by the physician responsible for the patient's care. When cholesterol test results are given directly to a person without also informing that person's physician, there's no guarantee that the person will contact his or her doctor for interpretation follow-up. People who interpret their own cholesterol test result may become unduly frightened or reassured. Screening agencies should refer screenees to their health-care provider. Follow-up methods such as letters or telephone calls are desirable.

Section 5.3

Questions and Answers about C-Reactive Protein

What is C-reactive protein? How does it relate to heart disease?

The body produces C-reactive protein (CRP) during the general process of inflammation. When a disease called atherosclerosis damages arteries around the heart, they become inflamed, which triggers CRP production. For years we thought that diseased arteries around the heart slowly narrow, then clog or collapse and cause a heart attack. While this does occur, it is much more rare than had been anticipated. And that theory didn't explain the patients who were fine one day, but had a heart attack the next week. We have since found that in some people inflamed, softened artery walls develop weak areas that can rupture suddenly, causing a heart attack. Also, plaque can build up quickly in inflamed arteries, increasing the risk of blood clots.

How do doctors test for CRP?

Physicians measure CRP with a simple, convenient blood test that does not require fasting. General CRP blood testing has been around for years, but only one kind, the high-sensitivity C-reactive protein (hs-CRP) test, helps determine heart disease risk. Patients should ask their doctors about hs-CRP specifically. With hs-CRP test results, a level above three raises major concern because it means a person's risk for heart attack is at least doubled. One to three merits some concern, but is not serious. Below one is where we want all patients. Readings of 50 and above are possible, but we generally attribute a level higher than 10 to an infection or other source of inflammation somewhere in the body, not arterial inflammation.

How does the hs-CRP test compare to other indicators, such as cholesterol and stress tests?

The exercise stress test tells us when narrowed arteries cause a shortage of blood going to the heart. It is still a vital risk indicator. LDL cholesterol is important to watch because it can narrow and clog arteries. LDL, or low density lipoprotein is the major carrier of "bad" cholesterol in the blood. There are two types of LDL, the bad kind and the really bad kind, which we call oxidized LDL. The available cholesterol test does not differentiate between these two types; it only tells a person's total LDL level. However, this bad, oxidized type, which hurts the arteries and speeds up plaque formation, is formed by inflammation and thus has a correlation to CRP levels. Hs-CRP testing offers a window into the degree of vascular inflammation, and therefore the ability to generate the especially bad form of LDL a person has.

How do people know if they need an hs-CRP test?

The American Heart Association recommends individuals at intermediate risk for developing heart disease (have two or more risk factors) should have hs-CRP testing as a screening test. There also is growing clinical data supporting that elevated hs-CRP—even in subjects with known heart disease—are at increased risk independent of their LDL cholesterol level. Some experts also recommend that people who have suffered a heart attack or stroke and those with at least one risk factor, such as family history, high blood pressure, high cholesterol, smoking, or diabetes, should be tested. While the American Heart Association and Centers for Disease Control just recently recommended hs-CRP testing as an option for those already at risk, The Cleveland Clinic has used the hs-CRP test routinely for at-risk patients for several years. Hs-CRP is an excellent test for people with one or two risk factors who wonder if they are really in jeopardy of a heart attack or a stroke. Having an elevated HS-CRP is associated with increased risk that otherwise might not have been identified. The test is probably less useful for people without any risk factors.

How often should CRP levels be tested?

There's no cookbook solution. In general the test is repeated in a couple months to see if levels remain high since even mild infections like colds, or even allergies or hay fever can cause mild elevations in hs-CRP. If someone comes in with high hs-CRP level, the Section of Preventive Cardiology at Cleveland Clinic recommends they work on lowering their CRP levels by losing weight, eating right, adopting a routine exercise program, and consider taking medications for elevated blood pressure and LDL cholesterol levels. In short—we re-double global preventive cardiovascular medicine efforts. If the initial level is low, they are not rechecked again for two-to-five years. It really depends on the patient and adoption of lifestyle changes or other treatments.

Is arterial inflammation the only cause of high CRP?

No. Many things can cause hs-CRP to be elevated, but inflammation in the body is the major thing (other than pregnancy). Inflammation may be a sign of infection, arthritis, or even periodontal disease. All of these are also associated with increased cardiac risks. Before getting an hs-CRP test, patients should tell their doctors if they are experiencing health problems that can cause general inflammation, for example, joint problems or a respiratory infection. If tested while ill or injured, and hs-CRP comes back elevated, it's important to get re-tested once healthy. But, pinpointing an alternative reason for a high hs-CRP reading doesn't eliminate the increased risk for heart disease or the value of the hs-CRP test. Inflammation anywhere in the body makes the arteries vulnerable because the cells and substances in the body that drive inflammation are thrown into high gear. Inflammation itself fuels further inflammation.

What can I do if my hs-CRP level is high?

Inflammation should be treated by lifestyle change, such as losing weight, exercising, controlling diabetes, stopping smoking, controlling high blood pressure, and reducing alcohol intake. Antithrombotic medications such as aspirin or clopidogrel may provide protection. Cholesterol-lowering statin drugs and ACE inhibitors may also reduce CRP. Your doctor will prescribe the correct medications and dosage to treat your condition.

Results

Less than 1.0 mg/L = Low risk for cardiovascular disease (CVD)

1.0–2.9 mg/L = Intermediate risk for CVD

Greater than 3.0 mg/L = High risk for CVD

Reference

AHA/CDC Scientific Statement: Markers of Inflammation and Cardiovascular Disease. *Circulation*. 2003;107:499–511. http://circ.ahajournals.org/cgi/content/full/107/3/499

Reviewed by Dr. Stanley Hazen M.D., Ph.D., Section Head of Preventive Cardiology at the Cleveland Clinic Heart & Vascular Institute

Section 5.4

Twelve-Step Screening May Help Reduce Sudden Death in Young Athletes

A 12-point screening process could help reduce sudden cardiac death in high school and college competitive athletes, according to an updated American Heart Association scientific statement.

The Recommendations for Preparticipation Cardiovascular Screening of Competitive Athletes, published in *Circulation: Journal of the American Heart Association*, revisits the original 1996 statement on this subject and makes no major changes to the mass screening process first recommended at that time.

The screening includes 12 questions about personal and family medical history and a physical examination to uncover aspects of a potential athlete's health that could signal a cardiovascular problem:

Personal History

- Chest pain/discomfort upon exertion
- Unexplained fainting or near-fainting
- Excessive and unexplained fatigue associated with exercise
- Heart murmur
- High blood pressure

Family History

- One or more relatives who died of heart disease (sudden/unexpected or otherwise) before age 50
- Close relative under age 50 with disability from heart disease
- Specific knowledge of certain cardiac conditions in family members: hypertrophic or dilated cardiomyopathy in which the heart cavity or wall becomes enlarged, long QT syndrome which affects the heart's electrical rhythm, Marfan syndrome in which the walls of the heart's major arteries are weakened, or clinically important arrhythmias or heart rhythms.

Physical Examination

- Heart murmur
- Femoral pulses to exclude narrowing of the aorta
- Physical appearance of Marfan syndrome
- Brachial artery blood pressure (taken in a sitting position)

Parents should verify this information, said members of the expert panel who wrote the statement. If any of the 12 screening elements has a "yes" answer, the participant would be referred for further cardiovascular examination.

The incidence of deaths is in the range of one in 200,000 high school-age athletes per year, based on a 12-year Minnesota study of 1.4 million student-athlete participations in 27 sports.

"Although the frequency of these deaths in young athletes appears to be relatively low, it is more common than previously thought and does represent a substantive public health problem," said Barry J. Maron, M.D., chair of the writing group.

In the United States, these deaths occur most commonly in basketball and football—high intensity sports with high levels of participation.

There is some debate whether mass prescreening of competitive athletes should also include an electrocardiogram (ECG) before they are allowed to participate in team sports. An ECG is a special test that reads the heart's electrical activity. Maron says current U.S. recommendations don't include ECGs, most notably due to a lack of policy mandate and infrastructure to support this.

"Recommendations of the European Society of Cardiology and International Olympic Committee include routine ECGs for all potential athletes," said Maron, who is director of the Hypertrophic Cardiomyopathy Center at the Minneapolis Heart Institute Foundation. "However, while advocating this kind of plan in the United States may seem simple, it's a much more complicated matter."

The statement cites several limitations for recommending such widespread, routine ECGs—including the high number of competitive athletes in this country, significantly higher than in other countries, such as Italy, where the tests are routinely conducted.

"Each year, there are probably more than five million competitive athletes at the high school level (grades 9–12), in addition to more than 500,000 collegiate (including NCAA [National Collegiate Athletic Association], NAIA [National Association of Intercollegiate Athletics], junior colleges) and 5,000 professional athletes," the panel wrote. "This figure does not include youth, middle school, and masters level (age 30 +) competitors for whom reliable numbers are not available. Therefore, the relevant athlete population available for mass screening may be as large as 10 million people per year."

Maron said the total estimated cost of mass screening for that many athletes, along with the follow-up required for abnormal findings, is more than $2 billion a year. Coupled with other limitations such as a lack of physicians and other medical resources for performing and reading ECGs and no laws to mandate the standards for pre-participation screening, he says the cost effectiveness and feasibility of such a program in the United States cannot justify such a recommendation at this time.

The panel does recommend the development of a national standard for cardiovascular screening of high school and college athletes and notes there has been significant improvement overall in the support and adherence to life-saving screening processes for youth participating in sports. In 1997, a study found 45 percent of states had inadequate screening processes in place, while a 2005 review found 81 percent of states now support adequate screening processes.

Other authors are co-chair Paul D. Thompson, M.D.; Michael J. Ackerman, M.D., Ph.D.; Gary Balady, M.D.; Stuart Berger, M.D.; David

Cohen, M.D.; Robert Dimeff, M.D.; Pamela S. Douglas, M.D., David W. Glover, M.D.; Adolph M. Hutter, Jr., M.D.; Michael D. Krauss, M.D.; Martin S. Maron, M.D.; Matthew J. Mitten, J.D.; William O. Roberts, M.D.; and James C. Puffer, M.D.

Chapter 6

Tests for Monitoring Diabetes and Kidney Disease

Chapter Contents

Section 6.1

Tests Used to Diagnose Diabetes

In diagnosing diabetes, physicians primarily depend upon the results of specific glucose tests. However, test results are just part of the information that goes into the diagnosis of diabetes. Doctors also take into account your physical exam, presence or absence of symptoms, and medical history. Some people who are significantly ill will have transient problems with elevated blood sugars which will then return to normal after the illness has resolved. Also, some medications may alter your blood glucose levels (most commonly steroids and certain diuretics, [water pills]). The two main tests used to measure the presence of blood sugar problems are the direct measurement of glucose levels in the blood during an overnight fast, and measurement of the body's ability to appropriately handle the excess sugar presented after drinking a high glucose drink.

Fasting Blood Glucose (Blood Sugar) Level

The "gold standard" for diagnosing diabetes is an elevated blood sugar level after an overnight fast (not eating anything after midnight). A value above 140 mg/dl on at least two occasions typically means a person has diabetes. Normal people have fasting sugar levels that generally run between 70–110 mg/dl.

The Oral Glucose Tolerance Test

An oral glucose tolerance test is one that can be performed in a doctor's office or a lab. The person being tested starts the test in a fasting state (having no food or drink except water for at least 10 hours but not greater than 16 hours). An initial blood sugar is drawn and then the person is given a "glucola" bottle with a high amount of sugar in it (75 grams of glucose or 100 grams for pregnant women).

The person then has their blood tested again 30 minutes, one hour, two hours and three hours after drinking the high glucose drink.

For the test to give reliable results, you must be in good health (not have any other illnesses, not even a cold). Also, you should be normally active (for example, not lying down or confined to a bed like a patient in a hospital) and taking no medicines that could affect your blood glucose. The morning of the test, you should not smoke or drink coffee. During the test, you need to lie or sit quietly.

The oral glucose tolerance test is conducted by measuring blood glucose levels five times over a period of three hours. In a person without diabetes, the glucose levels in the blood rise following drinking the glucose drink, but then fall quickly back to normal (because insulin is produced in response to the glucose, and the insulin has a normal effect of lowing blood glucose.) In a diabetic, glucose levels rise higher than normal after drinking the glucose drink and come down to normal levels much slower (insulin is either not produced, or it is produced but the cells of the body do not respond to it)

As with fasting or random blood glucose tests, a markedly abnormal oral glucose tolerance test is diagnostic of diabetes. However, blood glucose measurements during the oral glucose tolerance test can vary somewhat. For this reason, if the test shows that you have mildly elevated blood glucose levels, the doctor may run the test again to make sure the diagnosis is correct.

Glucose tolerance tests may lead to one of the following diagnoses:

Normal response: A person is said to have a normal response when the 2-hour glucose level is less than or equal to 110 mg/dl.

Impaired fasting glucose: When a person has a fasting glucose equal to or greater than 110 and less than 126 mg/dl, they are said to have impaired fasting glucose. This is considered a risk factor for future diabetes, and will likely trigger another test in the future, but by itself, does not make the diagnosis of diabetes.

Impaired glucose tolerance: A person is said to have impaired glucose tolerance when the 2-hour glucose results from the oral glucose tolerance test are greater than or equal to 140 but less than 200 mg/dl. This is also considered a risk factor for future diabetes. There has recently been discussion about lowering the upper value to 180 mg/dl to diagnose more mild diabetes to allow earlier intervention and hopefully prevention of diabetic complications.

Diabetes: A person has diabetes when oral glucose tolerance tests show that the blood glucose level at two hours is equal to or more than 200 mg/dl. This must be confirmed by a second test (any of the three) on another day. There has recently been discussion about lowering the upper value to 180 mg/dl to diagnose more people with mild diabetes to allow earlier intervention and hopefully prevention of diabetic complications.

Gestational diabetes: A woman has gestational diabetes when she is pregnant and has any two of the following: a fasting plasma glucose of more than 105 mg/dl, a 1-hour glucose level of more than 190 mg/dl, a 2-hour glucose level of more than 165 mg/dl, or a 3-hour glucose level of more than 145 mg/dl.

Section 6.2

Glucose Meters and Tests Used to Monitor Diabetes

Excerpted from "Glucose Meters and Diabetes Management,"
U.S. Food and Drug Administration, June 2005.

When people with diabetes can control their blood sugar (glucose), they are more likely to stay healthy. People with diabetes use two kinds of management devices: glucose meters and other diabetes management tests. Glucose meters help people with diabetes check their blood sugar at home, school, work, and play. Other blood and urine tests reveal trends in diabetes management and help identify diabetes complications.

Glucose Meters

Self-Monitoring of Blood Glucose

The process of monitoring one's own blood glucose with a glucose meter is often referred to as self-monitoring of blood glucose or "SMBG." Portable glucose meters are small battery-operated devices.

To test for glucose with a typical glucose meter, place a small sample of blood on a disposable "test strip" and place the strip in the meter. The test strips are coated with chemicals (glucose oxidase, dehydrogenase, or hexokinase) that combine with glucose in blood. The meter measures how much glucose is present. Meters do this in different ways. Some measure the amount of electricity that can pass through the sample. Others measure how much light reflects from it. The meter displays the glucose level as a number. Several new models can record and store a number of test results. Some models can connect to personal computers to store test results or print them out.

Choosing a Glucose Meter

At least 25 different meters are commercially available. They differ in several ways including the amount of blood needed for each test, testing speed, overall size, ability to store test results in memory, cost of the meter, and cost of the test strips used.

Newer meters often have features that make them easier to use than older models. Some meters allow you to get blood from places other than your fingertip. Some new models have automatic timing, error codes and signals, or barcode readers to help with calibration. Some meters have a large display screen or spoken instructions for people with visual impairments.

Learning to Use Your Glucose Meter

Not all glucose meters work the same way. Since you need to know how to use your glucose meter and interpret its results, you should get training from a diabetes educator. The educator should watch you test your glucose to make sure you can use your meter correctly. This training is better if it is part of an overall diabetes education program.

Instructions for Using Glucose Meters

The following are the general instructions for using a glucose meter:

1. Wash hands with soap and warm water and dry completely or clean the area with alcohol and dry completely.

2. Prick the fingertip with a lancet.

3. Hold the hand down and hold the finger until a small drop of blood appears; catch the blood with the test strip.

4. Follow the instructions for inserting the test strip and using the SMBG meter.

5. Record the test result.

The U.S. Food and Drug Administration (FDA) requires that glucose meters and the strips used with them have instructions for use. You should read carefully the instructions for both the meter and its test strips. Meter instructions are found in the user manual. Keep this manual to help you solve any problems that may arise. Many meters use "error codes" when there is a problem with the meter, the test strip, or the blood sample on the strip. You will need the manual to interpret these error codes and fix the problem.

You can get information about your meter and test strips from several different sources. Your user manual should include a toll free number in case you have questions or problems. If you have a problem and can't get a response from this number, contact your healthcare provider or a local emergency room for advice. Also, the manufacturer of your meter should have a website. Check this website regularly to see if it lists any issues with the function of your meter.

New devices are for sale such as laser lancets and meters that can test blood taken from "alternative sites" of the body other than fingertips. Since new devices are used in new ways and often have new use restrictions, you must review the instructions carefully.

Important Features of Glucose Meters

There are several features of glucose meters that you need to understand so you can use your meter and understand its results. These features are often different for different meters. You should understand the features of your own meter.

Measurement range: Most glucose meters are able to read glucose levels over a broad range of values from as low as zero to as high as 600 mg/dL. Since the range is different among meters, interpret very high or low values carefully. Glucose readings are not linear over their entire range. If you get an extremely high or low reading from your meter, you should first confirm it with another reading. You should also consider checking your meter's calibration.

Whole blood glucose vs. plasma glucose: Glucose levels in plasma (one of the components of blood) are generally 10–15% higher than glucose measurements in whole blood (and even more after eating).

This is important because home blood glucose meters measure the glucose in whole blood while most lab tests measure the glucose in plasma. There are many meters on the market now that give results as "plasma equivalent". This allows patients to easily compare their glucose measurements in a lab test and at home. Remember, this is just the way that the measurement is presented to you. All portable blood glucose meters measure the amount of glucose in whole blood. The meters that give "plasma equivalent" readings have a built in algorithm that translates the whole blood measurement to make it seem like the result that would be obtained on a plasma sample. It is important for you and your healthcare provider to know whether your meter gives its results as "whole blood equivalent" or "plasma equivalent."

Cleaning: Some meters need regular cleaning to be accurate. Clean your meter with soap and water, using only a dampened soft cloth to avoid damage to sensitive parts. Do not use alcohol (unless recommended in the instructions), cleansers with ammonia, glass cleaners, or abrasive cleaners. Some meters do not require regular cleaning but contain electronic alerts indicating when you should clean them. Other meters can be cleaned only by the manufacturer.

Display of high and low glucose values: Part of learning how to operate a meter is understanding what the meter results mean. Be sure you know how high and low glucose concentrations are displayed on your meter.

Factors That Affect Glucose Meter Performance

The accuracy of your test results depends partly on the quality of your meter and test strips and your training. Other factors can also make a difference in the accuracy of your results.

Hematocrit: Hematocrit is the amount of red blood cells in the blood. Patients with higher hematocrit values will usually test lower for blood glucose than patients with normal hematocrit. Patients with lower hematocrit values will test higher. If you know that you have abnormal hematocrit values you should discuss its possible effect on glucose testing (and HbA1C testing) with your health care provider. Anemia and Sickle Cell Anemia are two conditions that affect hematocrit values.

Other substances: Many other substances may interfere with your testing process. These include uric acid (a natural substance in the body that can be more concentrated in some people with diabetes), glutathione (an "anti-oxidant" also called "GSH"), and ascorbic acid (vitamin C). You should check the package insert for each meter to find what substances might affect its testing accuracy, and discuss your concerns with your health care provider.

Altitude, temperature, and humidity: Altitude, room temperature, and humidity can cause unpredictable effects on glucose results. Check the meter and test strip package insert for information on these issues. Store and handle the meter and test strips according to the instructions.

Third-party test strips: Third-party or "generic glucose reagent strips" are test strips developed as a less expensive option than the strips that the manufacturer intended the meter to be used with. They are typically developed by copying the original strips. Although these strips may work on the meter listed on the package, they could look like strips used for other meters. Be sure the test strip you use is compatible with your glucose meter.

Sometimes manufacturers change their meters and their test strips. These changes are not always communicated to the third-party strip manufacturers. This can make third-party strips incompatible with your meter without your knowledge. Differences can involve the amount, type or concentration of the chemicals (called "reagents") on the test strip, or the actual size and shape of the strip itself. Meters are sensitive to these features of test strips and may not work well or consistently if they are not correct for a meter. If you are unsure whether or not a certain test strip will work with you meter, contact the manufacturer of your glucose meter.

Making Sure Your Meter Works Properly

You should perform quality-control checks to make sure that your home glucose testing is accurate and reliable. Several things can reduce the accuracy of your meter reading even if it appears to still work. For instance, the meter may have been dropped or its electrical components may have worn out. Humidity or heat may damage test strips. It is even possible that your testing technique may have changed slightly. Quality control checks should be done on a regular basis according to the meter manufacturer's instructions.

- **Check using "Test Quality Control Solutions" or "Electronic Controls":** Test quality control solutions and electronic controls are both used to check the operation of your meter. Test quality control solutions check the accuracy of the meter and test strip. They may also give an indication of how well you use your system. Electronic controls only check that the meter is working properly.

- **Take your meter with you to the health care provider's office:** This way you can test your glucose while your health care provider watches your technique to make sure you are using the meter correctly. Your healthcare provider will also take a sample of blood and evaluate it using a routine laboratory method. If values obtained on the glucose meter match the laboratory method, you and your healthcare provider will see that your meter is working well and that you are using good technique. If results do not match the laboratory method results, then results you get from your meter may be inaccurate and you should discuss the issue with your healthcare provider and contact the manufacturer if necessary.

New Technologies: Alternative Site Testing

Some glucose meters allow testing blood from alternative sites, such as the upper arm, forearm, base of the thumb, and thigh.

Sampling blood from alternative sites may be desirable, but it may have some limitations. Blood in the fingertips show changes in glucose levels more quickly than blood in other parts of the body. This means that alternative site test results may be different from fingertip test results not because of the meter's ability to test accurately, but because the actual glucose concentration can be different. FDA believes that further research is needed to better understand these differences in test values and their possible impact on the health of people with diabetes.

Minimally Invasive and Non-Invasive Glucose Meters

Researchers are exploring new technologies for glucose testing that avoid fingersticks. One of these is based on near-infrared spectroscopy for measurement of glucose. Essentially, this amounts to measuring glucose by shining a beam of light on the skin. It is painless. There are increasing numbers of reports in the scientific literature on the challenges, strengths, and weaknesses of this and other new approaches to testing glucose without fingersticks.

FDA has approved one "minimally invasive" meter and one "non-invasive" glucose meter. Neither of these should replace standard glucose testing. They are used to obtain additional glucose values between fingerstick tests. Both devices require daily calibration using standard fingerstick glucose measurements and both remain the subject of continuing studies to find how they are best used as tools for diabetes management.

MiniMed continuous glucose monitoring system: The MiniMed system consists of a small plastic catheter (very small tube) inserted just under the skin. The catheter collects small amounts of liquid that is passed through a "biosensor" to measure the amount of glucose present.

MiniMed is intended for occasional use and to discover trends in glucose levels during the day. It does not give you readings for individual tests and therefore you can't use it for typical day-to-day monitoring. The device collects measurements over a 72-hour period and then must be downloaded by the patient or healthcare provider. Understanding trends over time might help patients know the best time to do their standard fingerstick tests. You need a prescription to buy MiniMed.

Cygnus GlucoWatch Biographer. GlucoWatch is worn on the arm like a wristwatch. It pulls tiny amounts of fluid from the skin and measures the glucose in the fluid without puncturing the skin. The device requires three hours to warm up after it is put on. After this, it can provide up to three glucose measurements per hour for 12 hours. Unlike the MiniMed device, the GlucoWatch displays results that can be read by the wearer, although like the MiniMed device, these readings are not meant to be used as replacements for fingerstick-based tests. The results are meant to show trends and patterns in glucose levels rather than report any one result alone. It is useful for detecting and evaluating episodes of hyperglycemia and hypoglycemia. However, you must confirm its results with a standard glucose meter before you take corrective action. You need a prescription to buy GlucoWatch.

Reporting Problems with Glucose Meters to FDA

FDA reviews all glucose meters and test strips before they can be marketed to the public. This FDA "premarket" review process requires the manufacturer of the meter to show that the meter system provides acceptable accuracy and consistency of glucose measurement at high, medium, and low levels of glucose as compared to glucose meters already being sold. The quality of software is an increasingly important feature of glucose meters since it controls the testing and data storage and controls the displays that the user sees and uses when testing.

FDA learns about problems with medical products through the MedWatch program. Consumers can report problems with medical devices, including glucose meters, through MedWatch.

- For general information about the MedWatch program and instructions for reporting problems with medical devices, go online to http://www.fda.gov/medwatch/how.htm.

- For further information about how medical device problems are reported to FDA, go online to http://www.fda.gov/cdrh/mdr.html.

Other Diabetes Management Tests

Glycosylated Hemoglobin

There is hemoglobin in all red blood cells. Hemoglobin is the part of the red blood cell that carries oxygen to the tissues and organs in the body. Hemoglobin combines with blood glucose to make glycosylated hemoglobin or hemoglobin A1c.

Red blood cells store glycosylated hemoglobin slowly over their 120-day life span. When you have high levels of glucose in your blood, your red blood cells store large amounts of glycosylated hemoglobin. When you have normal or near normal levels, your red blood cells store normal or near normal amounts of glycosylated hemoglobin. So, when you measure your glycosylated hemoglobin, you can find out your level of blood glucose, averaged over the last few months.

It is good to have your glycosylated hemoglobin tested at least two times a year if you meet your treatment goals or up to four times a year if you change therapy or do not meet your treatment goals. There are now many different ways to measure glycosylated hemoglobin. These tests vary in cost and convenience and you can do some at home. The values (glycosylated hemoglobin index) these tests give can vary too. Talk to your doctor about what your glycosylated hemoglobin index should be.

Glycosylated Serum Proteins

Serum proteins, like hemoglobin, combine with glucose to form glycosylated products. Testing these glycosylated products can give information about your glucose control over shorter periods of time than testing glycosylated hemoglobin.

One common test is the fructosamine test. It gives information on your glucose status over a one- to two-week period. High values mean your blood glucose was high over the past two weeks. This test is good for watching short-term changes in your glucose status during pregnancy or after major changes in your therapy. There is no general guideline for when to use this test. Talk to your doctor about whether this test is right for you.

Urine Glucose

Only patients who are unable to use blood glucose meters should use urine glucose tests. Testing urine for glucose, which was once the best way for patients to manage their diabetes, has mostly now been replaced by self-monitoring of blood glucose.

Urine and Blood Ketones

When the body does not have enough insulin, fats are used for fuel instead of glucose. A by-product of burning fats is the production of ketones. Ketones are passed in the urine and can be detected with a urine test.

If you do not have diabetes, you usually have only small amounts of ketones in your blood and urine. If you have diabetes, however, you may have high amounts of ketones and acid, a condition known as ketoacidosis. This condition can cause nausea, vomiting, or abdominal pain and can be life threatening.

You may use urine dipsticks to rapidly and easily measure the ketones in your urine. You dip a dipstick in your urine and follow the instruction on the package to see if you have a high amount of ketones.

Microalbumin

One common and extremely serious result of diabetes is kidney failure. Under normal conditions, the kidneys filter toxins from the blood. When the kidney's filtering processes begin to become impaired, protein (microalbumin) begins to spill into the urine. Testing urine for small, yet abnormal amounts of albumin (microalbuminuria) is a common way to detect this condition early, before it can damage your kidneys.

Many urine dipsticks are used to test for large amounts of albumin. To measure a small amount of albumin, which may show an early stage of kidney disease, your health care provider may use specific tests for low levels of albumin (microalbumin tests). To do this test, you may have to collect your urine for several 24-hour periods.

Cholesterol

If you have diabetes, you have a higher risk of heart and blood vessel disease (cardiovascular disease). One way to limit this risk is to measure your cholesterol routinely and control it by changing your lifestyle or taking prescription drugs. A cholesterol test usually shows your total cholesterol, total triglycerides, and high-density lipoproteins (HDLs).

Section 6.3

Tests Used to Monitor Kidney Function

Excerpted from "Your Kidneys and How They Work,"
National Kidney and Urologic Diseases Information Clearinghouse,
NIH Pub. No. 070-3195, August 2007.

What are the signs of kidney disease?

People in the early stages of kidney disease usually do not feel sick at all.

If your kidney disease gets worse, you may need to urinate more often or less often. You may feel tired or itchy. You may lose your appetite or experience nausea and vomiting. Your hands or feet may swell or feel numb. You may get drowsy or have trouble concentrating. Your skin may darken. You may have muscle cramps.

What medical tests will my doctor use to detect kidney disease?

Since you can have kidney disease without any symptoms, your doctor may first detect the condition through routine blood and urine tests. The National Kidney Foundation recommends three simple tests to screen for kidney disease: a blood pressure measurement, a spot check for protein or albumin in the urine (proteinuria), and a calculation of glomerular filtration rate (GFR) based on a serum creatinine measurement. Measuring urea nitrogen in the blood provides additional information.

Blood pressure measurement: High blood pressure can lead to kidney disease. It can also be a sign that your kidneys are already impaired. The only way to know whether your blood pressure is high is to have a health professional measure it with a blood pressure cuff. The result is expressed as two numbers. The top number, which is called the systolic pressure, represents the pressure when your heart is beating. The bottom number, which is called the diastolic pressure, shows the pressure when your heart is resting between beats. Your blood pressure is considered normal if it stays below 120/80 (expressed as "120 over 80"). The National Heart Lung and Blood Institute recommends that people with kidney disease use whatever therapy is necessary, including lifestyle changes and medicines, to keep their blood pressure below 130/80.

Microalbuminuria and proteinuria: Healthy kidneys take wastes out of the blood but leave protein. Impaired kidneys may fail to separate a blood protein called albumin from the wastes. At first, only small amounts of albumin may leak into the urine, a condition known as microalbuminuria, a sign of deteriorating kidney function. As kidney function worsens, the amount of albumin and other proteins in the urine increases, and the condition is called proteinuria. Your doctor may test for protein using a dipstick in a small sample of your urine taken in the doctor's office. The color of the dipstick indicates the presence or absence of proteinuria.

A more sensitive test for protein or albumin in the urine involves laboratory measurement and calculation of the protein-to-creatinine or albumin-to-creatinine ratio. This test should be used to detect kidney disease in people at high risk, especially those with diabetes. If your first laboratory test shows high levels of protein, another test should be done one to two weeks later. If the second test also shows high levels of protein, you have persistent proteinuria and should have additional tests to evaluate your kidney function.

Glomerular filtration rate (GFR) based on creatinine measurement: GFR is a calculation of how efficiently the kidneys are filtering wastes from the blood. A traditional GFR calculation requires an injection into the bloodstream of a substance that is later measured in a 24-hour urine collection. Recently, scientists found they could calculate GFR without an injection or urine collection. The new calculation requires only a measurement of the creatinine in a blood sample.

Creatinine is a waste product in the blood created by the normal breakdown of muscle cells during activity. Healthy kidneys take creatinine out of the blood and put it into the urine to leave the body. When kidneys are not working well, creatinine builds up in the blood.

In the lab, your blood will be tested to see how many milligrams of creatinine are in one deciliter of blood (mg/dL). Creatinine levels in the blood can vary, and each laboratory has its own normal range, usually 0.6 to 1.2 mg/dL. If your creatinine level is only slightly above this range, you probably will not feel sick, but the elevation is a sign that your kidneys are not working at full strength. One formula for estimating kidney function equates a creatinine level of 1.7 mg/dL for most men and 1.4 mg/dL for most women to 50 percent of normal kidney function. But because creatinine values are so variable and can be affected by diet, a GFR calculation is more accurate for determining whether a person has reduced kidney function.

The new GFR calculation uses the patient's creatinine measurement along with weight, age, and values assigned for sex and race. Some medical laboratories may make the GFR calculation when a creatinine value is measured and include it on their lab report.

Blood urea nitrogen (BUN): Blood carries protein to cells throughout the body. After the cells use the protein, the remaining waste product is returned to the blood as urea, a compound that contains nitrogen. Healthy kidneys take urea out of the blood and put it in the urine. If your kidneys are not working well, the urea will stay in the blood.

A deciliter of normal blood contains seven to 20 milligrams of urea. If your BUN is more than 20 mg/dL, your kidneys may not be working at full strength. Other possible causes of an elevated BUN include dehydration and heart failure.

Additional Tests for Kidney Disease: If blood and urine tests indicate reduced kidney function, your doctor may recommend additional tests to help identify the cause of the problem.

Renal imaging: Methods of renal imaging (taking pictures of the kidneys) include ultrasound, computed tomography (CT scan), and magnetic resonance imaging (MRI). These tools are most helpful in finding unusual growths or blockages to the flow of urine.

Renal biopsy: Your doctor may want to see a tiny piece of your kidney tissue under a microscope. To obtain this tissue sample, the doctor will perform a renal biopsy—a hospital procedure in which the doctor inserts a needle through your skin into the back of the kidney. The needle retrieves a strand of tissue about ½ to ¾ of an inch long. For the procedure, you will lie on your stomach on a table and receive local anesthetic to numb the skin. The sample tissue will help the doctor identify problems at the cellular level.

Chapter 7

Testing for Thyroid Dysfunction

Definition

What is the thyroid?

The thyroid gland is a butterfly-shaped endocrine gland that is normally located in the lower front of the neck. The thyroid's job is to make thyroid hormone, which is secreted into the blood and then carried to every tissue in the body. Thyroid hormone is essential to help each cell in each tissue and organ to work right. For example, thyroid hormone helps the body use energy, stay warm, and keep the brain, heart, muscles, and other organs working as they should.

Function

How does the thyroid gland function?

The major thyroid hormone secreted by the thyroid gland is thyroxine, also called T4 because it contains four iodine atoms. To exert its effects, T4 is converted to triiodothyronine (T3) by the removal of an iodine atom. This occurs mainly in the liver and in certain tissues where T3 acts, such as in the brain. The amount of T4 produced by the thyroid gland is controlled by another hormone, which is made in the pituitary gland located at the base of the brain, called thyroid

"Thyroid Function Tests," © 2005 American Thyroid Association (www.thyroid .org). Reprinted with permission.

stimulating hormone (abbreviated TSH). The amount of TSH that the pituitary sends into the blood stream depends on the amount of T4 that the pituitary sees. If the pituitary sees very little T4, then it produces more TSH to tell the thyroid gland to produce more T4. Once the T4 in the blood stream goes above a certain level, the pituitary's production of TSH is shut off. In fact, the thyroid and pituitary act in many ways like a heater and a thermostat. When the heater is off and it becomes cold, the thermostat reads the temperature and turns on the heater. When the heat rises to an appropriate level, the thermostat senses this and turns off the heater. Thus, the thyroid and the pituitary, like a heater and thermostat, turn on and off. This is illustrated in Figure 7.1.

Test

Tests to Evaluate Thyroid Function

Blood tests to measure TSH, T4, and T3 are readily available and widely used.

TSH tests: The best way to initially test thyroid function is to measure the TSH level in a blood sample. A high TSH level indicates that the thyroid gland is failing because of a problem that is directly affecting the thyroid (primary hypothyroidism). The opposite situation, in which the TSH level is low, usually indicates that the person

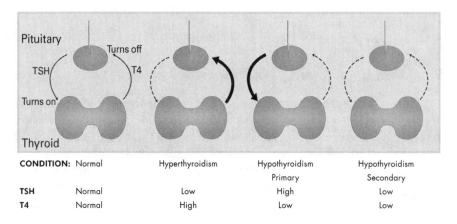

CONDITION:	Normal	Hyperthyroidism	Hypothyroidism Primary	Hypothyroidism Secondary
TSH	Normal	Low	High	Low
T4	Normal	High	Low	Low

Figure 7.1. The thyroid and the pituitary, like a heater and thermostat, turn on and off.

has an overactive thyroid that is producing too much thyroid hormone (hyperthyroidism). Occasionally, a low TSH may result from an abnormality in the pituitary gland, which prevents it from making enough TSH to stimulate the thyroid (secondary hypothyroidism). In most healthy individuals, a normal TSH value means that the thyroid is functioning normally.

T4 tests: T4 circulates in the blood in two forms: 1) T4 bound to proteins that prevent the T4 from entering the various tissues that need thyroid hormone and 2) free T4, which does enter the various target tissues to exert its effects. The free T4 fraction is the most important to determine how the thyroid is functioning, and tests to measure this are called the Free T4 (FT4) and the Free T4 Index (FT4I or FTI). Individuals who have hyperthyroidism will have an elevated FT4 or FTI, whereas patients with hypothyroidism will have a low level of FT4 or FTI. Combining the TSH test with the FT4 or FTI accurately determines how the thyroid gland is functioning. The finding of an elevated TSH and low FT4 or FTI indicates primary hypothyroidism due to disease in the thyroid gland. A low TSH and low FT4 or FTI indicates hypothyroidism due to a problem involving the pituitary gland. A low TSH with an elevated FT4 or FTI is found in individuals who have hyperthyroidism.

T3 tests: T3 tests are often useful to diagnosis hyperthyroidism or to determine the severity of the hyperthyroidism. Patients who are hyperthyroid will have an elevated T3 level. In some individuals with a low TSH, only the T3 is elevated and the FT4 or FTI is normal. T3 testing rarely is helpful in the hypothyroid patient, since it is the last test to become abnormal. Patients can be severely hypothyroid with a high TSH and low FT4 or FTI, but have a normal T3.

Thyroid antibody tests: The immune system of the body normally protects us from foreign invaders such as bacteria and viruses by destroying these invaders with substances called antibodies produced by blood cells known as lymphocytes. In many patients with hypothyroidism or hyperthyroidism, lymphocytes make antibodies against their thyroid that either stimulate or damage the gland. Two common antibodies that cause thyroid problems are directed against thyroid cell proteins: thyroid peroxidase and thyroglobulin. Measuring levels of thyroid antibodies may help diagnose the cause of the thyroid problems. For example, positive anti-thyroid peroxidase and/ or anti-thyroglobulin antibodies in a patient with hypothyroidism make a diagnosis of Hashimoto thyroiditis. If the antibodies are positive in a hyperthyroid patient, the most likely diagnosis is autoimmune thyroid disease.

Non-Blood Tests

Radioactive iodine uptake: Because T4 contains much iodine, the thyroid gland must pull a large amount of iodine out from the blood stream in order for the gland to make an appropriate amount of T4. The thyroid has developed a very active mechanism for doing this. Therefore, this activity can be measured by having an individual swallow a small amount of iodine, which is radioactive. The radioactivity allows the doctor to track where the iodine molecules go. By measuring the amount of radioactivity that is taken up by the thyroid gland (radioactive iodine uptake, RAIU), doctors may determine whether the gland is functioning normally. A very high RAIU is seen in individuals whose thyroid gland is overactive (hyperthyroidism), while a low RAIU is seen when the thyroid gland is underactive (hypothyroidism). In addition to the radioactive iodine uptake, a thyroid scan may be obtained, which shows a picture of the thyroid gland.

Chapter 8

Prenatal Tests

Every parent-to-be hopes for a healthy baby, but it can be hard not to worry: What if the baby has a serious or untreatable health problem? What would I do? Would it be my fault?

Concerns like these are completely natural. Fortunately, though, a wide array of tests for pregnant women can help to reassure them and keep them informed throughout their pregnancies.

Prenatal tests can help identify—and sometimes treat—health problems that could endanger both you and your unborn child. However, they do have limitations. As an expectant parent, it's important to educate yourself about these tests and to think about what you would do if a health problem is detected in either you or your baby.

Why Are Prenatal Tests Performed?

Prenatal tests can identify several different things:

- Treatable health problems in the mother that can affect the baby's health

- Characteristics of the baby, including size, sex, age, and placement in the uterus

- The chance that a baby has certain congenital, genetic, or chromosomal problems
- Certain types of fetal abnormalities, including heart problems

The last two items on this list may seem the same, but there's a key difference. Some prenatal tests are screening tests and only reveal the possibility of a problem. Other prenatal tests are diagnostic, which means they can determine—with a fair degree of certainty—whether a fetus has a specific problem. In the interest of making the more specific determination, the screening test may be followed by a diagnostic test.

Prenatal testing is further complicated by the fact that approximately 250 birth defects can be diagnosed in a fetus—many more than can be treated or cured.

What Do Prenatal Tests Find?

Among other things, routine prenatal tests can determine key things about the mother's health, including:

- her blood type;
- whether she has gestational diabetes;
- her immunity to certain diseases;
- whether she has a sexually transmitted disease (STD) or cervical cancer.

All of these conditions can affect the health of the fetus.

Prenatal tests also can determine things about the fetus's health, including whether it's one of the 2% to 3% of babies in the United States that the American College of Obstetricians and Gynecologists (ACOG) says have major congenital birth defects.

Categories of defects screened by prenatal tests include:

- dominant gene disorders;
- recessive gene disorders;
- X-linked disorders;
- chromosomal disorders;
- multifactorial disorders.

Dominant gene disorders: In dominant gene disorders, there's a 50-50 chance a child will inherit the gene from the affected parent and have the disorder. Dominant gene disorders include:

- Achondroplasia, a rare abnormality of the skeleton that causes a form of dwarfism;

- Huntington disease, a disease of the nervous system that causes a combination of mental deterioration and a movement disorder affecting people in their 30s and 40s.

Recessive gene disorders: Because there are so many genes in each cell, everyone carries some abnormal genes, but most people don't have a defect because the normal gene overrules the abnormal recessive one. But if a fetus has a pair of abnormal recessive genes (one from each parent), the child will have the disorder. It's more likely for this to happen in children born to certain ethnic groups. Recessive gene disorders include:

- Cystic fibrosis, a disease most common among people of northern European descent that is life threatening and causes severe lung damage and nutritional deficiencies;

- Sickle cell disease, a disease most common among people of African descent in which red blood cells form a "sickle" shape (rather than the typical donut shape), which can get caught in blood vessels and cause damage to organs and tissues;

- Tay-Sachs disease, a disorder most common among people of European (Ashkenazi) Jewish descent that causes mental retardation, blindness, seizures, and death;

- Beta thalassemia, a disorder most common among people of Mediterranean descent that causes anemia.

X-linked disorders: These disorders are determined by genes on the X chromosome. The X and Y chromosomes are the chromosomes that determine sex. These disorders are much more common in boys because the pair of sex chromosomes in males contains only one X chromosome (the other is a Y chromosome). If the disease gene is present on the one X chromosome, the X-linked disease shows up because there's no other paired gene to "overrule" the disease gene. One such X-linked disorder is hemophilia, which prevents the blood from clotting properly.

Chromosomal disorders: Some chromosomal disorders are inherited but most are caused by a random error in the genetics of the egg or sperm. The chance of a child having these disorders increases with the age of the mother. For example, according to ACOG, one in

1,667 live babies born to 20-year-olds have Down syndrome, which causes mental retardation and physical defects. That number changes to one in 378 for 35-year-olds and one in 106 for 40-year-olds.

Multifactorial disorders: This final category includes disorders that are caused by a mix of genetic and environmental factors. Their frequency varies from country to country, and some can be detected during pregnancy.

Multifactorial disorders include neural tube defects, which occur when the tube enclosing the spinal cord doesn't form properly. Neural tube defects, which often can be prevented by taking folic acid during the early part of pregnancy, include:

- *Spina bifida:* Also called "open spine," this defect happens when the lower part of the neural tube doesn't close during embryo development, leaving the spinal cord and nerve bundles exposed.

- *Anencephaly:* This defect occurs when the brain and head don't develop properly, and the top half of the brain is completely absent.

Other multifactorial disorders include:

- congenital heart defects;
- obesity;
- diabetes;
- cancer.

Who Has Prenatal Tests?

Certain prenatal tests are considered routine—that is, almost all pregnant women receiving prenatal care get them. Other non-routine tests are recommended only for certain women, especially those with high-risk pregnancies. These include women who:

- are age 35 or older;
- have had a premature baby;
- have had a baby with a birth defect—especially heart or genetic problems;
- have high blood pressure, diabetes, lupus, asthma, or a seizure disorder;

- have an ethnic background in which genetic disorders are common (or a partner who does);

- have a family history of mental retardation (or a partner who does).

Although your health care provider (which may be your OB-GYN, family doctor, or a certified nurse-midwife) may recommend these tests, it's ultimately up to you to decide whether to have them.

Also, if you or your partner have a family history of genetic problems, you may want to consult with a genetic counselor to help you construct a family tree going back as far as three generations.

To decide which tests are right for you, it's important to carefully discuss with your health care provider:

- what these tests are supposed to measure;

- how reliable they are;

- the potential risks;

- your options and plans if the results indicate a disorder or defect.

Prenatal Tests During the First Visit

During your first visit to your health care provider for prenatal care, you can expect to have a full physical, including a pelvic and rectal examination, and you'll undergo certain tests regardless of your age or genetic background.

Blood tests check for:

- your blood type and Rh factor. If your blood is Rh negative and your partner's is Rh positive, you may develop antibodies that prove dangerous to your fetus. This can be treated through a course of injections.

- anemia (a low red blood cell count) to make sure you're not iron deficient.

- hepatitis B, syphilis, and HIV/AIDS.

- immunity to German measles (rubella) and chickenpox (varicella).

- cystic fibrosis. Health care providers now routinely check for this even when there's no family history of the disorder.

Cervical tests (also called Pap smears) check for:

- STDs such as chlamydia and gonorrhea;
- cervical cancer.

To do a Pap smear, your health care provider uses what looks like a very long mascara wand or cotton swab to gently scrape the inside of your cervix (the opening to the uterus that's located at the very top of the vagina). This doesn't hurt at all; some women say they feel a little twinge, but it only lasts a second.

Prenatal Tests Performed Throughout or Later in Pregnancy

After the initial visit, your health care provider will order other tests based on, among other things, your personal medical history and needs. These tests may include:

- urine tests for sugar, protein, and signs of infection. The sugar in urine indicates gestational diabetes—diabetes that occurs during pregnancy; the protein can indicate preeclampsia—a condition that develops in late pregnancy and is characterized by a sudden rise in blood pressure and excessive weight gain, with fluid retention and protein in the urine.
- group B streptococcus (GBS) infection. GBS bacteria are found naturally in the vaginas of many women and can cause serious infections in newborns. This test involves swabbing the vagina, usually between the 35th and 37th weeks of pregnancy.
- sickle cell trait tests for women of African or Mediterranean descent, who are at higher risk for having sickle cell anemia—a chronic blood disease—or carrying the trait, which can be passed on to their children.

Other Tests

Other tests that might be performed during pregnancy include:

- ultrasound;
- glucose screening;
- chorionic villus sampling (CVS);
- maternal blood screening/triple screen/quadruple screen;
- amniocentesis;
- nonstress test;

86

- contraction stress test;
- percutaneous umbilical blood sampling (PUBS).

Ultrasound

Why is this test performed?

In this test, sound waves are bounced off the baby's bones and tissues to construct an image showing the baby's shape and position in the uterus. Ultrasounds were once used only in high-risk pregnancies but have become so common that they're often part of routine prenatal care.

Also called a sonogram, sonograph, echogram, or ultrasonogram, an ultrasound is used:

- to determine whether the fetus is growing at a normal rate;
- to verify the expected date of delivery;
- to record fetal heartbeat or breathing movements;
- to see whether there might be more than one fetus;
- to identify a variety of abnormalities that might affect the remainder of the pregnancy or delivery;
- to make sure the amount of amniotic fluid in the uterus is adequate;
- to indicate the position of the placenta in late pregnancy (which may be blocking the baby's way out of the uterus);
- to detect pregnancies outside the uterus;
- as a guide during other tests such as amniocentesis.

Ultrasounds also are used to detect:

- structural defects such as spina bifida and anencephaly;
- congenital heart defects;
- gastrointestinal and kidney malformations;
- cleft lip or palate.

Should I have this test?

Most women have at least one ultrasound. The test is considered to be safe; however, it is wise to find out from your health care provider if it's the most appropriate test for you.

When should I have this test?

An ultrasound is usually performed at 18 to 20 weeks to look at your baby's anatomy. If you want to know your baby's gender, you may be able to find out during this time—that is, if his or her genitals are in a visible position.

Ultrasounds also can be done sooner or later and sometimes more than once, depending on the health care provider. For example, some will order an ultrasound to date the pregnancy, usually during the first two months. And others may want to order one during late pregnancy to make sure the baby's turned the right way before delivery.

Women with high-risk pregnancies may need to have multiple ultrasounds using more sophisticated equipment. Results can be confirmed when needed using special three-dimensional (3-D) equipment that allows the technician to get a more detailed look at the baby.

How is this test performed?

Women need to have a full bladder for a transabdominal ultrasound (an ultrasound of the belly) to be performed in the early months—you may be asked to drink a lot of water and not urinate. You'll lie on an examining table and your abdomen will be coated with a special ultrasound gel. A technician will pass a wand-like instrument called a transducer back and forth over your abdomen. High-frequency sound waves "echo" off your body and create a picture of the fetus inside on a computer screen.

You may want to ask to have the picture interpreted for you, even in late pregnancy—it often doesn't look like a baby to the untrained eye.

Sometimes, if the technician isn't getting a good enough image from the ultrasound, he or she will determine that a transvaginal ultrasound is necessary. This is especially common in early pregnancy. For this procedure, your bladder should be empty. Instead of a transducer being moved over your abdomen, a slender probe called an endovaginal transducer is placed inside your vagina. This technique often provides improved images of the uterus and ovaries.

Some health care providers may have the equipment and trained personnel necessary to provide in-office ultrasounds, whereas others may have you go to a local hospital or radiology center. Depending on where you have the ultrasound done, you may be able to get a printed picture (or multiple pictures) of your baby and/or a disc of images you can view on your computer and even send to friends and family.

When are the results available?

Immediately, but a full evaluation may take up to one week. A radiologist (a physician experienced in obstetric ultrasound) will analyze the images and send a signed report with his or her interpretation to your doctor.

Depending on where you have the ultrasound done, the technician may be able to tell you that day whether everything looks OK. However, most radiology centers or health care providers prefer that technicians not comment until a specialist has taken a look—especially if an abnormality is detected, but even when everything is OK.

Glucose Screening

Why is this test performed?

Glucose screening checks for gestational diabetes, a short-term form of diabetes that develops in some women during pregnancy. Gestational diabetes occurs in 1% to 3% of pregnancies and can cause health problems for the baby.

Should I have this test?

Most women have this test.

When should I have this test?

Screening for gestational diabetes usually takes place at 12 weeks for women at higher risk of having the condition, including those who:

- have previously had a baby that weighs more than nine pounds (4.1 kilograms);
- have a family history of diabetes;
- are obese;
- are older than age 30.

All other pregnant women are tested for diabetes at around 24 to 28 weeks. But if you've had high sugar in two routine urine tests, your health care provider may order it earlier.

How is the test performed?

This test involves drinking a sugary liquid and then having your blood drawn after an hour. If the sugar level in the blood is high, you'll have a glucose-tolerance test, which means you'll drink a glucose solution on an empty stomach and have your blood drawn once every hour for three hours. The American Diabetes Association suggests that in order to confirm diabetes, these tests be performed at different times.

When are the results available?

The results are usually available within a day, although your health care provider probably won't call you unless the reading is high and you need to come in for another test.

Chorionic Villus Sampling (CVS)

Why is this test performed?

Chorionic villi are tiny finger-like units that make up the placenta (a disk-like structure that sticks to the inner lining of the uterus and provides nutrients from the mother to the fetus through the umbilical cord). They have the same chromosomes and genetic makeup as the fetus.

This newer alternative to an amniocentesis removes some of the chorionic villi and tests them for chromosomal abnormalities, such as Down syndrome. Its advantage over an amniocentesis is that it can be performed earlier, allowing more time for expectant parents to receive counseling and make decisions.

Should I have this test?

Your health care provider may recommend this test if you:

- are older than age 35;
- have a family history of genetic disorders (or a partner who does);
- have a previous child with a birth defect;
- have had an earlier screening test that indicates that there may be a concern.

Possible risks of this test include:

- between a 0.5% and 1% risk of miscarriage;
- prematurity;
- early labor;

- infection;
- spotting or bleeding (this is more common with the transcervical method).

When should I have this test?

At 10 to 12 weeks.

How is this test performed?

This test is done in one of two ways:

- *Transcervical:* Using ultrasound as a guide, a thin tube is passed from the vagina into the cervix. Gentle suction removes a sample of tissue from the chorionic villi. No anesthetic is used, although some women do experience a pinch and cramping.

- *Transabdominal:* A needle is inserted through the abdominal wall—this minimizes the chances of intrauterine infection, and in a woman whose uterus is in a bent position, reduces the chance of miscarriage. After the sample is taken, the doctor will check the fetus's heart rate. You should rest for several hours afterward.

When are the results available?

Less than one week for Down syndrome and about two weeks for a thorough analysis.

Maternal Blood Screening/Triple Screen/Quadruple Screen

Why is this test performed?

Doctors use this to test the mother's blood only for alpha-fetoprotein (AFP). AFP is the protein produced by the fetus, and it appears in varying amounts in the mother's blood and the amniotic fluid at different times during pregnancy. A certain level in the mother's blood is considered normal, but higher or lower levels may indicate a problem. The test typically is used to determine risk for Down syndrome.

This test has been expanded, however, to also detect two pregnancy hormones—estriol and human chorionic gonadotropin (HCG)—which is why it's now sometimes called a "triple screen" or "triple marker." The test is called a "quadruple screen" ("quad screen") or "quadruple marker" ("quad marker") when the level of an additional substance—inhibin-A—is also measured. The greater number of markers increases the accuracy of the screening and better identifies the possibility of a birth defect.

This test, which also is called a multiple-marker screening or maternal serum screening, calculates a woman's individual risk of birth defects based on the levels of the three (or more) substances plus:

- her age;
- her weight;
- her race;
- whether she has diabetes requiring insulin treatment.

It's important to note, though, that this screening test determines risk only—it doesn't diagnose a condition.

Should I have this test?

All women are offered this test. Remember that this is a screening, not a definitive test—it indicates whether a woman is likely to be carrying an affected fetus. It's also not foolproof—spina bifida may go undetected, and some women with high levels have been found to be carrying a healthy baby. Further testing is recommended to confirm a positive result.

When should I have this test?

At 16 to 18 weeks.

How is the test performed?

Blood is drawn from the mother.

When are the results available?

Three to five days, although it may take up two weeks.

Amniocentesis

Why is this test performed?

This test is most often used to detect:

- Down syndrome and other chromosome abnormalities;

- structural defects such as spina bifida and anencephaly;
- inherited metabolic disorders.

Late in the pregnancy, this test can reveal if a baby's lungs are strong enough to allow the baby to breathe normally after birth. This can help the health care provider make decisions about inducing labor or trying to prevent labor, depending on the situation. For instance, if a mother's water breaks early, the health care provider may want to try to hold off on delivering the baby as long as possible to allow for the baby's lungs to mature.

Other common birth defects, such as heart disorders and cleft lip and palate, can't be determined using this test.

Should I have this test?

Your health care provider may recommend this test if you:

- are older than age 35;
- have a family history of genetic disorders (or a partner who does);
- have a previous child with a birth defect.

This test can be very accurate—close to 100%—but only certain disorders can be detected. According to the Centers for Disease Control and Prevention (CDC), the rate of miscarriage with this procedure is between one in 400 and one in 200. The procedure also carries a low risk of uterine infection (less than one in 1,000), which can cause miscarriage.

When should I have this test?

At 16 to 18 weeks.

How is the test performed?

A needle is inserted through the abdominal wall into the uterus to remove some (about one ounce) of the amniotic fluid. A local anesthetic may be used. Some women report that they experience cramping when the needle enters the uterus or pressure while the doctor retrieves the sample.

The doctor will check the fetus's heartbeat after the procedure to make sure it's normal. Most doctors recommend rest for several hours after the procedure.

The cells in the withdrawn fluid are grown in a special culture and then analyzed (the specific tests conducted on the fluid depend on personal and family medical history).

When are the results available?

Timing varies; it can take up to one month, with the possibility that the lab will ask for a repeat. Tests of lung maturity are available immediately.

Nonstress Test

Why is this test performed?

A nonstress test (NST) can determine if the baby is responding normally to a stimulus. Used mostly in high-risk pregnancies or when a health care provider is uncertain of fetal movement, an NST can be performed at any point in the pregnancy after the 26th to 28th week when fetal heart rate can appropriately respond by accelerating and decelerating.

If you've gone beyond your due date, this test also uses external fetal monitoring to determine fetal movement. The NST can help a doctor make sure that the baby is receiving enough oxygen and that the nervous system is responding. However, a nonresponsive baby doesn't necessarily mean that the baby is in danger.

Should I have this test?

Your health care provider may recommend this if you have a high-risk pregnancy or if you have a low-risk pregnancy but are past your due date.

When should I have this test?

At one week after the due date.

How is the test performed?

The health care provider will measure the response of the fetus's heart rate to each movement the fetus makes as reported by the mother or observed by the doctor on an ultrasound screen. If the fetus doesn't move during the test, he or she may be asleep and the health care provider may use a buzzer to wake the baby.

When are the results available?

Immediately.

Contraction Stress Test

Why is this test performed?

This test stimulates the uterus with Pitocin, a synthetic form of oxytocin (a hormone secreted during childbirth), to determine the effect of contractions on fetal heart rate. It's usually recommended when a nonstress test indicates a problem and can determine whether the baby's heart rate remains stable during contractions.

Should I have this test?

This test is usually ordered if the nonstress test indicates a problem. It does have a high false-positive rate, though, and can induce labor.

When should I have this test?

Your doctor will schedule it if he or she is concerned about how the baby will respond to contractions or feels that it is the appropriate test to determine the fetal heart rate response to a stimulus.

How is the test performed?

Mild contractions are brought on either by injections of Pitocin or by squeezing the mother's nipples (which causes oxytocin to be secreted). The fetus's heart rate is then monitored.

When are the results available?

Immediately.

Percutaneous Umbilical Blood Sampling (PUBS)

Why is this test performed?

This test obtains fetal blood by guiding a needle into the umbilical vein. It's primarily used in addition to an ultrasound and amniocentesis if your health care provider needs to quickly check your baby's chromosomes for defects or disorders or if he or she is concerned that your baby may be anemic.

The advantage to this test is its speed. There are situations (such as when a fetus shows signs of distress) in which it's helpful to know whether the fetus has a fatal chromosomal defect. If the fetus is suspected to be anemic or to have a platelet disorder, this test is the only way to confirm this because it provides a blood sample rather than amniotic fluid. It also allows transfusion of blood or needed fluids into the baby while the needle is in place.

Should I have this test?

This test is used:

- after an abnormality has been noted on an ultrasound;
- when amniocentesis results aren't conclusive;
- if the fetus may have Rh disease;
- if you've been exposed to an infectious disease that could potentially affect fetal development.

When should I have this test?

Between 18 and 36 weeks.

How is the test performed?

A fine needle is passed through your abdomen and uterus into the fetal vein in the umbilical cord and blood is withdrawn for testing.

When are the results available?

In three days.

Talking to Your Health Care Provider

Some prenatal tests can be stressful, and because many aren't definitive, even a negative result may not ease any anxiety you may be experiencing. Because many women who have abnormal tests end up having healthy babies and because many of the problems that are detected can't be treated, some women decide not to have some of the tests.

One important thing to consider is what you'll do in the event that a birth defect is discovered. Your health care provider or a genetic counselor can help you establish priorities, give you the facts, and discuss your options.

It's also important to remember that tests are offered to women— they are not mandatory. You should feel free to ask your health care provider why he or she is ordering a certain test, what the risks and benefits are, and, most important, what the results will—and won't— tell you.

If you think that your health care provider isn't answering your questions adequately, you should say so. You don't have to accept the answer, "I do this test on all of my patients." Things you might want to ask include:

- How accurate is this test?
- What are you looking to get from these test results?/What do you hope to learn?
- How long before I get the results?
- Is the procedure painful?
- Is the procedure dangerous to me or the fetus?
- Do the potential benefits outweigh the risks?
- What could happen if I don't undergo this test?
- How much will the test cost?
- Will the test be covered by insurance?
- What do I need to do to prepare?

You also can ask your health care provider for literature about each type of test.

Preventing Birth Defects

The best thing that mothers-to-be can do to avoid birth defects is to take care of their bodies during pregnancy by:

- not smoking (and avoiding second-hand smoke);
- avoiding alcohol;
- eating a healthy diet;
- taking prenatal vitamins;
- getting exercise;
- getting plenty of rest;
- getting prenatal care.

Chapter 9

Infertility Testing

Female Fertility Testing

When a couple has been unsuccessful at achieving pregnancy after one year, both partners need to go through a comprehensive physical and medical assessment. Tests for female infertility and a semen analysis should start immediately. Because male factors account for approximately 50% of all infertility cases, it is important to examine both partners for possible infertility issues.

What is the process for female fertility testing?

Ideally, you will have already begun tracking your ovulation through fertility awareness or a fertility monitor. This will provide your reproductive specialists with valuable information about your ovulation. Usually the first question regarding female fertility is whether you are ovulating or not.

The first test performed by your fertility specialists involves measuring your follicle stimulating hormone (FSH) and luteinizing hormone (LH) to establish a baseline. This is performed on the third day of your cycle. This test is performed during your first visit.

This chapter includes "Female Infertility Testing," and "Male Fertility Testing," reprinted with permission from the American Pregnancy Association, (www.americanpregnancy.org), © 2007. All rights reserved.

Your second visit will occur on the day of the LH surge, which is before ovulation in most cases. During your first cycle, it is common for your fertility specialists to perform the following tests:

- **Cervical mucus tests**: This involves a postcoital test (PCT) which determines if the sperm is able to penetrate and survive in the cervical mucus. It also involves a bacterial screening.

- **Ultrasound tests:** This is used to assess the thickness of the lining of the uterus (endometrium), monitor follicle development, and check the condition of the uterus and ovaries. An ultrasound may be conducted two to three days later to confirm that an egg has been released.

- **Hormone tests:** These tests are done to assess the various hormone levels that contribute to the reproductive process. These hormone tests include the following:
  - Luteinizing Hormone
  - Follicle Stimulating Hormone
  - Estradiol
  - Progesterone
  - Prolactin
  - Free T3
  - Total Testosterone
  - Free Testosterone
  - DHEAS
  - Androstenedione

If both the semen analysis and the above testing return normal results, there is also additional testing that your fertility specialists may recommend. These tests include any of the following:

- **Hysterosalpingogram (HSG):** This is simply an x-ray of your uterus and fallopian tubes. A blue dye is injected through the cervix into the uterus and fallopian tubes. The dye enables the radiologist to see if there is blockage or any other problem.

- **Hysteroscopy:** This is a procedure that may be used if the HSG indicates that there may be problems. The hysteroscope is inserted through the cervix into the uterus, which allows your fertility specialist to see any abnormalities, growths, or scarring in the uterus.

The hysteroscope allows your physician to take pictures which may be used for future reference.

- **Laparoscopy:** This is a procedure which uses a narrow fiber optic telescope. The laparoscope is inserted through a woman's abdomen to look at the uterus, fallopian tubes, and ovaries. Your physician will be checking for endometriosis, scar tissue, or other adhesions. It is important to confirm that you are not pregnant before this test is performed.

- **Endometrial biopsy:** This is a procedure which involves scraping a small amount of tissue from the endometrium just prior to menstruation. This biopsy is performed to assess whether there is a hormonal imbalance or not. It is important to confirm that you are not pregnant before this test is performed.

These tests are not mandatory and your fertility specialists will know which tests best fit your situation.

Male Fertility Testing

Testing for male infertility is simple and routine. Male infertility is related to approximately 50% of all infertility cases, and male infertility alone accounts for approximately one-third of all cases. When a couple has not been able to conceive over the course of one year, both need to go through a comprehensive physical and medical history.

What types of tests are performed?

A semen analysis is the most common testing procedure for determining if there is a male infertility factor. Sperm is collected into a specimen jar and presented to a lab technician who examines the sperm under a microscope to evaluate the count, shape, appearance, and mobility.

When assessing sperm count, the technician will be checking to see whether the sperm concentration is above or below 20 million sperm cells per milliliter of ejaculation fluid.

If the sperm count is low, your fertility specialist will probably test the blood testosterone, FSH, LH, and prolactin levels.

A urinalysis may be used to look for white blood cells which may indicate an infection. The urinalysis will also determine if there is sperm in the urine, which would suggest that there is a problem with ejaculation known as retrograde ejaculation.

If the medical history, physical examination, and semen analysis are normal, attention should be directed to the female partner before further evaluation of the man.

Further male factor evaluation is unlikely to occur, but is sometimes needed. If so, additional laboratory and sperm analysis tests may be used. Here is a list of tests and a brief description of what each is examining:

- **Sperm agglutination:** This is a laboratory test which examines sperm under a microscope to determine whether the sperm are clumping together. Clumping prevents sperm from swimming through the cervical mucus.

- **Sperm penetration assay:** This is a laboratory test which uses hamster eggs to evaluate a sperms capability of penetrating the egg. This test is rarely used any more.

- **Hemizona assay:** This is a laboratory test that involves cutting a non-usable human egg in half. The purpose is to see if the sperm can penetrate the outermost protective layer of the egg.

- **Acrosome reaction:** This is a laboratory test which assesses whether sperm heads can go through the chemical changes necessary to dissolve an egg's tough outer shell.

- **Hypo-osmotic swelling:** This is a laboratory test that uses a special sugar and salt solution to evaluate the sperm's tail and ability to penetrate the egg. The tails of healthy sperm tend to swell in this solution whereas dead or abnormal sperm do not swell.

- **Testicular biopsy:** A small piece of tissue is removed from the tubules in the testes and examined to determine how well sperm are being produced.

- **Vasography:** An x-ray exam is used to determine if there is blockage or leakage of sperm in the vas deferens.

- **Ultrasonography:** This is an exam used to locate damage or blockages in the male reproductive tract, including the prostate, seminal vesicles, and ejaculatory ducts.

For further information about these testing procedures, consult with your fertility specialist.

Chapter 10

Tests for Osteoporosis

Osteoporosis is a disease of progressive bone loss associated with an increased risk of fractures. The term osteoporosis literally means "porous bone." Diagnosis of osteoporosis involves a measurement of bone mineral density (BMD).

Radiographic Measurement

The history of BMD measurement dates back to the 1940s. At that time, bone density was measured on plain radiographs (x-rays). However, because loss of bone density is not apparent on a plain x-ray until approximately 40% of the bone is lost, different methods of BMD measurement have been developed.

Singh index: The Singh index describes the trabecular patterns in the bone at the top of the thighbone (femur). X-rays are graded one through six according to the disappearance of the normal trabecular pattern. Studies have shown a link between a Singh index of less than three and fractures of the hip, wrist, and spine.

Radiographic absorptiometry: Radiographic absorptiometry was developed during the late 1980s as an easy way to determine BMD with plain x-ray. An x-ray of the hand is taken, incorporating an aluminum reference wedge. The x-ray is then analyzed, and the density of the bone is compared to the density of the reference wedge.

Single-Photon Absorptiometry

In the early 1960s, a new method of measuring BMD, called single-photon absorptiometry (SPA), was developed. In this method, a single-energy photon beam is passed through bone and soft tissue to a detector. The amount of mineral in the path is then quantified. The distal radius (wrist) is usually used as the site of measurement because the amount of soft tissue in this area is small.

SPA measurements are accurate, and the test usually takes about 10 minutes. The radioactive source gradually decays, however, and must be replaced after some time.

Dual-Photon Absorptiometry

Dual-photon absorptiometry (DPA) uses a photon beam that has two distinct energy peaks. One energy peak is absorbed more by the soft tissue. The other energy peak is absorbed more by bone. The soft-tissue component is subtracted to determine the BMD.

DPA allowed for the first time BMD measurements of the spine and proximal femur. However, although DPA is accurate for predicting fracture risk, the precision is poor because of decay of the isotope. In addition, the machine has limited usefulness in monitoring BMD changes over time.

Dual-Energy X-Ray Absorptiometry

Dual-energy x-ray absorptiometry (DXA) works in a similar fashion to DPA, but uses an x-ray source instead of a radioactive isotope. This measurement technique is superior to DPA because the radiation source does not decay and the energy stays constant over time. DXA has become the "gold standard" for BMD measurement today.

Scan times for DXA are much shorter than for DPA, and the radiation dose is very low. The skin dose for an anteroposterior spine scan is in the range of three millirem (mrem).

DXA scans are extremely precise. Precision in the range of 1% to 2% has been reported. DXA can be used as an accurate and precise method to monitor changes in bone density in patients undergoing treatments.

The first generation DXA machines used a pencil beam-type scanner. The x-ray source moved with a single detector. Second-generation machines use a fan-beam scanner that incorporates a group of detectors instead of a single detector. These machines are considerably faster and produce a higher resolution image.

Quantitative Computed Tomography

Measurement of BMD by quantitative computed tomography (QCT) can be performed with most standard CT scanners. QCT is unique in that it provides for true three-dimensional imaging and reports BMD as true volume density measurements.

The advantage of QCT is the ability to isolate an area of interest from surrounding tissues. QCT can, therefore, localize an area in a vertebral body of only trabecular bone, leaving out the elements most affected by degenerative change and sclerosis.

The radiation dose with QCT is about ten times that of DXA, and QCT tests may be more expensive than DXA.

Peripheral Bone Density Testing

Lower cost portable devices that can determine BMD at peripheral sites such as the radius, phalanges, or calcaneus are increasingly being used for osteoporosis screening. The advantage of using a portable device is the ability to bring BMD assessment to a population who otherwise would not be able to have the test. These machines are considerably less expensive than those that measure BMD in the hip and spine.

One of the problems with peripheral testing is that only one site is tested; thus, low bone density in the hip or spine may be missed. This may be a problem because of differences in bone density between different skeletal sites.

Although peripheral machines are considered accurate, doubts have been raised about their precision. Peripheral machines may not be good enough to monitor patients undergoing treatment for osteoporosis.

In postmenopausal women, differences in BMD between different skeletal sites are more common. BMD may be normal at one site and low at another site. In the early postmenopausal years, bone density in the spine decreases first because the bone turnover in this highly trabecular bone is greater than at other skeletal sites. Bone density becomes similar across the skeleton at approximately 70 years of age.

In early postmenopausal women—therefore, up to the age of 65 years—the most accurate site to measure BMD is probably the spine.

105

In women older than 65 years, BMD is similar across the skeleton; therefore, it may not make much difference which site is measured.

Caution must be used when interpreting spine scans in elderly patients because degenerative changes may falsely elevate BMD values. BMD measurements are, however, mostly site specific, and the most accurate predictor of fracture risk at any site is a BMD measurement of the spine.

At present, peripheral BMD testing machines are good screening devices because of their portability, availability, and lower cost. However, the following patients may still need central testing, even if peripheral testing is normal:

- Postmenopausal patients not on hormone replacement therapy (HRT) who would consider HRT, bisphosphonates, or selective estrogen receptor modulators (SERMs), if low bone mass is discovered

- Patients with a maternal history of hip fracture, smoking, tallness (more than 5' 7"), or thinness (less than 125 lb.)

- Patients on medications associated with bone loss

- Patients with secondary conditions associated with low bone mass, such as hyperthyroidism, posttransplantation, malabsorption, hyperparathyroidism, and alcoholism

- Patients found to have high urinary collagen crosslinks

- Patients with a history of previous fragility fracture

Interpreting a Bone Density Report

The main purpose of obtaining a bone density test is to determine fracture risk. BMD correlates very well with risk of fracture. It is more powerful in predicting fractures than cholesterol is in predicting myocardial infarction or blood pressure in predicting stroke.

T-Score

The T-score is the number of standard deviations (SD) above or below the young adult mean. The young adult mean is the expected normal value for the patient compared to others of the same sex and ethnicity. It is approximately what the patient should have been at their peak bone density at about age 20 years.

As a general rule, for every SD below normal the fracture risk doubles. Thus, a patient with a BMD of one SD below normal (a T-score of -1) has twice the risk of fracture as a person with a normal BMD. If the T-score is -2, the risk of fracture is four times normal. A T-score of -3 is eight times the normal fracture risk. Patients with a high fracture risk can be treated to prevent future fractures.

Other risk factors for fracture include a person's eyesight, balance, leg strength, and physical agility. Age itself is an independent risk factor for fracture, independent of bone density. Osteoporosis patients that have had a previous fragility fracture are considered to have severe osteoporosis and have a high risk for future fractures.

Z-Score

The Z-score is the number of SD the bone density measurement is above or below the value expected for the patient's age.

Primary osteoporosis is age-related osteoporosis, with no secondary causes.

Secondary osteoporosis occurs when underlying agents or conditions induce bone loss. Some common causes of secondary osteoporosis are thyroid or parathyroid abnormalities, malabsorption, alcoholism, smoking, and the use of certain medications especially corticosteroids.

A Z-score lower then -1.5 is suggestive of secondary osteoporosis. If secondary causes are suspected, laboratory testing should be performed to find out if there is an underlying reason for the osteoporosis. This is important because treating the underlying condition may be necessary to correct the low bone density.

Chapter 11

Testing for Infectious Diseases

Chapter Contents

Section 11.1

Testing for Sexually Transmitted Diseases

Excerpted from "Bacterial Vaginosis," "Chlamydia," "Genital Herpes," "Gonorrhea," "HIV/AIDS," "Human Papillomavirus and Genital Warts," "Pelvic Inflammatory Disease," "Syphilis," and "Trichomoniasis," National Institute of Allergy and Infectious Diseases, 2007.

Bacterial Vaginosis

According to the Centers for Disease Control and Prevention (CDC), bacterial vaginosis (BV) is the most common cause of vaginitis symptoms among women of childbearing age. It previously was called nonspecific vaginitis, or Gardnerella-associated vaginitis. Health experts are not sure what role sexual activity plays in developing BV.

Diagnosis

A health care provider can examine a sample of vaginal fluid under a microscope, either stained or in special lighting, to look for bacteria associated with BV. Then, they can diagnose BV based on the following:

- absence of lactobacilli
- presence of numerous "clue cells" (cells from the vaginal lining that are coated with BV germs)
- fishy odor
- change from normal vaginal fluid

Chlamydia

Chlamydia is a curable sexually transmitted infection (STI). You can get chlamydial infection during vaginal, oral, or anal sexual contact with an infected partner. It can cause serious problems in men and women, such as penile discharge and infertility respectively, as well as infections in newborn babies of infected mothers.

Chlamydia is one of the most widespread bacterial STIs in the United States. The Centers for Disease Control and Prevention (CDC) estimates 2.8 million people are infected each year.

Diagnosis

Chlamydia is easily confused with gonorrhea because the symptoms of both diseases are similar and the diseases can occur at the same time.

The most reliable ways to find out whether the infection is chlamydia are through laboratory tests.

A health care provider may collect a sample of fluid from the vagina or penis and send it to a laboratory that will look for the bacteria.

Another test looks for the bacteria in a urine sample and does not require a pelvic exam or swabbing of the penis. Results are usually available within 24 hours.

Genital Herpes

Genital herpes is a sexually transmitted infection (STI). According to the Centers for Disease Control and Prevention (CDC), one out of five American teenagers and adults is infected with genital herpes. Women are more commonly infected than men. In the United States, one out of four women has herpes.

Although at least 45 million people in the United States have genital herpes infection, there has been a substantial decrease in cases from 21 percent to 17 percent, according to a 1999 to 2004 CDC survey. Much of the decrease was in the 14 to 19 year age group, and continued through the young adult group.

Diagnosis

Your health care provider can diagnose typical genital herpes by looking at the sores. Some cases, however, are more difficult to diagnose.

The virus sometimes, but not always, can be detected by a laboratory test called a culture. A culture is done when your health care provider uses a swab to get and study material from a suspected herpes sore. You may still have genital herpes, however, even if your culture is negative (which means it does not show HSV).

A blood test called type-specific test can tell whether you are infected with HSV-1 or HSV-2. The type-specific test results plus the location of the sores will help your health care provider to find out whether you have genital infection.

Gonorrhea

Gonorrhea is a curable sexually transmitted infection (STI). It is the second most commonly reported bacterial STI in the United States following chlamydia. In 2004, 330,132 cases of gonorrhea were reported to the Centers for Disease Control and Prevention (CDC). When examining race and ethnicity, age, and gender, the highest rates of gonorrhea were found in African Americans, 15 to 24 years of age, and women, respectively.

Gonorrhea can spread into the uterus and fallopian tubes, resulting in pelvic inflammatory disease (PID). PID affects more than one million women in this country every year and can cause tubal (ectopic) pregnancy and infertility in as many as 10 percent of infected women. In addition to gonorrhea playing a major role in PID, some health researchers think it adds to the risk of getting HIV infection.

Diagnosis

Health care providers usually use three laboratory tests to diagnose gonorrhea.

- Staining samples directly for the bacteria
- Detecting bacterial genes or DNA in urine
- Growing the bacteria in laboratory cultures

Many providers prefer to use more than one test to increase the chance of an accurate diagnosis.

You usually can get the staining test results while in your doctor's office or in a clinic. This test is quite accurate for men but not so in women. Only one in two women with gonorrhea has a positive stain.

More often, health care providers use urine or cervical swabs for a new test that detects the genes of the bacteria. These tests are more accurate than culturing the bacteria.

The laboratory culture test involves placing a sample of the discharge onto a culture plate. The health care provider also can take a culture to detect gonorrhea in the throat. Culture also allows testing for drug-resistant bacteria.

HIV/AIDS

AIDS was first reported in the United States in 1981 and has since become a major worldwide epidemic. AIDS is caused by the human immunodeficiency virus, or HIV. By killing or damaging cells of the body's immune system, HIV progressively destroys the body's ability to fight infections and certain cancers. People diagnosed with AIDS may get life-threatening diseases called opportunistic infections. These infections are caused by microbes such as viruses or bacteria that usually do not make healthy people sick.

Since 1981, more than 980,000 cases of AIDS have been reported in the United States to the Centers for Disease Control and Prevention (CDC). According to CDC, more than 1,000,000 Americans may be infected with HIV, one-quarter of whom are unaware of their infection. The epidemic is growing most rapidly among minority populations and is a leading killer of African American males ages 25 to 44. According to CDC, AIDS affects nearly seven times more African Americans and three times more Hispanics than whites. In recent years, an increasing number of African American women and children are being affected by HIV/AIDS.

Diagnosis

Because early HIV infection often causes no symptoms, a healthcare provider usually can diagnose it by testing blood for the presence of antibodies (disease-fighting proteins) to HIV. HIV antibodies generally do not reach noticeable levels in the blood for one to three months after infection. It may take the antibodies as long as six months to be produced in quantities large enough to show up in standard blood tests. Hence, to determine whether a person has been recently infected (acute infection), a healthcare provider can screen blood for the presence of HIV genetic material. Direct screening of HIV is extremely critical to prevent transmission of HIV from recently infected individuals.

Anyone who has been exposed to the virus should get an HIV test as soon as the immune system is likely to develop antibodies to the virus—within six weeks to 12 months after possible exposure to the virus. By getting tested early, a healthcare provider can give advice to an infected person about when to start treatment to help the immune system combat HIV and help prevent the emergence of certain opportunistic infections. Early testing also alerts an infected person to avoid high-risk behaviors that could spread the virus to others.

Most healthcare providers can do HIV testing and will usually offer counseling at the same time. Of course, testing can be done anonymously at many sites if a person is concerned about confidentiality.

Healthcare providers diagnose HIV infection by using two different types of antibody tests: ELISA (enzyme-linked immunosorbent assay) and Western blot. If a person is highly likely to be infected with HIV but has tested negative for both tests, a healthcare provider may request additional tests. A person also may be told to repeat antibody testing at a later date, when antibodies to HIV are more likely to have developed.

Diagnosis in Babies

Babies born to mothers infected with HIV may or may not be infected with the virus, but all carry their mothers' antibodies to HIV for several months. If these babies lack symptoms, healthcare providers cannot make a definitive diagnosis of HIV infection using standard antibody tests. Instead, they are using new technologies to detect HIV and more accurately determine HIV infection in infants between ages three months and 15 months. Researchers are evaluating a number of blood tests to determine which ones are best for diagnosing HIV infection in babies younger than three months.

Human Papillomavirus and Genital Warts

Human Papillomavirus

Human papillomavirus (HPV) is one of the most common causes of sexually transmitted infection (STI) in the world. Health experts estimate there are more cases of genital HPV infection than any other STI in the United States. According to the Centers for Disease Control and Prevention (CDC), approximately 6.2 million new cases of sexually transmitted HPV infections are reported every year. At least 20 million people in this country are already infected.

Genital Warts

Genital warts (sometimes called condylomata acuminata or venereal warts) are the most easily recognized sign of genital HPV infection. Many people, however, have a genital HPV infection without genital warts.

Genital warts are soft, moist, or flesh colored and appear in the genital area within weeks or months after infection. They sometimes appear in clusters that resemble cauliflower-like bumps, and are either raised or flat, small or large. Genital warts can show up in women on the vulva and cervix, and inside and surrounding the vagina and anus. In men, genital warts can appear on the scrotum or penis. There are cases where genital warts have been found on the thigh and groin.

Diagnosis

Your health care provider usually diagnoses genital warts by seeing them.

If you are a woman with genital warts, you also should be examined for possible HPV infection of the cervix. Your health care provider can diagnose HPV infection based on results from an abnormal Pap smear, a primary cancer-screening tool for cervical cancer or precancerous changes of the cervix. In some cases, a health care provider will take a small piece of tissue from the cervix and examine it under the microscope.

Another test to diagnose HPV infection detects HPV DNA, which may indicate possible infection.

Your provider may be able to identify some otherwise invisible warts in your genital tissue by applying vinegar (acetic acid) to areas of your body that might be infected. This solution causes infected areas to whiten, which makes them more visible.

Pelvic Inflammatory Disease

Pelvic inflammatory disease (PID) is a general term that refers to infection and inflammation of the upper genital tract in women. It can affect the uterus (womb), fallopian tubes (tubes that carry eggs from the ovaries to the uterus), ovaries, and other organs related to reproduction. The scarring that results on these organs can lead to infertility, tubal (ectopic) pregnancy, chronic pelvic pain, abscesses (sores containing pus), and other serious problems. PID is the most common preventable cause of infertility in the United States.

Women at greater risk for PID include those at risk for sexually transmitted infections (STIs) and those with a prior episode of PID. Sexually active women under age 25 are at risk as well because the cervix (opening to the uterus) of teens and young women has greater susceptibility to STIs. This may be because the cervix of teenage girls and young women is not fully matured, increasing their risk for STIs linked to PID.

Other potential risk factors include douching, which women should avoid. In some women, using an intrauterine device (IUD) to prevent pregnancy can also cause PID. Rarely, PID results from gynecological procedures or surgeries.

In the United States, more than one million women seek treatment for acute PID each year, according to the Centers for Disease Control and Prevention (CDC). A similar or greater number of women may have PID and not know it. PID is more common among teenage than adult women. It is also more common among African American and Hispanic women.

Every year, more than 100,000 women become infertile and more than 150 women die from PID or its complications.

Diagnosis

PID can be difficult for your health care provider to diagnose because symptoms can be subtle and mild and similar to those of some other diseases. If you think you might have PID, you should get medical care promptly because early treatment can limit long-term complications such as infertility and chronic pelvic pain.

If you have symptoms such as lower abdominal pain, your health care provider will perform a physical exam, including a pelvic (internal) exam, to find out the nature and location of the pain. Your health care provider also will check for the following:

- abnormal vaginal or cervical discharge
- masses near your ovaries and tubes
- tenderness or pain of your abdomen, cervix, uterus, and ovaries

Health experts have found that about 70 percent and 50 percent of chlamydial and gonococcal infections, respectively, are asymptomatic (without symptoms) in women. These infections were found first through screening. You should get regular laboratory tests for chlamydia, gonorrhea, urinary tract infection, and if appropriate, pregnancy. Your health care provider may suggest these tests as part of a routine annual exam as well as tests for HIV infection and syphilis.

If necessary, your health care provider may do other tests such as an ultrasound (sonogram), endometrial (uterine) biopsy, or laparoscopy to distinguish between PID and other serious problems that can mimic PID.

Laparoscopy is a surgical procedure in which a tube is inserted through a small incision near your navel. This allows your health care provider to view the internal abdominal and pelvic organs and to take specimens to examine in the laboratory.

Syphilis

Syphilis is a sexually transmitted bacterial infection (STI) that initially causes genital ulcers (sores). If untreated, these ulcers can then lead to more serious symptoms of infection.

An ancient disease, syphilis is still of major importance today. Although syphilis rates in the United States declined by almost 90 percent from 1990 to 2000, the number of cases rose from 5,979 in 2000 to 7,980 in 2004. In a single year, from 2003 to 2004, the number of syphilis cases jumped eight percent.

There also was a dramatic change in whom the disease affects. Between 2002 and 2003, the number of cases in men increased 13.5 percent, reflecting an increase in syphilis in men who have sex with men. During the same time the number of cases in women declined by 27.3 percent.

Syphilis also disproportionately affects African Americans, who represent 41 percent of all cases reported to the Centers for Disease Control and Prevention (CDC).

HIV infection and syphilis are linked. Syphilis increases the risk of transmitting as well as getting infected with HIV.

Diagnosis

It can be very difficult for your health care provider to diagnose syphilis based on symptoms. This is because symptoms and signs of the disease might be absent, go away without treatment, or be confused with those of other diseases. Because syphilis can be hard to diagnose, you should:

- visit your health care provider if you have a lesion (sore) in your genital area or a widespread rash,
- get tested periodically for syphilis if your sexual behaviors put you at risk for STIs, and
- get tested to be sure you do not also have syphilis if you have been treated for another STI such as gonorrhea or HIV infection.

Your health care provider can diagnose early syphilis by seeing a chancre or rash and then confirming the diagnosis with laboratory tests. Because latent syphilis has no symptoms, it is diagnosed only by laboratory tests.

There are two laboratory methods for making the diagnosis.

- Identifying the bacteria under a microscope in a sample taken from a lesion
- Performing a blood test for syphilis

If your doctor thinks you might have neurosyphilis, your spinal fluid will be tested as well.

117

Trichomoniasis

Trichomoniasis is one of the most common curable sexually trans-mitted infections (STIs), especially in young, sexually active women. According to the Centers for Disease Control and Prevention (CDC), an estimated 7.4 million new cases occur in men and women every year in the United States.

Diagnosis

A health care provider can diagnose trichomoniasis by performing laboratory tests on fluid samples from the vagina or penis.

When women are infected with trichomoniasis, a pelvic examina-tion reveals red sores on the cervix (opening to the womb) or inside the vagina.

Section 11.2

Frequently Asked Questions about HIV Testing

"Frequently Asked Questions," an undated document produced by Na-tional HIV Testing Resources, a service of the Centers for Disease Con-trol and Prevention, available online at http://www.hivtest.org.subindex .cfm?FuseAction=faq; accessed December 15, 2007.

Should I get tested?

The following are behaviors that increase your chances of getting HIV. If you answer yes to any of them, you should definitely get an HIV test. If you continue with any of these behaviors, you should be tested every year. Talk to a health care provider about an HIV test-ing schedule that is right for you.

- Have you injected drugs or steroids or shared equipment (such as needles, syringes, works) with others?

- Have you had unprotected vaginal, anal, or oral sex with men who have sex with men, multiple partners, or anonymous part-ners?

- Have you exchanged sex for drugs or money?

- Have you been diagnosed with or treated for hepatitis, tuberculosis (TB), or a sexually transmitted infection (STI), like syphilis?

- Have you had unprotected sex with someone who could answer yes to any of the above questions?

If you have had sex with someone whose history of sex partners or drug use is unknown to you or if you or your partner has had many sex partners, then you have more of a chance of being infected with HIV. Both you and your new partner should get tested for HIV, and learn the results, before having sex for the first time.

For women who plan to become pregnant, testing is even more important. If a woman is infected with HIV, medical care and certain drugs given during pregnancy can lower the chance of passing HIV to her baby. All women who are pregnant should be tested during each pregnancy.

How long after a possible exposure should I wait to get tested for HIV?

Most HIV tests are antibody tests that measure the antibodies your body makes against HIV. It can take some time for the immune system to produce enough antibodies for the antibody test to detect and this time period can vary from person to person. This time period is commonly referred to as the "window period." Most people will develop detectable antibodies within two to eight weeks (the average is 25 days). Even so, there is a chance that some individuals will take longer to develop detectable antibodies. Therefore, if the initial negative HIV test was conducted within the first three months after possible exposure, repeat testing should be considered more than three months after the exposure occurred to account for the possibility of a false-negative result. Ninety seven percent will develop antibodies in the first three months following the time of their infection. In very rare cases, it can take up to six months to develop antibodies to HIV.

Another type of test is an RNA test, which detects the HIV virus directly. The time between HIV infection and RNA detection is nine to 11 days. These tests, which are more costly and used less often than antibody tests, are used in some parts of the United States.

For information on HIV testing, you can talk to your health care provider or you can find the location of the HIV testing site nearest to you by calling CDC-INFO 24 Hours/Day at 800-CDC-INFO (232-4636),

888-232-6348 (TTY), in English, en Español. Both of these resources are confidential.

How do HIV tests work?

Once HIV enters the body, the immune system starts to produce antibodies—chemicals that are part of the immune system that recognize invaders like bacteria and viruses and mobilize the body's attempt to fight infection. In the case of HIV, these antibodies cannot fight off the infection, but their presence is used to tell whether a person has HIV in his or her body. In other words, most HIV tests look for the HIV antibodies rather than looking for HIV itself. There are tests that look for HIV's genetic material directly, but these are not in widespread use.

The most common HIV tests use blood to detect HIV infection. Tests using saliva or urine are also available. Some tests take a few days for results, but rapid HIV tests can give results in about 20 minutes. All positive HIV tests must be followed up by another test to confirm the positive result. Results of this confirmatory test can take a few days to a few weeks.

What are the different HIV screening tests available in the United States?

In most cases the EIA (enzyme immunoassay), used on blood drawn from a vein, is the most common screening test used to look for antibodies to HIV. A positive (reactive) EIA must be used with a follow-up (confirmatory) test such as the Western blot to make a positive diagnosis. There are EIA tests that use other body fluids to look for antibodies to HIV. These include oral fluid tests and urine tests:

- **Oral fluid tests:** Use oral fluid (not saliva) that is collected from the mouth using a special collection device. This is an EIA antibody test similar to the standard blood EIA test. A follow-up confirmatory Western Blot uses the same oral fluid sample.

- **Urine tests:** Use urine instead of blood. The sensitivity and specificity (accuracy) are somewhat less than that of the blood and oral fluid tests. This is also an EIA antibody test similar to blood EIA tests and requires a follow-up confirmatory Western Blot using the same urine sample.

Rapid tests: A rapid test is a screening test that produces very quick results, in approximately 20 minutes. Rapid tests use blood from a vein or from a finger stick, or oral fluid to look for the presence of antibodies to HIV. As is true for all screening tests, a reactive rapid HIV test result must be confirmed with a follow-up confirmatory test before a final diagnosis of infection can be made. These tests have similar accuracy rates as traditional EIA screening tests.

Home testing kits: Consumer-controlled test kits (popularly known as "home testing kits") were first licensed in 1997. Although home HIV tests are sometimes advertised through the internet, currently only the Home Access HIV-1 Test System is approved by the Food and Drug Administration. (The accuracy of other home test kits cannot be verified). The Home Access HIV-1 Test System can be found at most local drug stores. It is not a true home test, but a home collection kit. The testing procedure involves pricking a finger with a special device, placing drops of blood on a specially treated card, and then mailing the card in to be tested at a licensed laboratory. Customers are given an identification number to use when phoning in for the results. Callers may speak to a counselor before taking the test, while waiting for the test result, and when the results are given. All individuals receiving a positive test result are provided referrals for a follow-up confirmatory test, as well as information and resources on treatment and support services.

RNA tests: RNA tests look for genetic material of the virus and can be used in screening the blood supply and for detection of very early infection rare cases when antibody tests are unable to detect antibodies to HIV.

If I test HIV negative, does that mean that my sex partner is HIV negative also?

No. Your HIV test result reveals only your HIV status. Your negative test result does not indicate whether or not your partner has HIV. HIV is not necessarily transmitted every time you have sex. Therefore, your taking an HIV test should not be seen as a method to find out if your partner is infected.

Ask your partner if he or she has been tested for HIV and what risk behaviors he or she has engaged in, both currently and in the past. Think about getting tested together.

It is important to take steps to reduce your risk of getting HIV. Not having (abstaining from) sex is the most effective way to avoid HIV. If you choose to be sexually active, having sex with one person who only has sex with you and who is uninfected is also effective. If you are not sure that both you and your partner are HIV negative, use a latex condom to help protect both you and your partner from HIV and other STIs. Studies have shown that latex condoms are very effective, though not 100%, in preventing HIV transmission when used correctly and consistently. If either partner is allergic to latex, plastic (polyurethane) condoms for either the male or female can be used.

What if I test positive for HIV?

If you test positive for HIV, the sooner you take steps to protect your health, the better. Early medical treatment and a healthy lifestyle can help you stay well. Prompt medical care may delay the onset of AIDS and prevent some life-threatening conditions. There are a number of important steps you can take immediately to protect your health:

- See a licensed health care provider, even if you do not feel sick. Try to find a health care provider who has experience treating HIV. There are now many medications to treat HIV infection and help you maintain your health. It is never too early to start thinking about treatment possibilities.

- Have a TB (tuberculosis) test. You may be infected with TB and not know it. Undetected TB can cause serious illness, but it can be successfully treated if caught early.

- Smoking cigarettes, drinking too much alcohol, or using illegal drugs (such as methamphetamines) can weaken your immune system. There are programs available that can help you stop or reduce your use of these substances.

- Get screened for other sexually transmitted infections (STIs). Undetected STIs can cause serious health problems. It is also important to practice safe-sex behaviors so you can avoid getting STIs.

There is much you can do to stay healthy. Learn all that you can about maintaining good health.

Not having (abstaining from) sex is the most effective way to avoid transmitting HIV to others. If you choose to have sex, use a latex condom to help protect your partner from HIV and other STIs. Studies have shown that latex condoms are very effective, though not 100%, in preventing HIV transmission when used correctly and consistently.

If either partner is allergic to latex, plastic (polyurethane) condoms for either the male or female can be used.

I'm HIV positive. Where can I get information about treatment?

CDC recommends that you be in the care of a licensed health care provider, preferably one with experience treating people living with HIV. Your health care provider can assist you with treatment information and guidance.

Detailed information on specific treatments is available from the Department of Health and Human Services' AIDSinfo. Information on enrolling in clinical trials is also available at AIDSinfo. You may contact AIDSinfo by phone at 800-448-0440 (English and Spanish) or 888-480-3739 (TTY).

Why does CDC recommend HIV screening for all pregnant women?

HIV testing during pregnancy is important because antiviral therapy can improve the mother's health and greatly lower the chance that an HIV-infected pregnant woman will pass HIV to her infant before, during, or after birth. The treatment is most effective for babies when started as early as possible during pregnancy. However, there are still great health benefits to beginning treatment even during labor or shortly after the baby is born.

CDC recommends HIV screening for all pregnant women because risk-based testing (when the health care provider offers an HIV test based on the provider's assessment of the pregnant woman's risk) misses many women who are infected with HIV. CDC does recommend providing information on HIV (either orally or by pamphlet) and, for women with risk factors, referrals to prevention counseling. Refer to the Public Health Service Task Force Recommendations for Use of Antiretroviral Drugs in Pregnant HIV-1-Infected Women for Maternal Health and Interventions to Reduce Perinatal HIV-1 Transmission in the United States for more information.

HIV testing provides an opportunity for infected women to find out that they are infected and to gain access to medical treatment that may help improve their own health. It also allows them to make informed choices that can prevent transmission to their infant. For some uninfected women with risks for HIV, the prenatal care period could be an ideal opportunity for HIV prevention and subsequent behavior change to reduce risk for acquiring HIV infection.

Section 11.3

Understanding Test Results for Hepatitis B

Understanding your hepatitis B blood test results can be confusing. It is important to discuss your test results with your health care provider so that you can clearly understand whether you have a new infection, chronic infection, or have recovered from an infection. You may want to take this information with you to your appointment as a reference guide. In addition, it is helpful if you request a written copy of your blood tests so that you can be sure you know which tests are positive or negative.

Before explaining the tests, there are two basic medical terms that you should be familiar with:

- **Antigen:** A foreign substance in the body, such as the hepatitis B virus.

- **Antibody:** A protein that your immune system makes in response to a foreign substance. Antibodies can be produced in response to a vaccine or to a natural infection. Antibodies usually protect you against future infections.

The test that is used to help you understand your hepatitis B status is called the hepatitis B blood panel. This is a simple 3-part blood test that your doctor can order. Your results can be returned within seven to ten days.

The 3-part hepatitis B blood panel includes the following:

1. **Hepatitis B surface antigen (HBsAg):** The "surface antigen" is part of the hepatitis B virus that is found in the blood of someone who is infected. If this test is positive, then the hepatitis B virus is present.

2. **Hepatitis B surface antibody (HBsAb or anti-HBs):** The "surface antibody" is formed in response to the hepatitis B virus. Your body can make this antibody if you have been vaccinated,

or if you have recovered from a hepatitis B infection. If this test is positive, then your immune system has successfully developed a protective antibody against the hepatitis B virus. This will provide long-term protection against future hepatitis B infection. Someone who is surface antibody positive is not infected, and cannot pass the virus on to others.

3. **Hepatitis B core antibody (HBcAb or anti-HBc):** This antibody does not provide any protection or immunity against the hepatitis B virus. A positive test indicates that a person may have been exposed to the hepatitis B virus. This test is often used by blood banks to screen blood donations. However, all three test results are needed to make a diagnosis.

Use Table 11.1 to help you and your doctor interpret your blood panel results.

What is hepatitis B?

Hepatitis B is the world's most common serious liver infection. It is caused by the hepatitis B virus (HBV) that attacks liver cells and can lead to liver failure, cirrhosis (scarring), or cancer of the liver later in life. Approximately 90% of healthy adults who are exposed to the

Table 11.1. Blood Panel Results

Tests	Results	Interpretation	Recommendation
HBsAg HBsAb HBcAb	Negative (-) Negative (-) Negative (-)	NOT IMMUNE—has not been infected but is still at risk for possible future infection—needs vaccine	Get the vaccine
HBsAg HBsAb HBcAb	Negative (-) Positive (+) Negative or positive (-/+)	IMMUNE—has been vaccinated or recovered from previous infection—cannot infect others	Vaccine is not needed
HBsAg HBsAb HBcAb	Positive (+) Negative (-) Negative or Positive (-/+)	ACUTE infection or CHRONIC infection—hepatitis B virus is present—can spread the virus to others	Find a knowledgeable doctor for further evaluation
HBsAg HBsAb HBcAb	Negative (-) Negative (-) Positive (+)	UNCLEAR—several interpretations are possible—all 3 tests should be repeated	Find a knowledgeable doctor for further evaluation

hepatitis B virus (HBV) recover on their own and develop the protective surface antibody. However, 10% of infected adults, 50% of infected children and 90% of infected babies are unable to get rid of the virus and develop chronic infection. These people need further evaluation by a liver specialist or doctor knowledgeable about hepatitis B.

Who should be tested?

HBV is transmitted through contact with blood or infected bodily fluids, through unprotected sex, unsterile needles, and from an infected mother to her newborn during the delivery process. HBV is not transmitted casually, through the air, or from casual social contact (hugging, coughing, sneezing).

The following groups are especially at high-risk for infection and should be tested:

- Health care workers and emergency personnel
- Partners or individuals living in close household contact with someone who is infected
- Individuals who have had multiple sex partners or who have been diagnosed with an STI
- Injection drug users
- Men who have sex with men
- Individuals who received a blood transfusion prior to 1972
- Individuals who have tattoos or body piercings
- Individuals who travel to countries where hepatitis B is common (Asia, Africa, South America, the Pacific Islands, Eastern Europe, and the Middle East)
- Individuals emigrating from countries where hepatitis B is common, or who are born to parents who emigrated from these countries (see above)
- ALL pregnant women should be tested for hepatitis B infection

Is there a vaccine for hepatitis B?

The good news is that there is a safe and effective vaccine for hepatitis B that lasts a lifetime. It is recommended in the U.S. and other countries for all infants and children up to age 18 and adults at high risk for infection.

Additional Diagnostic Tests

Liver function tests (LFTs): These are a group of blood tests that help your doctor find out how well your liver is working. The most important test is the following:

Alanine aminotransferase (ALT): This is an enzyme that is released from liver cells into the bloodstream when the liver is injured. An ALT level above normal may indicate liver damage. ALT levels are included in the regular monitoring of all chronic hepatitis B patients; this test can also be useful in deciding whether a patient would benefit from therapy, or for evaluating how well a current treatment is working.

Liver biopsy: This involves the removal of a small piece of tissue from the liver using a special needle. The tissue is examined under a microscope to look for inflammation or liver damage.

Hepatitis B DNA test: This is a highly sophisticated blood test that checks for the presence of hepatitis B virus DNA in the bloodstream. The DNA test indicates how much virus is present in the blood.

E-antigen: This is a protein that is made by the virus. If this test is positive, it indicates that there is a lot of virus in the blood, which means that you can more easily spread the virus to others.

E-antibody: Often as the virus stops replicating in the body and the e-antigen disappears from the blood, the e-antibody appears. This can happen spontaneously or after treatment.

More Information

For more information about HBV diagnostic tests, please visit the following websites:

- Hepatitis B Foundation website at www.hepb.org
- HIV & Hepatitis Treatment Advocates at www.hivandhepatitis.com/tests.html
- University of Maryland Medical Center at www.umm.edu/liver

Section 11.4

Hepatitis C Test Results

Reprinted from "The Importance of Laboratory Test Results in Hepatitis C Infection," by David E. Bernstein, MD. © 2003 David Bernstein, MD. Reprinted with permission.

Most people with hepatitis C feel well and have no specific findings on physical examination that would lead a health care provider to suspect liver disease. Even the vast majority of people with liver disease that has advanced to cirrhosis have a normal physical examination. Therefore, the evaluation and treatment of liver disease, in particular hepatitis C, places a large emphasis on laboratory tests results to diagnose, stage, and predict and evaluate response to therapy.

The liver has several general functions and it is often called both the body's manufacturing center and its filtering plant. Blood tests used to evaluate the liver can be divided into those representing liver cell damage, cholestasis, or liver function. The serum aminotransaminases, alanine aminotransferase (ALT or SGPT), and aspartate aminotransferase (AST or SGOT) are part of most automated blood chemistry panels. Elevation of these enzymes is caused by damage to the hepatocyte or liver cell. The degree of elevation may be important in acute disease but is unimportant in chronic disease. The most common causes of elevated aminotransaminases are fatty liver, viral hepatitis, medication induced hepatitis, autoimmune hepatitis, and alcoholic liver disease. The tests are a reflection of cell damage and death but are not liver function tests. Although many patients and physicians refer to these tests as "liver function tests", this term is incorrect and they do not reflect the liver's ability to either synthesize or metabolize various chemicals. Therefore, an abnormality in these tests does not mean that the liver is not functioning. In fact, the vast majority of patients with elevated aminotransaminases, regardless of degree, have normal liver function.

Cholestatic liver disease is any condition leading to the obstruction of bile ducts in either the liver or biliary tree. Elevation of the enzymes alkaline phosphatase and gamma-glutamyl transpeptidase are indicative of this type of disease. Conditions that commonly lead to the elevation of these enzymes include primary biliary cirrhosis, primary sclerosing cholangitis, and gallstone disease.

Bilirubin is the final breakdown product of heme, the majority of which comes from hemoglobin. Bilirubin can be elevated in many liver-related and non-liver-related conditions and it may be elevated in conditions which lead to liver cell damage and cholestasis. The level of serum bilirubin is not a sensitive indicator of liver function and it may not accurately reflect the degree of liver damage.

Albumin and blood clotting factors are proteins made in the liver. Blood tests such as the serum albumin and prothrombin time are measures of these proteins. As these tests evaluate the functional integrity of the liver, they can be correctly called "liver function tests". Abnormalities of these tests are of concern and are indicative of extensive liver damage.

The most common laboratory abnormality seen in chronic hepatitis C infection is an isolated, elevated alanine aminotransferase (ALT) although as many as 60% of hepatitis C infected patients will have a normal ALT level. The level of serum ALT elevation does not correlate with histological disease and may be normal in any stage of chronic hepatitis C. Therefore, patients with minimal ALT elevations should be evaluated for the presence of chronic hepatitis. In advanced disease, an increase in alkaline phosphatase and total bilirubin as well as thrombocytopenia (low platelets) may be seen.

In the patient with risk factors for hepatitis C or an abnormal ALT, the most practical method of diagnosing HCV infection is by obtaining a second generation enzyme linked immunosorbent assay (EIA) antibody to hepatitis C (anti-HCV). False-positive results may occur at a rate of 10–20% and are usually seen in the presence of autoimmune disease, hypergammaglobulinemia, and low-risk blood donors. False negative results may occur in immunosuppressed patients, including people infected with the human immunodeficiency virus. In early infection, anti-HCV testing may be negative, as antibodies may not develop until four to six weeks after exposure. Unfortunately, a positive hepatitis C antibody does not distinguish acute from chronic disease or active from past infection nor is it a sign of immunity or protection. Therefore, a positive EIA anti-HCV test is a marker that hepatitis C may be present and it must be followed by confirmatory viral load testing.

The recombinant immunoblot assay (RIBA) is another type of antibody test with limited utility. As with EIA antibody tests, it does not distinguish between acute or chronic disease or between past and active infection. Therefore, it adds little to the care of a patient with a positive hepatitis C antibody by the EIA method and known risk factors except extra expense. The NIH consensus conference on hepatitis C has recommended that it be used as a confirmatory test in patients without known risk factors who test positive for the EIA anti-HCV to eliminate the possibility of a false positive EIA. RIBA testing is not influenced by the presence of autoimmune disease or hypergammaglobulinemia. In clinical practice, this test has little if any utility and, except for rare exceptions, it should not be obtained.

Confirmatory tests for the presence of hepatitis C infection are those tests that determine the presence of hepatitis C viral particles (HCV-RNA) in the blood. A positive HCV-RNA in the serum confirms the diagnosis of active hepatitis C. This type of viral testing may be either qualitative or quantitative. Qualitative testing is more sensitive and specific than quantitative testing and results are reported as either positive or negative. Quantitative testing reports on the actual measured amount of viral particles in the serum and the viral levels are usually expressed as thousands or millions of international units. Of note, quantitative viral testing may be falsely negative if viral levels are below the lower limit of detection of the assay being used. Therefore, qualitative HCV-RNA testing is used for diagnosis while quantitative testing should be reserved for use during treatment. It is important to note that the level of virus does not correlate with prognosis, underlying liver histology, or how ill a person feels. Therefore, a patient with a viral level of 3,000,000 international units does not have a worse prognosis nor is the person any sicker than someone with a viral count of 200,000 international units. Small fluctuations in HCV-RNA level are equally unimportant. A patient whose viral level has decreased from five to one million international units has shown no significant change in viral level and should not be rejoicing. The converse is also true and an elevation from one to five million international units should not lead a patient to be upset. It is important to understand the relative lack of importance of viral level in the untreated hepatitis C patient. Misconceptions about viral levels often lead to tremendous angst among patients who insist on comparing numbers in the waiting room, are upset by the initial level of viremia or feel falsely relieved or upset with small changes in HCV-RNA viral load. Recently, however, it has been suggested that in the population co-infected with hepatitis C and HIV, a higher hepatitis C viral load is associated with a more rapid progression to advanced disease. As regards viral level and its significance, the co-infected patient appears to behave differently that the HCV mono-infected person. Quantitative viral load testing should not be repeated yearly or more often as it adds little to the care of the untreated patient other than increased expense and anxiety. These tests, however, should be followed serially in someone undergoing anti-viral therapy, as the goal of therapy is the loss of detectable serum HCV-RNA.

Several other liver tests are frequently obtained in patients with hepatitis C. The serum alpha-fetoprotein is a marker of liver cancer but it may be mildly elevated in patients with chronic hepatitis C in the absence of liver cancer. If it is elevated, this test should be followed closely. Autoimmune markers may be present in as many as 25% patients with hepatitis C without the presence of autoimmune disease. These markers include an anti-nuclear antibody, smooth muscle antibody, anti-mitochondrial antibody or anti-thyroid antibodies. The presence of these antibodies does not appear to influence disease progression. Patients in whom autoimmune disease is suspected should be adequately evaluated before the presence of autoantibodies is attributed to HCV infection.

The adequate interpretation of laboratory test results is very important to understand the evaluation of hepatitis C infection. Unfortunately, in the majority of cases, these blood tests are unable to accurately predict current disease stage or possible disease progression. Therefore, despite all these advanced tests, the performance of a liver biopsy cannot be emphasized enough as this is the best test to accurately stage the disease and predict disease progression.

Section 11.5

Testing for Respiratory Infections

This section includes two documents produced by the U.S. Food and Drug Administration (FDA): "First Quick Test for Deadly, Drug-Resistant MRSA Bacterium," January 10, 2008; and, "FDA Clears for Marketing Real-Time Test for Respiratory Viruses," January 18, 2008.

First Quick Test for Deadly, Drug-Resistant MRSA Bacterium

The U.S. Food and Drug Administration (FDA) has cleared for marketing the first rapid blood test for a deadly and drug-resistant staph bacterium known as MRSA (methicillin-resistant *Staphylococcus aureus*).

Methicillin is an antibiotic that has been used successfully to treat infections from the Staphylococcus aureus bacterium. Over the years, the staph bacterium mutated and spawned MRSA, a strain that is resistant to methicillin and has a higher rate of being fatal. The MRSA bacterium can cause potentially life-threatening conditions such as blood stream infections, surgical site infections, and pneumonia.

The blood test, called the BD GeneOhm StaphSR Assay, can identify whether a blood sample contains genetic material from the MRSA bacterium or the more common, less dangerous staph bacterium that can still be treated with methicillin.

"Rather than waiting more than two days for test results, health care personnel will be able to identify the source of a staph infection in only two hours, allowing for more effective diagnosis and treatment," said Daniel Schultz, M.D., Director of FDA's Center for Devices and Radiological Health.

The BD GeneOhm StaphSR test is manufactured by BD Diagnostics, a subsidiary of BD of Franklin Lakes, New Jersey.

Who is at risk for staph infections?

Staph infections occur most frequently among people in hospitals and health care facilities (such as nursing homes and dialysis centers) who have weakened immune systems. But they can also occur in healthy people.

FDA Clears for Marketing Real-Time Test for Respiratory Viruses

The U.S. Food and Drug Administration has cleared for marketing a test that simultaneously detects four common respiratory viruses, including the flu, in a patient's respiratory secretions. The ProFlu+ test provides results in as few as three hours. Other diagnostic tests for respiratory viruses are fast but not as accurate or are accurate but not as rapid.

The real-time test employs a multiplex platform that allows several tests to be processed using the same sample to detect influenza A virus, influenza B virus, and respiratory syncytial virus A and B (RSV).

These viruses can cause influenza, an infection of the airways called bronchiolitis, and pneumonia. All are among the leading causes of lower respiratory tract infections.

"Antiviral drugs are most effective when initiated within the first two days of symptoms," said Daniel Schultz, M.D., director of FDA's Center for Devices and Radiological Health. "This new test, which is part of the new era of molecular medicine, can help the medical community quickly determine whether a respiratory illness is caused by one of these four viruses and initiate the appropriate treatment."

ProFlu+ uses a molecular biology process to isolate and amplify viral genetic material present in secretions taken from the back of the throat in patients.

While ProFlu+ is faster than conventional tests, it is specific to the four viruses, and is more accurate when used with other diagnostics, such as patient data, bacterial, or viral cultures, and x-rays, in diagnosing a patient. Positive results do not rule out other infection or co-infection and the virus detected may not be the specific cause of the disease or patient symptoms.

An estimated five percent to 20 percent of the U.S. population contracts influenza each year, resulting in more than 200,000 hospitalizations and up to 36,000 deaths. Influenza A, one of three types of human influenza, is the most severe and has been the cause of major epidemics. Influenza B is less severe than influenza A.

Bronchiolitis usually affects children under the age of two, and is a common, sometimes severe illness. A common cause of the disease is RSV.

Pneumonia is a common illness that affects millions of people each year in the United States and is usually caused by an infection. People most at risk are older than 65 or younger than two years of age, or already have health problems.

ProFlu+ is manufactured by Prodesse, Inc. of Milwaukee.

Chapter 12

Allergy Testing

Definition

Allergy tests are any of several tests used to determine the substances to which a person is allergic.

How the Test Is Performed

There are many methods of allergy testing. Among the more common are:

- skin tests,
- elimination-type tests, and
- radioallergosorbent test (RAST).

Skin Tests

Skin tests are the most common. Specific methods vary. The scratch test, one of the most common methods, involves placing a small amount of suspected allergy-causing substances on the skin, usually the forearm, upper arm, or the back. Then, the skin is scratched or pricked so the allergen goes under the skin's surface. The health care provider closely watches the skin for signs of a reaction, usually swelling and redness of the site. Results are usually obtained within about 20 minutes, and a number of allergens can be tested at the same time.

A similar method involves injecting a small amount of allergen under the surface of the skin and watching for a reaction at the site.

Skin tests are most useful for diagnosing:

- insect bite allergies,

- penicillin allergy, and

- respiratory allergies.

Penicillin and closely related medications are the only drugs that can be tested using skin tests. Skin tests for other drugs are at best non-informative and can be dangerous.

Elimination Tests

An elimination diet can be used to check for food allergies. An elimination diet is one in which the suspected foods are avoided for several weeks and then gradually re-introduced one at a time while the person is observed for signs of an allergic reaction.

Another version of this diet is the double-blind test. This method involves giving suspected foods and harmless substances in a disguised form. The person being tested and the provider are both unaware of whether the substance tested in that session is the harmless substance or the suspected food. A third party knows the identity of the substances and identifies them with some sort of code. This test requires several sessions if more than one substance is under investigation.

While the double-blind strategy is useful and practical for mild allergic reactions, it must be done carefully in individuals with suspected severe reactions to foods. Blood tests may be a safer first approach. Skin testing is almost never performed to detect food allergies because of the higher risk of causing a severe allergic reaction.

Blood Tests

RAST measures the amount of specific IgE antibodies in the blood. These antibodies are present if there is a true allergic reaction.

Other blood tests include:

- absolute eosinophil count,

- blood differential, and

- serum immunoglobulin electrophoresis.

Provocation

Provocation (challenge) testing involves exposing a person to a suspected allergen under controlled circumstances. This may be done in the diet or by breathing in the suspected allergen. This type of test may provoke severe allergic reactions. Challenge testing should only be done by a doctor.

How to Prepare for the Test

Before any allergy testing, the health care provider will ask for a very detailed medical history. This may include questions about such things as illnesses, emotional and social conditions, work, entertainment, lifestyle, foods, and eating habits.

If skin testing will be performed, you should not take antihistamines before the test. This may lead to a false-negative result, falsely reassuring you that a substance is unlikely to cause a severe allergic reaction. Your doctor will tell you which medicines to avoid and when to stop taking them before the test.

How the Test Will Feel

Skin tests may cause very mild discomfort when the skin is scratched or pricked. Itching may accompany a positive reaction to the allergen.

Why the Test Is Performed

Allergy tests are used to determine the specific substances that cause an allergic reaction in an individual.

They may also be used to determine if a group of symptoms is a true allergic reaction, which involves antibodies and histamine release. Some food intolerances, in which there is an inability to digest a food because of lack of appropriate enzymes, produce symptoms similar to allergies. Some drugs, such as aspirin, can cause allergy-like symptoms without the formation of antibodies or the release of histamine.

Additional conditions under which the test may be performed:

- allergic rhinitis
- angioedema
- contact dermatitis
- nasal obstruction

Normal Results

In a nonallergic person, allergy tests should be negative (no response to the allergen).

What Abnormal Results Mean

Most often, a positive test means you are allergic to the substance in question. The skin tests are most reliable when testing for airborne substances (such as animal dander or pollen). However, if the dose of allergen is excessive, a positive reaction will occur even in persons who are not allergic.

Risks

Risks related to skin and food allergy tests may include:

• allergic reaction and

• life-threatening anaphylactic reaction.

Considerations

The accuracy of allergy testing varies quite a bit. Even the same test performed at different times on a person may give different results. A person may react to a substance during testing, but never react during normal exposure. A person may also have a negative allergy test and yet still be allergic to the substance.

References

Adkinson NF Jr. *Middleton's Allergy: Principles and Practice.* 6th ed. Philadelphia, Pa: Mosby; 2003.

Rakel RE. *Textbook of Family Medicine.* 7th ed. Philadelphia, Pa: WB Saunders; 2007.

Chapter 13

Hearing Assessments

Individuals throughout their lives have their hearing assessed on the basis of self-referral, family/caregiver referral, failure of an audiologic screening, follow-up to previous audiologic assessment, case history for risk indicators, or referral from other professionals.

Purpose

The purpose of audiological assessment is to quantify and qualify hearing in terms of the degree of hearing loss, the type of hearing loss and the configuration of the hearing loss.

With regard to degree of hearing loss, the audiologist is looking for quantitative information. Hearing levels are expressed in decibels based on the pure tone average for the frequencies 500 to 4000 Hz and discussed using descriptors related to severity: normal hearing (zero to 20 dB HL), mild hearing loss (20 to 40 dB HL), moderate hearing loss (40 to 60 dB HL), severe (60 to 80 dB HL) and profound hearing loss (80 dB HL or greater).

With regard to the type of hearing loss, the audiologist is looking for information that suggests the point in the auditory system where the loss is occurring. The loss may be conductive (a temporary or permanent hearing loss typically due to abnormal conditions of the outer or middle ear), sensorineural (typically a permanent hearing loss due to disease, trauma, or inherited conditions affecting the nerve cells in the cochlea, the inner ear, or the eighth cranial nerve), mixed (a combination of conductive and sensorineural components), or a central auditory processing disorder (a condition where the brain has difficulty processing auditory signals that are heard).

With regard to the configuration of the hearing loss, the audiologist is looking at qualitative attributes such as bilateral versus unilateral hearing loss; symmetrical versus asymmetrical hearing loss; high-frequency versus low frequency hearing loss; flat versus sloping versus precipitous hearing loss; progressive vs. sudden hearing loss; and stable vs. fluctuating hearing loss.

Audiological evaluation is also carried out for purposes of monitoring an already identified hearing loss. Once a particular hearing loss has been identified, a treatment and management plan is put into place. The plan may include medical or surgical intervention, prescription of personal hearing aids, prescription/ provision of assistive listening devices, skills development through aural (audiologic) habilitation/ rehabilitation, or simply monitoring of the condition through periodic assessment.

Once a treatment and management plan is in place, it is still important for an individual's hearing loss to be checked periodically to determine its stability. Is it fluctuating? Has it improved as a result of medical intervention? Is it progressing? Have new conditions come into play that have affected the original condition?

It is also important that a person's ability to hear using amplification (that is, personal hearing aids and any assistive listening devices that are used in place of, or in conjunction with, personal amplification) be monitored and documented. This monitoring would include functional gain assessment, real ear measurement, electroacoustic analysis, listening check, and even informal "functional" assessment in the person's typical listening environment (that is, the classroom, the workplace, the home).

The Assessment Itself

An audiologic evaluation is sometimes thought of as "just a hearing test," but more than "just" the ability to hear sounds is involved. The audiologic evaluation consists of a battery of tests each providing specific stand alone information. Yet, the tests are complementary to one another. The audiologic evaluation consists of several different components.

Case History

The audiologist will ask several questions during the case history. For example:

- What brought you here today?
- Have you noticed difficulty with your hearing? What have you noticed? For how long? When do you think the hearing loss began?
- Does your hearing problem affect both ears or just one ear?
- Has your difficulty with hearing been gradual or sudden?
- Do you have ringing (tinnitus) in your ears?
- Do you have a history of ear infection?
- Have you noticed any pain in your ears or any discharge from your ears?
- Do you experience dizziness?
- Is there a family history of hearing loss?
- Do you have greater difficulty hearing women's, men's, or children's voices?
- Do people comment on the volume setting of your television?
- Has someone said that you speak too loudly in conversation?
- Do you frequently have to ask people to repeat?
- Do you hear people speaking, but can't understand what is being said?
- Do you have any history of exposure to noise in recreational activities, at work. or in the military?
- Are there situations where it is particularly difficult for you to follow conversation? Noisy restaurant? Theater? Car? Large groups?

For children, questions will also be asked regarding:

- speech and language development;
- health history;
- recognition of and response to familiar sounds;
- the startle response to loud, unexpected sounds;

141

- the presence of other disabilities;
- any previous hearing screening or testing results.

Physical Examination

The audiologist will look at the outer ear (the pinna) checking for any misformation. The audiologist will use an otoscope, an instrument that contains a light and a magnifying lens, to examine the ear canal and eardrum. The ear canal is examined for the presence of excessive wax (cerumen), or foreign objects (food, toys, pieces of cotton swabs, etc.). The eardrum (tympanic membrane) is examined for any perforation and signs of fluid or infection. The audiologist will look for any indicators suggesting the need for referral for a medical evaluation or treatment.

Tests of Hearing and Listening

The audiologist will conduct tests of hearing tones. This is called pure-tone audiometry. The results are recorded on a graph called an audiogram. The audiologist will also determine speech reception threshold or the faintest speech that can be heard half the time. Then the audiologist will determine word recognition or ability to recognize words at a comfortable loudness level.

Tests of Middle Ear Function

The audiologist may also take measurements that will provide information about the status of the outer and middle ear. These are called acoustic immittance measures. Tympanometry, one aspect of immittance testing, can assist in the detection of fluid in the middle ear, perforation of the eardrum, or wax blocking the ear canal. Acoustic reflex measurement, another aspect of immittance testing, can add diagnostic information about middle ear function and hearing loss.

After the test battery is completed, the audiologist will review each component of the audiologic evaluation to obtain a profile of hearing abilities and needs. Additional specialized testing may be indicated and recommended on the initial test results. Audiological evaluation may result in recommendations for further follow-up such as medical referral, educational referral, hearing aid/sensory aid assessment, assessment for assistive listening devices, audiologic rehabilitation assessment, speech and language assessment, or counseling.

As you can see, an audiologic evaluation is much more than "just a hearing test."

Pure-Tone Audiometry

Pure-tone audiometry is completed in a soundproof booth—a room with special treatment to the walls, ceiling, and floor to ensure that background noise does not affect test results. Only those sounds that the audiologist introduces into the room, either through earphones or through speakers located in the room, will be heard. Sounds may also be sent through a special headset "vibrator" that has been placed just behind the ear or on the forehead.

In testing hearing for tones, a pure tone air conduction hearing test is given to find out the faintest tones a person can hear at selected pitches (frequencies) from low to high. During this test, earphones are worn and the sound travels through the air in the ear canal to stimulate the eardrum and then the auditory nerve. The person taking the test is instructed to give some type of response such as raising a finger or hand, pressing a button, pointing to the ear where the sound was received, or saying "yes" to indicate that the sound was heard.

Sometimes children are given a more play-like activity (conditioned play audiometry) to indicate response. They may be instructed to string a peg, drop a block in a bucket, or place a ring on a stick in response to hearing the sound. Infants and toddlers are observed for changes in their behavior such as sucking a pacifier, quieting, or searching for the sound and are rewarded for the correct response by getting to watch an animated toy (visual reinforcement audiometry).

The audiologist uses a calibrated machine called an audiometer to present tones at different frequencies (pitches) and at different intensity (loudness) levels. A signal of a particular frequency (something like a piano note) is presented to one ear, and its intensity is raised and lowered until the person no longer responds consistently. Then another signal of a different frequency is presented to the same ear, and its intensity is varied until there is no consistent response. This procedure is done for at least six frequencies. Then the other ear is tested in the same way.

The frequency or pitch of the sound is referred to in hertz (Hz). The intensity or loudness of the sound is measured in decibels (dB). The responses are recorded on a chart called an audiogram that provides a graph of intensity levels for each frequency tested.

In some cases, it is necessary to give a pure tone bone conduction hearing test. In this test, the tone is introduced through a small vibrator placed on the temporal bone behind the ear (or on the forehead). This method "by-passes" blockage, such as wax or fluid, in the outer or middle ears and reaches the auditory nerve through vibration of skull bones. This testing can measure functionality of the inner ear independent of the functionality of the outer and middle ears.

Air conduction test results indicate hearing losses that are either conductive or sensorineural. Bone conduction test results reflect only the sensorineural component. By comparing air conduction and bone conduction test results, the audiologist can determine whether there is a hearing loss due to a problem in the outer or middle ear. If air and bone conduction thresholds are the same, the loss is sensorineural. If there is a difference between air and bone thresholds (an air-bone gap), the loss is conductive or mixed.

Speech Audiometry

Speech audiometry includes determining speech reception threshold (SRT) and testing of word recognition. Speech reception threshold testing determines the faintest level at which a person can hear and correctly repeat easy-to-distinguish two-syllable (spondaic) words. Examples of spondaic words are "baseball", "ice cream", "hot dog", "outside", and "airplane". Spondaic words have equal stress on each syllable. The individual repeats words (or points to pictures) as the audiologist's voice gets softer and softer. The faintest level, in decibels, at which 50% of the two-syllable words are correctly identified, is recorded as the speech reception threshold (SRT). A separate SRT is determined for each ear.

Tests of word recognition attempt to evaluate how well a person can distinguish words at a comfortable loudness level. It relates to how clearly one can hear single-syllable (monosyllabic) words when speech is comfortably loud. Examples of words used in this test are "come", "high", "knees", "chew". In this test, the audiologist's voice (or a recording) stays at the same loudness level throughout. The individual being tested repeats words (or points to pictures). The percentage of words correctly repeated is recorded for each ear.

Thus, a score of 100% would indicate that every word was repeated correctly. A score of 0% would suggest no understanding.

Word recognition is typically measured in quiet. For specific purposes, word recognition may also be measured in the presence of recorded background noise that can also be delivered through the audiometer.

How to Interpret an Audiogram

The audiogram is a graph showing the results of the pure-tone hearing tests.

Pitch or Frequency

Each line from left to right represents a pitch or frequency in hertz (Hz) starting with the lowest pitches on the left side to the very highest frequencies tested on the right side. The range of frequencies tested by the audiologist are 125 Hz, 250 Hz, 500 Hz, 1000 Hz, 2000 Hz, 4000 Hz and 8000 Hz. If you are familiar with a piano keyboard with the low notes at the left end and the high notes at the right end, the audiogram is similar. 250 Hz on the audiogram is the same as the "middle C" key on the piano.

Examples of sounds in everyday life that would be considered "low frequency" are: bass drum, tuba, vowel sounds such as "oo" in "who".

Examples of sounds in everyday life that would be considered "high frequency" are: a bird chirping, a triangle playing, consonant sounds such as "s" in "sun".

If we were to compare a flute playing and a tuba playing, we'd say the flute was primarily high frequency (high pitches) and the tuba was primarily low frequency (low pitches).

If we were to compare the sound of "f" as in "fly" to the sound of "m" as in "moon," we'd say the "f" was primarily high frequency (high pitch) and the "m" was primarily low frequency (low pitch).

Loudness or Intensity

Each line on the audiogram from top to bottom represents loudness or intensity in units of decibels (dB). Lines at the top of the chart (small numbers starting at minus 10 dB and 0 dB) represent soft sounds. Lines at the bottom of the chart represent very loud sounds.

Examples of sounds in everyday life that would be considered "soft" are: a clock ticking, whispering, or the consonant sound "t" in the word "too".

Examples of sounds in everyday life that would be considered "loud" are: a lawnmower, a car horn, or the vowel sound "o" as in the word "poke".

If we were to compare the sound of a jackhammer to the sound of a vacuum cleaner, we'd say the jackhammer was "loud" and the vacuum cleaner was "soft".

If we were to compare the sound of "s" as in "spot" to the sound of "ah" as in "spot", we'd say the "s" was "soft" in comparison to the vowel "ah".

If we were to compare "normal conversational loudness level" (typically 60 dB) to "whispering" (typically 30 dB), we'd say that whispering is soft and conversation is loud.

Some audiograms are also divided into sections showing the severity of hearing loss.

As the audiologist tests your hearing, the results are recorded on the graph. At each frequency tested, the "O" represents the softest tone you can hear in your right ear and the "X" represents the softest tone you can hear in your left ear.

If the "X's" and "O's" all fall in the -10 dB to 15 dB range, your hearing lies in the normal range. If the "X's" and "O's" all fall in the 16 dB to 25 dB range, you have a slight/minimal loss. If the "X's" and "O's" all fall in the 31 dB to 51 dB range, you have a moderate loss. If the "X's" and "O's" all fall in the 91 dB and above range, you have a profound loss.

The audiogram configuration may be flat; sloping down showing better hearing in the low frequencies; rising showing better hearing in the high frequencies. The configuration may be symmetrical, showing the same hearing loss for both ears; or, asymmetrical, showing a different hearing loss configuration for each ear.

Once the audiogram is completed, the audiologist computes the pure tone average for each ear. It is the average of hearing thresholds at 500, 1000, and 2000 Hz, which are considered to be the major frequencies for speech. The pure-tone average represents the degree of hearing loss in decibels. It is not a percentage.

Table 13.1. Example of Pure Tone Average for Each Ear

Frequency	Right Ear Threshold	Left Ear Threshold
500 Hz	20 dB	40 dB
1000 Hz	30 dB	45 dB
2000 Hz	35 dB	50 dB

Average loss = 28 dB (mild loss)

45 dB (moderate loss)

Other Audiologic Procedures

There are a variety of other audiologic procedures that assess the auditory system and determine the presence of hearing loss. They are sometimes used independently and sometimes used to complement the standard audiologic test battery. They help to supplement information from behavioral testing or to resolve conflicting information from behavioral testing. They are auditory evoked potentials, otoacoustic emissions testing, and acoustic immittance measures.

Auditory Evoked Potentials

Electrodiagnostic test procedures give information about the status of neural pathways. These procedures are used with individuals who are difficult to test by conventional behavioral methods. They are also indicated for a person with signs, symptoms, or complaints suggesting a nervous system disease or disorder.

Auditory brainstem response (ABR) is an auditory evoked potential that originates from the auditory nerve. It is often used with babies. Electrodes are placed on the head (similar to electrodes placed around the heart when an electrocardiogram is run), and brain wave activity in response to sound is recorded.

Otoacoustic Emissions (OAE)

Otoacoustic emissions (OAE) are inaudible sounds emitted by the cochlea when the cochlea is stimulated by a sound. When sound stimulates the cochlea, the outer hair cells vibrate. The vibration produces an inaudible sound that echoes back into the middle ear. The sound can be measured with a small probe inserted into the ear canal. Persons with normal hearing produce emissions. Those with hearing loss greater than 25–30 dB do not.

Acoustic Immittance Measures

Acoustic immittance measures are a battery of tests including tympanometry, acoustic reflex, and static acoustic impedance.

Tympanometry introduces air pressure into the ear canal making the eardrum move back and forth. The test measures the mobility of the eardrum. Tympanograms or graphs are produced which show stiffness, flaccidity, or normal eardrum movement.

We all have an acoustic reflex to sounds. A tiny muscle in the ear contracts when a loud sound occurs. The loudness level in decibels at which the acoustic reflex occurs, or the absence of the acoustic reflex, gives diagnostic information that aids in identifying location of the problem along the auditory pathway.

Through static acoustic measures, the physical volume of air in the ear canal is measured. This test is useful in identifying a perforated eardrum or the openness of ventilation tubes.

Balance Assessment

Our sense of balance is determined by our visual system, the inner ear, and our sense of movement via muscles (kinesthetic sense). When these systems don't work together and function properly, we become dizzy.

Dizziness is a symptom. Any disturbance in the inner ear, with or without hearing loss or ringing in the ears (tinnitus), may cause a feeling of dizziness. Dizziness can be caused by disease such as Ménière's Disease, by small calcium deposits in the inner ear, drugs which are toxic to the vestibular (balance) system, head trauma, and other conditions not necessarily related to the vestibular system.

Balance system assessment is conducted to detect pathology with the vestibular or balance system; to determine site of lesion; to monitor changes in balance function; or, to determine the contribution of visual, vestibular, and proprioceptive systems to functional balance.

Vestibular or balance system assessment is indicated when a person has nystagmus (rapid involuntary eye movement), complaints of vertigo (dizziness) balance dysfunction, gait abnormalities, or when pathology/disease of the vestibular system is suspected.

Chapter 14

Vision Screening

Chapter Contents

Section 14.1

The Importance of Regular Eye Exams

Early diagnosis and treatment are important for maintaining good vision.

Periodic optometric examinations are an important part of routine preventive health care. Many eye and vision conditions present no obvious symptoms. Therefore, individuals are often unaware that a problem exists. Early diagnosis and treatment are important for maintaining good vision and, when possible, preventing permanent vision loss.

The need for and frequency of optometric examinations vary with age, race, medical history, family history, occupation, and other factors. Individuals with ocular signs or symptoms require prompt examination. In addition, the presence of certain risk factors may necessitate more frequent evaluations based on professional judgment. The following are the recommendations of the American Optometric Association for regular eye care.

Infants and Children

Newborns are typically screened at birth for congenital eye disorders and disease. In addition, all infants should receive an evaluation for vision problems and eye disease by a doctor of optometry by six months of age or sooner if abnormalities or risk factors are present. Early diagnosis and treatment are important to assure proper visual development, to prevent vision loss due to eye disease and to manage hereditary or congenital eye disorders such as lazy eye or crossed eyes.

In the absence of specific problems or symptoms, re-examinations at age three and prior to entry into school are recommended. These examinations provide the opportunity to evaluate the level of a child's visual development and can provide early diagnosis and intervention to prevent visual impairment due to various conditions.

At risk: Infants born prematurely, with low birth weight, or whose mother had rubella, venereal disease, AIDS-related infection, or a history of substance abuse or other medical problems during pregnancy are at a particularly high risk for the development of eye and vision problems. Also, the presence of high refractive error or a family history of eye disease, crossed eyes, or congenital eye disorders places infants and children at risk.

School-Age Children

Vision may change frequently during the school years. The most common problems are due to the development and progression of nearsightedness. In addition, the existence of eye focusing and/or eye coordination problems may affect school performance. Periodic examinations are recommended.

At risk: Children failing to progress educationally or exhibiting reading and/or learning disabilities should receive an optometric examination as part of a multidisciplinary evaluation.

Adults

During the adult years, the increased visual demands of our technological society bring about the need for regular optometric care. While the incidence of ocular disease is low for young adults, vocational and recreational visual demands are significant. To maintain visual efficiency, productivity, and optimum eye health, periodic examinations are recommended.

Adults, beginning in their early to mid-40s, can experience changes in their ability to see clearly at close distances. This normal aging change in the eye's focusing ability will continue during the 40s and 50s. In addition, increases in the incidence of eye health problems occur during these years. Therefore, periodic eye examinations are recommended.

At risk: Individuals diagnosed with diabetes or hypertension, or who have a family history of glaucoma, particularly African Americans, those who work in highly visually demanding or eye hazardous occupations, those taking certain systemic medications with ocular side effects or those with other health concerns or conditions.

Older Adults

Individuals age 61 or older have an increasing risk for the development of cataracts, glaucoma and macular degeneration, and other sight threatening or visually disabling eye conditions as well as systemic health conditions. Therefore, annual eye examinations are recommended.

At risk: Individuals diagnosed with diabetes or hypertension, or who have a family history of glaucoma or cataracts, and those taking systemic medications with ocular side effects or those with other health concerns or conditions.

Table 14.1. Frequency of Examination

Patient Age	Examination Interval for:	
	Asymptomatic/Risk Free	At Risk
Birth to 24 Months	By 6 months of age	By 6 months of age or as recommended
2 to 5 years	At 3 years of age	At 3 years of age or as recommended
6 to 18 years	Before first grade and every two years thereafter	Annually or as recommended
18 to 40 years	Every two to three years	Every one to two years or as recommended
41 to 60 years	Every two years	Every one to two years or as recommended
61 and older	Annually	Annually or as recommended

Section 14.2

When Should My Child Have an Eye Exam?

"When should my child have an eye exam?" Health Tips for Parents, Mattel Children's Hospital at UCLA, May 2007. © 2007 University of California Los Angeles. Reprinted with permission.

Visual difficulties can affect a child's overall well-being. Children with poor visual skills often struggle in school, which in turn, may lead to a short attention span and low self-esteem. Regular eye screenings can detect vision problems early so that corrective therapies can be initiated.

"Pediatricians are well trained to screen for eye problems," says Heide Woo, M.D., a pediatrician at Mattel Children's Hospital at UCLA. During a child's annual physical exam, a standard eye-chart test measures sharpness of vision. A 20/20 reading means a child sees what an average person sees at a distance of 20 feet. The vision test screens for nearsightedness but does not rule out farsightedness. Nearsighted or farsighted children may need glasses or contacts to help correct blurry vision.

When to Get an Eye Exam

While a pediatrician's eye chart can help catch common problems, it may not detect other conditions. According to Arthur Rosenbaum, M.D., chief of the pediatric ophthalmology at the Jules Stein Eye Institute at UCLA, children should receive a comprehensive exam with an ophthalmologist—a medical doctor who specializes in treating eye diseases—if there is a family history of eye disease, such as hereditary retinal disease, large refractive errors, or amblyopia. If a child has eye misalignment or has an eye that wanders, this may be a sign of strabismus, another serious condition.

Parents who notice problems in school or who are concerned about their child's reading abilities should schedule a comprehensive eye examination. If the exam is normal, Dr. Rosenbaum suggests that a child be seen by an educational therapist or tutor to improve learning skills.

Glasses or Contacts?

Glasses are usually the best option for children who need corrective lenses. While contact lenses are medically acceptable for children, Dr. Rosenbaum cautions parents to consider their child's habits before agreeing to this option. "Most of the time, children are not mature enough until age 11 or 12 years to accept the responsibility of cleaning, storing, and inserting contact lenses," he notes. Dr. Rosenbaum adds that popular refractive surgeries are not appropriate for children, whose eyes are still growing and maturing, and should be delayed until adulthood.

Caring for Young Eyes

In addition to regular vision screenings and parental diligence, parents should make sure their child uses ample light for reading and wears sunglasses to protect their eyes from sun damage. When buying sunglasses for children, UV protection is the most important factor; look for glasses that offer 99 percent or 100 percent protection from UVA and UVB rays. While children today spend a great deal of time in front of a computer screen or television, Dr. Rosenbaum notes that these activities are generally not going to harm a child's vision.

Section 14.3

Tests for Glaucoma

Early detection, through regular and complete eye exams, is the key to protecting your vision from damage caused by glaucoma.

It is important to have your eyes examined regularly. Your eyes should be tested at:

- ages 35 and 40;

- age 40 to age 60, get tested every two to four years; and

- after age 60, every one to two years.

Anyone with high risk factors, should be tested every year or two after age 35.

Four Common Tests for Glaucoma

Regular glaucoma check-ups include two routine eye tests: tonometry and ophthalmoscopy.

Tonometry: The tonometry test measures the inner pressure of the eye. Usually drops are used to numb the eye. Then the doctor or technician will use a special device that measures the eye's pressure.

Ophthalmoscopy: Ophthalmoscopy is used to examine the inside of the eye, especially the optic nerve. In a darkened room, the doctor will magnify your eye by using an ophthalmoscope (an instrument with a small light on the end). This helps the doctor look at the shape and color of the optic nerve.

If the pressure in the eye is not in the normal range, or if the optic nerve looks unusual, then one or two special glaucoma tests will be done. These two tests are called perimetry and gonioscopy.

Perimetry: The perimetry test is also called a visual field test. During this test, you will be asked to look straight ahead and then indicate when a moving light passes your peripheral (or side) vision. This helps draw a "map" of your vision.

Gonioscopy: Gonioscopy is a painless eye test that checks if the angle where the iris meets the cornea is open or closed, showing if either open angle or closed angle glaucoma is present.

Optic Nerve Computer Imaging

In recent years three new techniques of optic nerve imaging have become widely available. These are scanning laser polarimetry (GDx), confocal laser ophthalmoscopy (Heidelberg retinal tomography or HRT II), and optical coherence tomography (OCT).

The GDx machine does not actually image the optic nerve but rather it measures the thickness of the nerve fiber layer on the retinal surface just before the fibers pass over the optic nerve margin to form the optic nerve. The HRT II scans the retinal surface and optic nerve with a laser. It then constructs a topographic (3-D) image of the optic nerve including a contour outline of the optic cup. The nerve fiber layer thickness is also measured. The OCT instrument utilizes a technique called optical coherence tomography which creates images by use of special beams of light. The OCT machine can create a contour map of the optic nerve, optic cup, and measure the retinal nerve fiber thickness. Over time all three of these machines can detect loss of optic nerve fibers.

Your intraocular eye pressure (IOP) is important to determining your risk for glaucoma. If you have high IOP, careful management of your eye pressure with medications can help prevent vision loss. Recent discoveries about the cornea, the clear part of the eye's protective covering, are showing that corneal thickness is an important factor in accurately diagnosing eye pressure. In response to these findings, the Glaucoma Research Foundation has put together this brief guide to help you understand how your corneal thickness affects your risk for glaucoma, and what you can do to make sure your diagnosis is accurate.

Corneal Thickness

In 2002, the five-year report of the Ocular Hypertension Study (OHTS) was released. The study's goal was to determine if early intervention with pressure lowering medications could reduce the number of ocular hypertensive (OHT) patients that develop glaucoma. During the study, a critical discovery was made regarding corneal thickness and its role in intraocular eye pressure and glaucoma development.

Why is corneal thickness important?

Corneal thickness is important because it can mask an accurate reading of eye pressure, causing doctors to treat you for a condition that may not really exist or to treat you unnecessarily when are normal. Actual IOP may be underestimated in patients with thinner central corneal thickness (CCT), and overestimated in patients with thicker CCT. This may be important to your diagnosis; some people originally diagnosed with normal tension glaucoma may in fact be more accurately treated as having regular glaucoma; others diagnosed with ocular hypertension may be better treated as normal based on accurate CCT measurement. In light of this discovery, it is important to have your eyes checked regularly and to make sure your doctor takes your CCT into account for diagnosis.

A Thin Cornea—The Danger of Misreading Eye Pressure

Many times, patients with thin corneas (less than 555 μm) show artificially low IOP readings. This is dangerous because if your actual IOP is higher than your reading shows, you may be at risk for developing glaucoma and your doctor may not know it. Left untreated, high IOP can lead to glaucoma and vision loss. It is important that your doctor have an accurate IOP reading to diagnose your risk and decide upon a treatment plan.

A Thicker Cornea May Mean Less Reason to Worry about Glaucoma

Those patients with thicker CCT may show a higher reading of IOP than actually exists. This means their eye pressure is lower than thought, a lower IOP means that risk for developing glaucoma is lowered. However, it is still important to have regular eye exams to monitor eye pressure and stay aware of changes.

Pachymetry—A Simple Test to Determine Corneal Thickness

A pachymetry test is a simple, quick, painless test to measure the thickness of your cornea. With this measurement, your doctor can better understand your IOP reading, and develop a treatment plan that is right for your condition. The procedure takes only about a minute to measure both eyes.

Section 14.4

Diagnosing Macular Degeneration

Excerpted from "Age-Related Macular Degeneration,"
National Eye Institute (www.nei.nih.gov), March 2008.

What is age-related macular degeneration?

Age-related macular degeneration (AMD) is a disease associated with aging that gradually destroys sharp, central vision. Central vision is needed for seeing objects clearly and for common daily tasks such as reading and driving.

AMD affects the macula, the part of the eye that allows you to see fine detail. AMD causes no pain.

In some cases, AMD advances so slowly that people notice little change in their vision. In others, the disease progresses faster and may lead to a loss of vision in both eyes. AMD is a leading cause of vision loss in Americans 60 years of age and older.

AMD occurs in two forms: wet and dry.

What is wet AMD?

Wet AMD occurs when abnormal blood vessels behind the retina start to grow under the macula. These new blood vessels tend to be very fragile and often leak blood and fluid. The blood and fluid raise the macula from its normal place at the back of the eye. Damage to the macula occurs rapidly.

With wet AMD, loss of central vision can occur quickly. Wet AMD is also known as advanced AMD. It does not have stages like dry AMD.

An early symptom of wet AMD is that straight lines appear wavy. If you notice this condition or other changes to your vision, contact your eye care professional at once. You need a comprehensive dilated eye exam.

What is dry AMD?

Dry AMD occurs when the light-sensitive cells in the macula slowly break down, gradually blurring central vision in the affected eye. As dry AMD gets worse, you may see a blurred spot in the center of your vision. Over time, as less of the macula functions, central vision is gradually lost in the affected eye.

The most common symptom of dry AMD is slightly blurred vision. You may have difficulty recognizing faces. You may need more light for reading and other tasks. Dry AMD generally affects both eyes, but vision can be lost in one eye while the other eye seems unaffected.

Symptoms and Detection

What are the symptoms?

Both dry and wet AMD cause no pain.

For dry AMD: The most common early sign is blurred vision. As fewer cells in the macula are able to function, people will see details less clearly in front of them, such as faces or words in a book. Often this blurred vision will go away in brighter light. If the loss of these light-sensing cells becomes great, people may see a small—but growing—blind spot in the middle of their field of vision.

For wet AMD: The classic early symptom is that straight lines appear crooked. This results when fluid from the leaking blood vessels gathers and lifts the macula, distorting vision. A small blind spot may also appear in wet AMD, resulting in loss of one's central vision.

How is AMD detected?

Your eye care professional may suspect AMD if you are over age 60 and have had recent changes in your central vision. To look for signs of the disease, he or she will use eye drops to dilate, or enlarge, your pupils. Dilating the pupils allows your eye care professional to view the back of the eye better.

AMD is detected during a comprehensive eye exam that includes the following:

- **Visual acuity test:** This eye chart test measures how well you see at various distances.

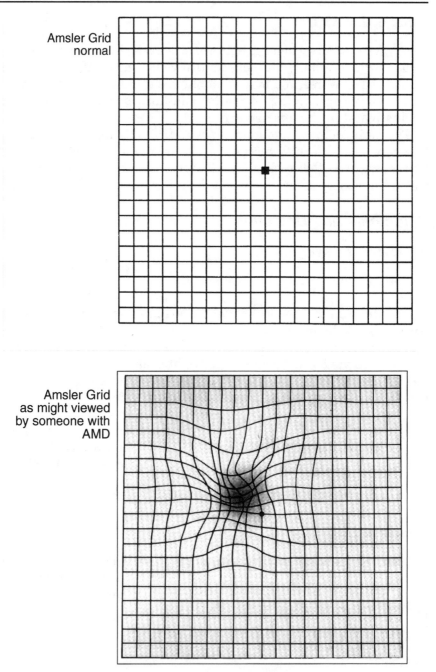

Amsler Grid
normal

Amsler Grid
as might viewed
by someone with
AMD

Figure 14.1. *Amsler grid, normal and as might be viewed by a person with age-related macular degeneration.*

- **Dilated eye exam:** Drops are placed in your eyes to widen, or dilate, the pupils. Your eye care professional uses a special magnifying lens to examine your retina and optic nerve for signs of AMD and other eye problems. After the exam, your close-up vision may remain blurred for several hours.

- **Tonometry:** An instrument measures the pressure inside the eye. Numbing drops may be applied to your eye for this test.

Your eye care professional also may do other tests to learn more about the structure and health of your eye.

During an eye exam, you may be asked to look at an Amsler grid. The pattern of the grid resembles a checkerboard. You will cover one eye and stare at a black dot in the center of the grid. While staring at the dot, you may notice that the straight lines in the pattern appear wavy. You may notice that some of the lines are missing. These may be signs of AMD.

Do NOT depend on the grids in Figure 14.1 for any diagnoses—check with your eye care professional.

If your eye care professional believes you need treatment for wet AMD, he or she may suggest a fluorescein angiogram. In this test, a special dye is injected into your arm. Pictures are taken as the dye passes through the blood vessels in your retina. The test allows your eye care professional to identify any leaking blood vessels and recommend treatment.

Part Three

Laboratory Tests of
Body Fluids and Specimens

Chapter 15

Understanding Laboratory Tests

Chapter Contents

Section 15.1

Questions and Answers about Lab Tests

"Lab Tests," Office of In Vitro Diagnostic Device Evaluation
and Safety (OIVD), U.S. Food and Drug Administration,
February 3, 2005.

This section provides information about lab tests your doctor may use to screen for certain diseases or conditions.

What are lab tests?

Laboratory tests are medical procedures that involve testing samples of blood, urine, or other tissues or substances in the body.

Why does your doctor use lab tests?

Your doctor uses laboratory tests to help with the following:

- Identify changes in your health condition before any symptoms occur
- Diagnose a disease or condition before you have symptoms
- Plan your treatment for a disease or condition
- Evaluate your response to a treatment
- Monitor the course of a disease over time

How are lab tests analyzed?

After your doctor collects a sample from your body, it is sent to a laboratory. Laboratories perform tests on the sample to see if it reacts to different substances. Depending on the test, a reaction may mean you do have a particular condition or it may mean that you do not have the particular condition. Sometimes laboratories compare your results to results obtained from previous tests, to see if there has been a change in your condition.

What do lab tests show?

Lab tests show whether or not your results fall within normal ranges. Normal test values are usually given as a range, rather than as a specific number, because normal values vary from person to person. What is normal for one person may not be normal for another person.

Some laboratory tests are precise, reliable indicators of specific health problems, while others provide more general information that gives doctors clues to your possible health problems. Information obtained from laboratory tests may help doctors decide whether other tests or procedures are needed to make a diagnosis or to develop or revise a previous treatment plan. All laboratory test results must be interpreted within the context of your overall health and should be used along with other exams or tests.

What factors affect your lab test results?

Many factors can affect test results, including the following:

- Sex
- Age
- Race
- Medical history
- General health
- Specific foods
- Drugs you are taking
- How closely your follow preparatory instructions
- Variations in laboratory techniques
- Variation from one laboratory to another

How can you get more information about lab tests?

The American Association for Clinical Chemistry (AACC) and other prominent laboratory associations have created a detailed website about clinical lab testing (www.labtestsonline.org). You can use this website to learn general information about lab tests as well as specific information about lab tests your doctor may prescribe.

Section 15.2

Interpreting Laboratory Results

A Fact Sheet produced by the National Cancer Institute
(www.cancer.gov), January 15, 2003.

A laboratory test is a medical procedure in which a sample of blood, urine, or other tissues or substances in the body is checked for certain features. Such tests are often used as part of a routine checkup to identify possible changes in a person's health before any symptoms appear. Laboratory tests also play an important role in diagnosis when a person has symptoms. In addition, tests may be used to help plan a patient's treatment, evaluate the response to treatment, or monitor the course of the disease over time.

Laboratory test samples are analyzed to determine whether the results fall within normal ranges. They also may be checked for changes from previous tests. Normal test values are usually given as a range, rather than as a specific number, because normal values vary from person to person. What is normal for one person may not be normal for another person. Many factors (including the patient's sex, age, race, medical history, and general health) can affect test results. Sometimes, test results are affected by specific foods, drugs the patient is taking, and how closely the patient follows pre-test instructions. That is why a patient may be asked not to eat or drink for several hours before a test. It is also common for normal ranges to vary somewhat from laboratory to laboratory.

Some laboratory tests are precise, reliable indicators of specific health problems. Others provide more general information that simply gives doctors clues to possible health problems. Information obtained from laboratory tests may help doctors decide whether other tests or procedures are needed to make a diagnosis. The information may also help the doctor develop or revise a patient's treatment plan. All laboratory test results must be interpreted in the context of the overall health of the patient and are generally used along with other exams or tests. The doctor who is familiar with the patient's medical history and current condition is in the best position to explain test results and their implications. Patients are encouraged to discuss questions or concerns about laboratory test results with the doctor.

Section 15.3

Reference Ranges and What They Mean

The "Normal" or Reference Range

"Your test was out of the normal range," your doctor says to you,
handing you a sheet of paper with a set of test results, numbers on a
page. Your heart starts to race in fear that you are really sick. But what
does this statement mean, "Out of the normal range"? Is it cause for
concern? The brief answer is that a result out of the normal range is a
signal that further investigation is needed.

Tests results—all medical data—can only be understood once all the
pieces are together. Take one of the simplest medical indicators of all—
your heart rate. You can take your resting heart rate right now by put-
ting your fingers on your pulse and counting for a minute. Most people
know that the "average" heart rate is about 70 beats per minute. How
do you know what a "normal" heart rate is? We know this on the basis
of taking the pulse rate of millions of people over time.

You probably also know that if you are a regular runner or are otherwise in good physical condition, your pulse rate could be considerably lower—so a pulse rate of 55 could also be "normal". Say you walk
up a hill—your heart rate is now 120 beats a minute. That would be
high for a resting heart rate but "normal" for the rate during this kind
of activity.

Your heart rate, like any medical observation, must be considered
in context. Without the proper context, any observation or test result
is meaningless. To understand what is normal for you, your doctor must
know what is the normal heart rate of most other people of your age,
and what activity you are doing at the time—or just before—your heart
rate is measured.

The interpretation of any clinical laboratory test involves an important concept in comparing the patient's results to the test's "reference range." It's also commonly called the "normal range" but today

reference range or reference interval is considered more appropriate, for reasons explained on the next page. The term reference interval is increasing in use and is often used interchangeably with reference range. For simplicity, we use the term reference range in this section.

What is a reference range?

Some tests provide a simple yes or no answer. Was the culture positive for strep throat? Did the test find antibodies to a virus that indicates an infection?

But for many more tests, the meaning of the results depends on their context. A typical lab report will provide your results followed by a reference range. For example, your results for a thyroid-stimulating hormone (TSH) test might look something like: 2.0 mIU/L, ref range 0.5–5.0 mIU/L. The test results indicate that it falls within the "normal" range.

How was that reference range established? The short answer is: by testing a large number of healthy people and observing what appears to be "normal" for them.

The first step in determining a given reference range is to define the population to which the reference range will apply, for example, healthy females between 20 and 30 years old. A large number of individuals from this category would be tested for a specific laboratory test. The results would be averaged and a range (plus or minus two standard deviations of the average) of normal values would be established.

The term "reference range" is preferred over "normal range" because the reference population can be clearly defined. Rather than implying that the test results are being compared with some ill-defined concept of "normal," the reference range means the results are being considered in the most relevant context. When you examine test results from different populations, you quickly discover that what is "normal" for one group is not necessarily normal for another group. For example, pregnancy changes many aspects of the body's chemistry, so pregnant women have their own set of reference ranges.

Effects of Age and Sex

For many tests, there is no single reference range that applies to everyone because the tests performed may be affected by the age and sex of the patient, as well as many other considerations.

Alkaline phosphatase is an enzyme found in the cells that make bone, so its concentration in the body rises in proportion to new bone cell production. In a child or adolescent, a high alkaline phosphatase level is not only normal but desirable—the child should be growing healthy bones. But these same levels found in an adult are a sign of trouble—osteoporosis, metastatic bone disease (extra bone growth associated with tumors), or other conditions. It is because of these significant variations due to age that the few reference ranges that you may see on this site do not include ranges for children or adolescents. Experience from testing large numbers of people has led to different reference ranges by age group.

Hemoglobin and hematocrit (a red blood cell measure) both decline as a natural part of the aging process.

The patient's sex is another important consideration for many tests:

- Creatinine is produced as a natural by-product of muscle activity and then removed from your bloodstream by your kidneys. It is often measured as a gauge of how well your kidneys are functioning. Because males have greater muscle mass than females, the reference range for males is higher than for females.

- The form of the enzyme creatine kinase called CK-MB presents a similar situation. It is released into the bloodstream by damaged muscles, and a high level of CK-MB indicates damage to the heart muscle, so this enzyme is one of the indicators used to diagnose heart attacks. Because of their greater muscle mass, men tend to have higher CK levels. When the test first came into use, many elderly women demonstrated considerably lower levels of CK-MB and, thus, did not pass the threshold level believed to indicate a heart attack, so heart attacks were often missed in this age group of women.

As another example, blood loss through menstruation may cause lower hemoglobin and hematocrit levels in pre-menopausal women. These are examples of tests with reference ranges keyed to both age and sex.

Other Factors Affecting Test Results

Laboratories will generally report your test results accompanied by a reference range keyed to your age and sex. Your physician then will still need to interpret the results based on personal knowledge of your particulars, including any medications or herbal remedies you may be taking. A plethora of additional factors can affect your test results: your intake of caffeine, tobacco, alcohol, and vitamin C; your diet (vegetarian vs. carnivorous); stress or anxiety; or a pregnancy. Even your posture when the sample is taken can affect some results, as can recent heavy exertion. For example, albumin and calcium levels may increase when shifting from lying down to an upright position.

Such exotic factors as occupation, altitude, and distance from the ocean have been known to affect results. Regular exercise can also affect values—in particular, levels of creatine phosphokinase (CK), aspartate aminotransferase (AST), and lactate dehydrogenase (LDH) will increase. Additionally, testosterone, luteinizing hormone (LH), and platelet levels can increase in people who participate for months and years in strenuous exercise such as distance running and weightlifting.

All these considerations underscore the significance of taking blood or urine samples in a standardized fashion for performing and interpreting laboratory tests (and home tests as well). It's important to comply with your doctor's instructions in preparing for the test, such as coming in first thing in the morning, before you eat anything, to get your blood drawn. That compliance makes your sample as close as possible to others; it keeps you within the parameters of your reference group.

When "Normal" Doesn't Matter

For some tests, such as cholesterol, rather than worry about the "normal" range, the vast majority of people need only be concerned if their test result falls above or below a cut-off value that is sometimes referred to as a "decision point." If, for example, as studies have shown, a cholesterol level of 200 milligrams per deciliter is the cut-off where heart disease risk should trigger medical intervention, then it doesn't really matter if this result falls into a statistically "normal" range.

There are additional tests for which the "normal" range is irrelevant. In testing for the amount of a drug in the blood of an unconscious person, for example, the doctor will interpret the result in terms of the likely effects of the drug at the tested level, not in terms of a reference range.

In addition, clinically significant, dramatic changes in a person's test values, even if those values remain within the reference range for that test, should be brought to the doctor's attention.

What Does it Mean if My Test Result Is out of the Reference Range?

First, there are a few reasons why a test result could fall outside of the established reference range despite the fact that you are in good health:

- **Statistical variability:** Even when performing the same test on the same sample multiple times, one out of 20 (or 5%) determinations will fall outside an established range, based on the laws of probability. Sometimes, if the test is repeated on this same sample, the result will then be within range.

- **Biological variability:** If a doctor runs the same test on you on several different occasions, there's a good chance that one result will fall outside a reference range even though you are in good health. For biological reasons, your values can vary from day to day. That's why a doctor may repeat a test on you and why he may look at results from other times that you have the same test performed.

References ranges are usually established by collecting results from a large population and determining from the data an expected average (mean) result and expected differences from that average (standard deviation). There are individuals who are healthy but whose tests results, which are normal for them, do not always fall within the expected range of the overall population.

Thus, a test value that falls outside of the established reference range supplied by the laboratory may mean nothing significant. Generally, the test value may be only slightly higher or lower than the reference range, and you may indeed be healthy.

Second, a result outside the range may indicate a problem and warrants further investigation. Your doctor will evaluate your test results in the context of your medical history, physical examination, and other relevant factors to determine whether a result that falls outside of the reference range means something significant for you.

The first thing your doctor is likely to do is to re-run the test on the same sample, or he may request that you submit another sample for testing. Perhaps the analyte being measured happened to be high that day due to one of the reasons stated previously or perhaps something went awry with the sample (the blood specimen was not refrigerated, or the serum was not separated from the red cells, or it was exposed to heat). Your doctor may also compare the latest test result to previous results if you have been tested for the same thing in the past to get a better idea of what is normal for you.

Laboratories will generally report the findings based on age and sex when appropriate and leave it to the physician to interpret the results based on factors such as diet, your level of activity, or medications you are taking. If you have a result that falls outside the reference range,

173

talk to your doctor about what it means for you and what steps need to be taken next.

If you know of any special circumstances that could affect a test, mention them to your doctor; don't assume your doctor has thought of every possible circumstance.

Common Misconceptions

There are two main misconceptions about test results and reference ranges:

Myth: "An abnormal test result is a sign of a real problem."

Truth: A test result outside the reference range may or may not indicate a problem—the only sure signal it sends is that your doctor should investigate it further. You can have an abnormal value and have nothing wrong—but your doctor should try to determine the cause.

It's possible that your result falls in that 5% of healthy people who fall outside the statistical reference range. In addition, there are many things that could throw off a test without indicating a major problem: High blood sugar could be diet-related rather than caused by diabetes. A lipid result could be high because you didn't fast before the test. High liver enzymes can be the temporary result of a recent drinking binge rather than a sign of cirrhosis. New drugs come on the market constantly, faster than laboratories can evaluate whether they might interfere with test results. It is not uncommon for many of these drugs to interfere with certain laboratory tests, resulting in falsely high or low values.

Most likely, your doctor will want to re-run the test. Some abnormal results may disappear on their own, especially if they are on the border of the reference range. Your doctor will also seek explanations for an abnormal result, such as those above. A key point your doctor will address is, how far out of the reference range is the result?

If these investigations point to a problem, then your doctor will address it. But there are very few medical questions that can be answered by a single test.

Myth: "If all my test results are normal, I have nothing to worry about."

Truth: It's certainly a good sign, but it's only one set of tests, not a guarantee. There is a large overlap among results from healthy

174

people and those with diseases, so there is still a small chance that there is an undetected problem. Just as some healthy people's results fall outside the reference range, lab test results in some people with disease fall within the reference range.

If you're trying to follow a healthy lifestyle, take it as a good sign, and keep it up. But if you're engaging in high-risk behavior, such as drug and alcohol abuse or a poor diet, it only means "so far so good," and the potential consequences haven't caught up with you yet. A good test result is not a license for an unhealthy lifestyle.

If you had abnormal results previously, normal results certainly provide good news. But your doctor may want to conduct follow-up tests some months later to make sure you're still on track and to document any trends.

Chapter 16

Blood Tests

Chapter Contents

Section 16.1

Overview of Blood and Blood Components

Excerpted from *Blood Groups and Red Cell Antigens*, by Laura Dean, M.D., National Center for Biotechnology Information, National Library of Medicine (www.ncbi.nlm.nih.gov); accessed February 20, 2008.

The average human adult has more than five liters (six quarts) of blood in his or her body. Blood carries oxygen and nutrients to living cells and takes away their waste products. It also delivers immune cells to fight infections and contains platelets that can form a plug in a damaged blood vessel to prevent blood loss.

Through the circulatory system, blood adapts to the body's needs. When you are exercising, your heart pumps harder and faster to provide more blood and hence oxygen to your muscles. During an infection, the blood delivers more immune cells to the site of infection, where they accumulate to ward off harmful invaders.

All of these functions make blood a precious fluid. Each year in the United States, 30 million units of blood components are transfused to patients who need them. Blood is deemed so precious that is also called "red gold" because the cells and proteins it contains can be sold for more than the cost of the same weight in gold.

This section introduces the components of blood.

Blood Contains Cells, Proteins, and Sugars

If a test tube of blood is left to stand for half an hour, the blood separates into three layers as the denser components sink to the bottom of the tube and fluid remains at the top.

The straw-colored fluid that forms the top layer is called plasma and forms about 60% of blood. The middle white layer is composed of white blood cells (WBCs) and platelets, and the bottom red layer is the red blood cells (RBCs). These bottom two layers of cells form about 40% of the blood.

Plasma is mainly water, but it also contains many important substances such as proteins (albumin, clotting factors, antibodies, enzymes, and hormones), sugars (glucose), and fat particles.

All of the cells found in the blood come from bone marrow. They begin their life as stem cells, and they mature into three main types of cells—RBCs, WBCs, and platelets. In turn, there are three types of WBC—lymphocytes, monocytes, and granulocytes—and three main types of granulocytes (neutrophils, eosinophils, and basophils).

A sample of blood can be further separated into its individual components by spinning the sample in a centrifuge. The force of the spinning causes denser elements to sink, and further processing enables the isolation of a particular protein or the isolation of a particular type of blood cell. With the use of this method, antibodies and clotting factors can be harvested from the plasma to treat immune deficiencies and bleeding disorders, respectively. Likewise, RBCs can be harvested for blood transfusion.

Red Blood Cells Transport Oxygen

Every second, two to three million RBCs are produced in the bone marrow and released into the circulation. Also known as erythrocytes, RBCs are the most common type of cell found in the blood, with each cubic millimeter of blood containing four to six million cells. With a diameter of only six μm, RBCs are small enough to squeeze through the smallest blood vessels. They circulate around the body for up to 120 days, at which point the old or damaged RBCs are removed from the circulation by specialized cells (macrophages) in the spleen and liver.

In humans, as in all mammals, the mature RBC lacks a nucleus. This allows the cell more room to store hemoglobin, the oxygen-binding protein, enabling the RBC to transport more oxygen. RBCs are also biconcave in shape; this shape increases their surface area for the diffusion of oxygen across their surfaces. In non-mammalian vertebrates such as birds and fish, mature RBCs do have a nucleus.

If a patient has a low level of hemoglobin, a condition called anemia, they may appear pale because hemoglobin gives RBCs, and hence blood, their red color. They may also tire easily and feel short of breath because of the essential role of hemoglobin in transporting oxygen from the lungs to wherever it is needed around the body.

White Blood Cells Are Part of the Immune Response

WBCs come in many different shapes and sizes. Some cells have nuclei with multiple lobes, whereas others contain one large, round nucleus. Some contain packets of granules in their cytoplasm and so are known as granulocytes.

Despite their differences in appearance, all of the various types of WBCs have a role in the immune response. They circulate in the blood until they receive a signal that a part of the body is damaged. Signals include interleukin 1 (IL-1), a molecule secreted by macrophages that contributes to the fever of infections, and histamine, which is released by circulating basophils and tissue mast cells, and contributes to allergic reactions. In response to these signals, the WBCs leave the blood vessel by squeezing through holes in the blood vessel wall. They migrate to the source of the signal and help begin the healing process.

Individuals who have low levels of WBCs may have more and worse infections. Depending upon which WBCs are missing, the patient is at risk for different types of infection. For example, macrophages are especially good at swallowing bacteria, and a deficiency in macrophages leads to recurrent bacterial infections. In contrast, T cells are particularly skilled in fighting viral infections, and a loss of their function results in an increased susceptibility to viral infections.

Neutrophils Digest Bacteria

Neutrophils are also known as polymorphonuclear cells because they contain a nucleus whose shape (morph) is irregular and contains many (poly) lobes. They also belong to a group of WBCs known as granulocytes because their cytoplasm is dotted with granules that contain enzymes that helps them digest pathogens.

Monocytes Become Macrophages

Monocytes are young WBCs that circulate in the blood. They develop into macrophages after they have left the blood and migrated into tissue. There they provide an immediate defense because they can engulf (phagocytose) and digest pathogens before other types of WBCs reach the area.

In the liver, tissue macrophages are called Kupffer cells, and they specialize in removing harmful agents from blood that has left the gut. Alveolar macrophages are in the lungs and remove harmful agents that may have been inhaled. Macrophages in the spleen remove old or damaged red blood cells and platelets from the circulation.

Macrophages are also "antigen-presenting cells", presenting the foreign proteins (antigens) to other immune cells, triggering an immune response.

Lymphocytes Consist of B Cells and T Cells

Lymphocytes are round cells that contain a single, large round nucleus. There are two main classes of cells, the B cells that mature in the bone marrow, and the T cells that mature in the thymus gland.

Once activated, the B cells and T cells trigger different types of immune response. The activated B cells, also known as plasma cells, produce highly specific antibodies that bind to the agent that triggered the immune response. T cells, called helper T cells, secrete chemicals that recruit other immune cells and help coordinate their attack. Another group, called cytotoxic T cells, attacks virally infected cells.

Platelets Help Blood to Clot

Platelets are irregularly shaped fragments of cells that circulate in the blood until they are either activated to form a blood clot or are removed by the spleen. Thrombocytopenia is a condition of low levels of platelets and carries an increased risk of bleeding. Conversely, a high level of platelets (thrombocythemia) carries an increased risk of forming inappropriate blood clots. These could deprive essential organs such as the heart and brain, of their blood supply, causing heart attacks and strokes, respectively.

As with all the cells in the blood, platelets originate from stem cells in the bone marrow. The stem cells develop into platelet precursors (called megakaryocytes) that "shed" platelets into the bloodstream. There, platelets circulate for about nine days. If they encounter damaged blood vessel walls during this time, they stick to the damaged area and are activated to form a blood clot. This plugs the hole. Otherwise, at the end of their life span they are removed from the circulation by the spleen. In a diverse number of diseases where the spleen is overactive, for example rheumatoid arthritis and leukemia, the spleen removes too many platelets, leading to increased bleeding.

Section 16.2

Lipid Profile: Cholesterol and Triglycerides

"Your Lipid Profile," © 2007 Medical College of Wisconsin.
Reprinted with permission of Medical College of Wisconsin HealthLink,
www.healthlink.mcw.edu.

When doctors order a lab test called a lipid profile (sometimes called a lipid panel), they are looking for information about the amounts of four types of fats in the blood. You will be asked to give a small sample of blood from your arm. The results can help your doctor evaluate your risk for heart disease.

- Cholesterol helps the body form hormones, vitamin D, and other important substances, but too much of it in the blood can clog and damage the blood vessels. Because it is a fat-like substance that doesn't mix with blood, cholesterol has to combine with proteins to form lipoproteins. Lipoproteins can travel in the blood to all the organs and tissues of the body.

- Low-density lipoproteins (LDLs, or "bad" cholesterol) build up in the blood and increase your risk of heart disease.

- High-density lipoproteins (HDLs, or "good" cholesterol) carry cholesterol to the liver, where it is removed from the body.

- Triglycerides store energy for your body to use when it is needed. If there is too much, it can block blood vessels and cause other health problems such as abdominal pain and pancreatitis.

It's important to know that the ranges listed here are the most common results, and apply mainly to people without existing medical problems. The ideal range for each person depends on individual risk factors, including conditions such as diabetes or heart disease. Your doctor will help you determine the levels that are healthiest for you.

Mg/dl means milligrams per deciliter. This is a way to measure tiny amounts of substances (a milligram is one-thousandth of a gram) in one deciliter (one-tenth of a liter) of your blood. The symbol < means "less than." The symbol > means "more than."

Total cholesterol: Lower is better:

- Best = < 200 mg/dL
- Borderline high = 200–239 mg/dL
- High = 240 mg/dL or higher

Triglycerides: Lower is better:

- Best = < 150 mg/dL
- Borderline high = 150–199 mg/dL
- High = 200–499 mg/dL
- Very high = 500 mg/dl or higher

LDL cholesterol: Lower is better:

- Best = < 100 mg/dL
- Good = 100–129 mg/dL
- Borderline high = 130–159 mg/dL
- High = 160–189 mg/dL
- Very high = 190 mg/dL or higher

HDL cholesterol: Higher is better:

- Low = < 40 mg/dL
- Best = 60 mg/dL or higher

Risk Factors

Certain conditions or behaviors will increase your risk for heart disease. The major risk factors include:

- Smoking;
- High blood pressure or on blood pressure medication;
- Low HDL cholesterol;
- Family history of early heart disease (heart disease in father or brother before age 55; heart disease in mother or sister before age 65);
- Age (men 45 years or older; women 55 years or older).

Some of these can be changed (like smoking or diet) and some cannot (like age or family history). You can ask your doctor for advice on how to change what you can.

If you already have some risk factors, your doctor might ask you to make changes to your lifestyle—like losing weight and exercising more—and/or recommend medications to lower your cholesterol.

Your doctor will most likely recommend lifestyle changes and consider drug therapy when:

- You are considered high risk because you already have heart disease.

- You are considered at moderately high risk of heart disease because you have two or more major risk factors in addition to other health conditions, and you have an LDL of 100 or more.

- You are considered at moderate risk of heart disease because you have two or more major risk factors and your LDL is 160 or more. (If your LDL is 130–159, only lifestyle changes—not drug therapy—might be recommended.)

- You are considered at lower risk of heart disease because you have zero or one risk factors and your LDL is 190 or more. (If your LDL is 160–189, lifestyle changes will be recommended and drug therapy might be considered.)

Section 16.3

Basic Blood Chemistry Tests

Doctors order basic blood chemistry tests to assess a wide range of conditions and the function of organs. Often, blood tests check electrolytes, the minerals that help keep the body's fluid levels in balance, and are necessary to help the muscles, heart, and other organs work properly. To assess kidney function and blood sugar, blood tests measure other substances.

Tests for Electrolytes

Typically, tests for electrolytes measure levels of sodium, potassium, chloride, and bicarbonate in the body.

Sodium plays a major role in regulating the amount of water in the body. Also, the passage of sodium in and out of cells is necessary for many body functions, like transmitting electrical signals in the brain and in the muscles. The sodium levels are measured to detect whether there's the right balance of sodium and liquid in the blood to carry out those functions.

If a child becomes dehydrated because of vomiting, diarrhea, or inadequate fluid intake, the sodium levels can be abnormally high or low, which can cause a child to feel confused, weak and lethargic, and even to have seizures.

Potassium is essential to regulate how the heart beats. When potassium levels are too high or too low, it can increase the risk of an abnormal heartbeat. Low potassium levels are also associated with muscle weakness.

Chloride, like sodium, helps maintain a balance of fluids in the body. If there's a large loss of chloride, the blood may become more acidic and prevent certain chemical reactions from occurring in the body that are necessary it to keep working properly.

Bicarbonate prevents the body's tissues from getting too much or too little acid. The kidney and lungs balance the levels of bicarbonate in the body. So if bicarbonate levels are too high or low, it might indicate that there's a problem with those organs.

Other Substances Measured

Other blood substances measured in the basic blood chemistry test include blood urea nitrogen and creatinine, which tell how well the kidneys are functioning, and glucose, which indicates whether there is a normal amount of sugar in the blood.

Blood urea nitrogen (BUN) is a measure of how well the kidneys are working. Urea is a nitrogen-containing waste product that's created when the body breaks down protein. If the kidneys are not working properly, the levels of BUN will build up in the blood. Dehydration and excessive bleeding can also elevate the BUN levels in the blood.

Creatinine levels in the blood that are too high can indicate that the kidneys aren't working properly. The kidneys filter and excrete creatinine. So if they are not functioning properly, creatinine can build up in the bloodstream. Both dehydration and muscle damage also can raise creatinine levels.

Glucose is the main type of sugar in the blood. It comes from the foods we eat and is the major source of energy needed to fuel the body's functions. Glucose levels that are too high or too low can cause problems. The most common cause of high blood glucose levels is diabetes.

Section 16.4

Understanding Your Complete Blood Count

Excerpted from a Patient Information publication produced by
the NIH Clinical Center, National Institutes of Health, April 2000.
Reviewed by David A. Cooke, M.D., June 2008.

What is a complete blood count?

A complete blood count, often referred to as a CBC, is a common
blood test. A CBC provides detailed information about three types of
cells in your blood: red blood cells, white blood cells, and platelets.
These blood cells are made in the bone marrow, the spongy tissue filling the center of your bones. Bone marrow in the skull, sternum (breast
bone), ribs, vertebral column (backbone), and pelvis produces these
blood cells.

Each type of blood cell plays an important role in your body's normal function.

What does a complete blood count measure?

A complete blood count includes five major measurements:

- **White blood cell (WBC) count:** White blood cells fight infections. They are measured in thousands per cubic milliliter (K/
  mm^3) of blood.

- **Red blood cell (RBC) count:** Red blood cells carry oxygen to
  and remove waste products from the body's tissues. These cells
  also contain hemoglobin. Red blood cells are measured in millions per cubic millimeter (mil/mm^3) of blood.

- **Hemoglobin (HGB) value:** Hemoglobin gives red blood cells
  their color. Hemoglobin carries oxygen from the lungs to the
  tissues and takes carbon dioxide (the waste products) from the
  tissues to the lungs. From the lungs, carbon dioxide is exhaled.
  Hemoglobin is measured in grams per deciliter (g/dL) of blood.

- **Hematocrit (HCT) value:** The hematocrit is the percentage of
  red blood cells in relation to your total blood volume.

187

- **Platelet count:** Platelets help to stop bleeding by forming blood clots. They are measured in thousands per cubic millimeter (K/mm^3) of blood.

What are the normal ranges of these measurements?

Each measurement in a complete blood count has a normal range:

- WBC: 3.4–9.6 K/mm^3
- RBC: 3.58–4.99 mil/mm^3
- HGB: 11.1–15.0 g/dL
- HCT: 31.8–43.2%
- Platelets: 162–380 K/mm^3.

You will see these ranges on your complete blood count.

A More Detailed Look at What the Complete Blood Count Measures

White blood cells: These cells are the mobile units of the body's infection-fighting system. White blood cells travel in the bloodstream to areas of infection and destroy the responsible bacteria. However, the WBC lab value is not meaningful unless the "differential" is also known.

Differential: The differential measures each of the five types of white blood cells:

- neutrophils (polys and bands)
- basophils
- eosinophils
- lymphocytes
- monocytes

The differential is usually based on 100 cells counted in a laboratory sample.

Neutrophils: Neutrophils are the most numerous white blood cells. They make up about 56 percent of white blood cells. Neutrophils are the "soldiers" that fight infections. They eat or gobble up the infectious particles (bacteria) in your body.

On your lab sheet, you will see the words "polys" and "bands." Polys are mature neutrophils; bands are young polys, which also fight infections.

ANC or AGC: The absolute neutrophil count (ANC), also called absolute granulocyte count (AGC), is the measure of the number of infection-fighting white blood cells in your blood.

To calculate the ANC, the number of white blood cells and the percentage of polys and bands must be known. Then, the number of white blood cells is multiplied by the percentage of polys and bands.

For example, let the number of white blood cells be 300. (This number would be 0.3 on the lab sheet. To get this number, move the decimal three places to the right.) Let the number of polys be 10 percent (0.10), and bands 5 percent (0.05). The ANC is found by doing the following:

$$300 \times (0.10 + 0.05) = 300 \times 0.15 = 45 \text{ The ANC is 45.}$$

The normal ranges shown are based on adult women; adult men's and children's ranges will be slightly different.

Section 16.5

Blood Cultures

"Blood Culture," June 2006, reprinted with permission from www
.kidshealth.org. Copyright © 2006 The Nemours Foundation. This information was provided by KidsHealth, one of the largest resources online for medically reviewed health information written for parents, kids, and teens. For more articles like this one, visit www.KidsHealth.org, or www
.TeensHealth.org.

A blood culture is a test to detect germs such as bacteria or fungi in the blood. One may be ordered when a child has symptoms of an infection—such as a high fever or chills—and the doctor suspects bacteria or fungi have spread into the blood. The culture can disclose what type of germ is causing the infection, which will determine how it is treated.

To do the test, the doctor will take a blood sample and send it to a lab for testing. Results are ready in a few days, but if the child is severely ill, the doctor may start treatment before the results are complete. Treatment will be based on the most likely cause of the infection, but can be changed to be specific for the microbe found when the culture is completed and the antibiotic sensitivity of the bacteria or fungi has been determined.

Why do a blood culture?

During some illnesses, certain infection-causing bacteria and fungi can invade the bloodstream and spread into other parts of the body, away from the original infection site. Their presence in the blood usually means that a child has a serious infection. Such infections usually cause a more rapid heart rate and high fever with an increase in the white blood cell count.

A blood culture can reveal a number of infections or problems, such as endocarditis, a severe and potentially life-threatening problem that occurs when bacteria in the bloodstream stick to the heart valves. A blood culture might also detect meningitis, an infection of the outer lining of the brain, osteomyelitis, a bone infection often caused by Staphylococcus aureus, and cellulitis, a skin infection that involves areas of tissue just below the skin's surface.

How is a blood culture done?

The blood culture is done with a simple blood draw performed after the skin is wiped with an alcohol pad, then smeared with a special antibacterial solution. This careful skin sterilization is important because it prevents contamination of the blood that's being drawn. It kills bacteria that may be on the surface of the skin so that they don't appear in the blood culture and interfere with identification of the germ causing the infection.

Sometimes it seems like a lot of blood is drawn for the test, but it's important that enough blood be drawn for the culture to be accurate. This may be less than a teaspoon (five milliliters) in babies and one to two teaspoons (five to ten milliliters) in older children, depending on their size. The amount of blood drawn is tiny compared with the amount of blood in the body, and it's quickly replenished—usually within 24 to 48 hours.

Section 16.6

Liver Function Tests

What are Liver Function Tests?

LFTs (liver function tests) are a group of blood tests that can help to show how well a person's liver is working. LFTs include measurements of albumin, various liver enzymes (ALT, AST, GGT, and ALP), bilirubin, prothrombin time, cholesterol, and total protein. All of these tests can be performed at the same time.

Measuring Liver Proteins

Total protein testing (also called TP or serum total protein) measures the amount of proteins in the bloodstream. Many different things can cause abnormally high or low protein levels. A doctor may order total protein testing to help diagnose kidney or liver disease, blood cancer, malnutrition, or abnormal body swelling. Normal protein levels in the bloodstream range from 6.5 to 8.2 grams per deciliter. Two of the main proteins found in the bloodstream are albumin and globulin.

Globulins are made by various liver cells and the immune system. They help to fight off infections. Low globulin levels can have many causes other than liver damage.

Albumin is a protein made in the liver. If the liver is badly damaged, it can no longer produce albumin. Albumin maintains the amount of blood in the veins and arteries. When albumin levels become very low, fluid can leak out from the blood vessels into nearby tissues, causing swelling in the feet and ankles. Very low levels of albumin may be a sign of liver damage. The normal albumin range is from 3.9 grams/deciliter to 5.0 grams/deciliter.

Prothrombin (also called factor II) is a protein that helps to clot blood. Prothrombin is made in the liver. A prothrombin time test measures how much time it takes for a person's blood to clot. The normal time needed for blood to clot is between 10 and 15 seconds. A person with an abnormally long prothrombin time may be at risk for excessive bleeding. A longer prothrombin time can be caused by serious liver disease or:

- A lack of vitamin K,
- Blood-thinning medicines,
- Other medications that can interfere with the test,
- Certain bleeding disorders.

Measuring Liver Enzymes

ALT and AST are enzymes made in the liver. They are also known as transaminases. The liver uses these enzymes to metabolize amino acids and to make proteins. When liver cells are damaged or dying, ALT and AST leak into the bloodstream. Many different things can cause liver enzymes to rise above normal levels, including:

- viral hepatitis,
- excessive alcohol intake/Alcoholic liver disease,
- liver inflammation from medications and certain herbs,
- auto-immune hepatitis—a condition where a person's immune system mistakes the liver for an invader and attacks it,
- fatty liver-fat build-up in liver cells, called steatohepatitis when the fatty liver is inflamed,
- inherited liver diseases,
- liver tumors,
- heart failure.

ALT (also called alanine aminotransferase or SGPT) is found in the liver only. High levels of ALT in the bloodstream mean that there may be liver inflammation and/or damage. This test cannot predict liver damage or disease progression. It is simply a direct measurement of the amount of ALT in the person's bloodstream at the time of the test. The normal range of ALT levels is between 5 IU/L to 60 IU/L (International Units per Liter). ALT levels in people with HCV often rise and fall over time, so additional testing such as HCV RNA, HCV genotyping, and a liver biopsy may be needed to help determine the cause and extent of liver damage.

AST (also called aspartate aminotransferase or SGOT) is found in other organs besides the liver. High AST levels in the bloodstream can be a sign of liver trouble. AST testing measures the level of AST in a person's bloodstream at a given time. The normal range for AST levels in the bloodstream are 5 IU/L to 43 IU/L. Like ALT levels, AST levels in people with HCV often vary over time and can't be used to forecast disease progression or specifically measure liver damage.

Cholestatic Liver Enzymes

GGT and ALP are also called cholestatic liver enzymes. Cholestasis is a term used for partial or full blockage of the bile ducts. Bile ducts bring bile from the liver into the gallbladder and the intestines. Bile is a green fluid produced in liver cells. Bile helps the body to break down fat, process cholesterol and get rid of toxins. If the bile duct is inflamed or damaged, GGT and ALP can get backed up and spill out from the liver into the bloodstream.

ALP metabolizes phosphorus and brings energy to the body. GGT brings oxygen to tissues.

Causes of elevated ALP and GGT levels include:

- scarring of the bile ducts (called primary biliary cirrhosis),
- fatty liver (steatosis),
- alcoholic liver disease,
- liver inflammation from medications and certain herbs,
- liver tumors,
- gallstones or gall bladder problems.

ALP (also called alkaline phosphatase) is found in the bones, intestines, kidneys, and placenta as well as the liver. Abnormally high ALP can have many causes other than liver damage, including: bone disease, congestive heart failure, and hyperthyroidism. A rise in ALP levels can indicate liver trouble if GGT levels are also elevated. The normal range of ALP is from 30 IU/L to 115 IU/L.

GGT (gamma-glutamyltranspeptidase) is found in the liver. Obesity, PBC, heavy drinking, fatty liver, and certain medications or herbs that are toxic to the liver can cause GGT levels to rise the normal range of GGT is from 5 IU/L to 80 IU/L.

Bilirubin

Bilirubin is a yellow fluid produced in the liver when worn-out red blood cells are broken down. Bilirubin can leak out from the liver into the bloodstream if the liver is damaged. When bilirubin builds up, it can cause jaundice—a yellowing of the eyes and skin, dark urine, and light colored feces. The causes of abnormal bilirubin levels include:

- viral hepatitis,
- blocked bile ducts,
- other liver diseases,
- liver scarring (cirrhosis).

Total bilirubin testing measures the amount of bilirubin in the bloodstream. Normal total bilirubin levels range from .20 mg/dl to 1.50 (milligrams per deciliter). Direct bilirubin testing measures bilirubin made in the liver. The normal level of direct bilirubin range from .00 to .03 mg/dl.

Chapter 17

Sweat Test

The sweat test has been the "gold standard" for diagnosing cystic fibrosis (CF) for more than 40 years. When it is performed by trained technicians, and evaluated in an experienced, reliable laboratory, the sweat test is still the best test to diagnose CF.

It is recommended that the sweat test be performed in a Cystic Fibrosis Foundation-accredited care center where strict guidelines are followed to ensure the accuracy of the results. The test can be performed on individuals of any age. However, some infants may not make enough sweat for the laboratory to analyze. If an infant does not produce enough sweat on the first sweat test, the test should be repeated.

What happens during a sweat test?

The sweat test determines the amount of chloride in the sweat. here are no needles involved in the procedure. In the first part of the test, a colorless, odorless chemical, known to cause sweating, is applied to a small area on an arm or leg. An electrode is then attached to the arm or leg, which allows the technician to apply a weak electrical current to the area to stimulate sweating. Individuals may feel a tingling sensation in the area, or a feeling of warmth. This part of the procedure lasts approximately five minutes.

The second part of the test consists of cleaning the stimulated area and collecting the sweat on a piece of filter paper or gauze or in a plastic coil. Thirty minutes later, the collected sweat is sent to a hospital laboratory for analysis. The entire collection procedure takes approximately one hour.

What does the sweat test reveal?

Your doctor has asked that this test be performed to rule out the presence of CF, an inherited disorder of the lungs, intestines, and sweat glands. Children and adults with CF have an increased amount of chloride (salt) in their sweat. In general, sweat chloride concentrations less than 40 mmol/L are normal (does not have CF); values between 40 to 60 mmol/L are borderline, and sweat chloride concentrations greater than 60 mmol/L are consistent with the diagnosis of CF.

For individuals who have CF, the sweat chloride test will be positive from birth. Once a test result is positive, it is always positive. Sweat test values do not change from positive to negative or negative to positive, as a person grows older. Sweat test values also do not vary when individuals have colds or other temporary illnesses.

Is there any preparation for the sweat test?

There are no restrictions on activity or diet or special preparations before the test. However, one should not apply creams or lotions to the skin 24 hours before the test. All regular medications may be continued and will have no effect on the test results.

When are sweat test results made available?

Sweat test results are usually available to your doctor on the next working day after the test is performed. In a small number of cases, the quantity of sweat obtained is not sufficient to give an accurate result, and the test may need to be repeated.

Can the test results be inconclusive?

Yes. In a small number of cases, the test results fall into "borderline" range between not having CF and indicative of CF. In these situations, repeat sweat tests, as well as other diagnostic procedures, may need to be carried out. These will only be done after consultation with a doctor.

Chapter 18

Biopsies

Chapter Contents

Section 18.1

What Is a Biopsy?

"The Biopsy Report," Surveillance, Epidemiology, and End Results (SEER), National Cancer Institute, 2000. Available online at http://training.seer .cancer.gov/module_abstracting/unit03_sec04_part01_page01_biopsy _rep.html; accessed April 21, 2008.

The term biopsy refers to the removal and examination, gross and microscopic, of tissue or cells from the living body for the purpose of diagnosis. A variety of techniques exist for performing a biopsy of which the most common ones are the following:

- **Aspiration biopsy or bone marrow aspiration:** Biopsy of material (fluid, cells or tissue) obtained by suction through a needle attached to a syringe.

- **Bone marrow biopsy:** Examination of a piece of bone marrow by needle aspiration, can also be done as an open biopsy using a trephine (removing a circular disc of bone).

- **Curettage:** Removal of growths or other material by scraping with a curette.

- **Excisional biopsy (total):** The removal of a growth in its entirety by having a therapeutic as well as diagnostic purpose.

- **Incisional biopsy:** Incomplete removal of a growth for the purpose of diagnostic study.

- **Needle biopsy:** Same as aspiration biopsy.

- **Percutaneous biopsy:** A needle biopsy with the needle going through the skin.

- **Punch biopsy:** Biopsy of material obtained from the body tissue by a punch technique.

- **Sponge (gel foam) biopsy:** Removal of materials (cells, particles of tissue, and tissue juices) by rubbing a sponge over a lesion or over a mucous membrane for examination.

- **Surface biopsy:** Scraping of cells from surface epithelium, especially from the cervix, for microscopic examination.

- **Surgical biopsy:** Removal of tissue from the body by surgical excision for examination.

- **Total biopsy:** See excisional biopsy.

Section 18.2

Sentinel Lymph Node Biopsies

"Sentinel Lymph Node Biopsy: Questions and Answers,"
National Cancer Institute (www.cancer.gov), April 27, 2005.

What is a lymph node?

A lymph node is part of the body's lymphatic system. In the lymphatic system, a network of lymph vessels carries clear fluid called lymph. Lymph vessels lead to lymph nodes, which are small, round organs that trap cancer cells, bacteria, or other harmful substances that may be in the lymph. Groups of lymph nodes are found in the neck, underarms, chest, abdomen, and groin.

What is a sentinel lymph node (SLN)?

The sentinel lymph node is the first lymph node to which cancer is likely to spread from the primary tumor. Cancer cells may appear in the sentinel node before spreading to other lymph nodes. In some cases, there can be more than one sentinel lymph node.

What is SLN biopsy?

SLN biopsy is a procedure in which the sentinel lymph node is removed and examined under a microscope to determine whether cancer cells are present. SLN biopsy is based on the idea that cancer cells spread (metastasize) in an orderly way from the primary tumor to the sentinel lymph node(s), then to other nearby lymph nodes.[1, 2]

A negative SLN biopsy result suggests that cancer has not spread to the lymph nodes. A positive result indicates that cancer is present in the SLN and may be present in other lymph nodes in the same area (regional lymph nodes). This information may help the doctor determine the stage of cancer (extent of the disease within the body) and develop an appropriate treatment plan.[2]

What happens during the SLN biopsy procedure?

In SLN biopsy, one or a few lymph nodes (the sentinel node or nodes) are removed. To identify the sentinel lymph node(s), the surgeon injects a radioactive substance, blue dye, or both near the tumor. The surgeon then uses a scanner to find the sentinel lymph node(s) containing the radioactive substance or looks for the lymph node(s) stained with dye. Once the SLN is located, the surgeon makes a small incision (about ½ inch) in the skin overlying the SLN and removes the lymph node(s).

The sentinel node(s) is/are checked for the presence of cancer cells by a pathologist (a doctor who identifies diseases by studying cells and tissue under a microscope). If cancer is found, the surgeon will usually remove more lymph nodes during the biopsy procedure or during a follow-up surgical procedure. SLN biopsy may be done on an outpatient basis or require a short stay in the hospital.

What are the possible benefits of SLN biopsy?

To understand the possible benefits of SLN biopsy, it helps to know about standard lymph node removal. Standard lymph node removal involves surgery to remove most of the lymph nodes in the area of the tumor (regional lymph nodes). For example, breast cancer surgery may include removing most of the axillary lymph nodes, the group of lymph nodes under the arm. This is called axillary lymph node dissection (ALND).

If SLN biopsy is done and the sentinel node does not contain cancer cells, the rest of the regional lymph nodes may not need to be removed. Because fewer lymph nodes are removed, there may be fewer side effects. When multiple regional lymph nodes are removed, the patient may experience side effects such as lymphedema (swelling caused by excess fluid build-up), numbness, a persistent burning sensation, infection, and difficulty moving the affected body area.[1, 3]

What are the side effects and disadvantages of SLN biopsy?

Side effects of SLN biopsy can include pain or bruising at the biopsy site and the rare possibility of an allergic reaction to the blue dye used to find the sentinel node. Patients may find that their urine is discolored or that their skin has been stained the same color as the dye. These problems are temporary.[2]

Although some surgeons consider SLN biopsy to be the standard of care for some cancers, its role and benefit are yet to be determined.[2] We do not know whether SLN biopsy improves a patient's survival or reduces the chance that the cancer will recur (come back). That is why studies are being conducted to compare SLN biopsy with standard lymph node dissection.

What research has been done with SLN biopsy?

The concept of mapping (finding) the SLN was first reported in 1977 by a researcher studying cancer of the penis.[2, 3, 4] In the 1980s, researchers at the University of California, Los Angeles (UCLA) developed the technique of lymphatic mapping to identify the SLN in patients with melanoma.[3] SLN mapping for breast cancer was first reported in 1994.[1, 3] Since then, researchers have improved methods for finding the SLN. Several studies have shown that when the sentinel node is negative, the remaining nodes are usually negative.[1, 3] However, these studies were done in a small number of centers and overall survival was not examined.

Other research has focused on the identification of the SLN in patients with cancer of the vulva, cervix, prostate, bladder, thyroid, head and neck, colon, rectum, stomach, as well as non-small-cell lung cancer, and Merkel cell cancer[2, 3, 4, 5] Clinical studies continue to examine the accuracy of SLN biopsy and its effect on survival of people with various cancers.

What clinical trials (research studies) are being conducted with SLN biopsy?

The National Cancer Institute (NCI) recently sponsored two large randomized clinical trials (research studies) for breast cancer comparing SLN biopsy with conventional axillary lymph node dissection. The trials were conducted by the National Surgical Adjuvant Breast and Bowel Project (NSABP) and the American College of Surgeons Oncology Group (ACOSOG). NSABP and ACOSOG are both NCI-sponsored Clinical Trials Cooperative Groups, which are networks of institutions and physicians across the country who jointly conduct trials. Although several studies have examined the correlation between the sentinel node and the remaining axillary nodes, these are the first two randomized trials that will compare the long-term results of SLN removal with full axillary node dissection. Both of these large trials are now closed.

Where can people find more information about clinical trials with SLN biopsy?

The NCI's website provides general information about clinical trials at http://www.cancer.gov/clinicaltrials on the internet. It also links to PDQ®, the NCI's cancer information database. PDQ contains detailed information about specific ongoing clinical trials in the United States, Europe, and elsewhere.

Information about clinical trials with SLN biopsy is also available from the NCI's Cancer Information Service (CIS). The CIS, a national information and education network, is a free public service of the NCI, the Nation's primary agency for cancer research. The toll-free phone number for the CIS is 800-4-CANCER (800-422-6237). For callers with TTY equipment, the number is 800-332-8615. The CIS also offers online assistance through the Help link at http://www.cancer.gov on the internet.

Selected References

1. Harris JR, Lippman ME, Morrow M, Osborne CK, editors. *Diseases of the Breast. 3rd ed*. Philadelphia: Lippincott Williams & Wilkins, 2004.

2. DeVita VT Jr., Hellman S, Rosenberg SA, editors. *Cancer: Principles and Practice of Oncology*. Vol. 1 and 2. 6th ed. Philadelphia: Lippincott Williams and Wilkins, 2001.

3. Cochran AJ, Roberts AA, Saida T. The place of lymphatic mapping and sentinel node biopsy in oncology. *International Journal of Clinical Oncology* 2003; 8:139–150.

4. Gipponi M, Solari N, Di Somma FC, Bertoglio S, Cafiero F. New fields of application of the sentinel lymph node biopsy in the pathologic staging of solid neoplasms: Review of literature and surgical perspectives. *Journal of Surgical Oncology* 2004; 85:171–179.

5. Ota DM. What's new in general surgery: Surgical oncology. *Journal of the American College of Surgeons* 2003; 196(6):926–932.

Section 18.3

Breast Biopsies

Breast Biopsy Overview

A breast biopsy involves removing a sample of breast tissue to determine whether it is cancerous or benign (non-cancerous). There are several different types of breast biopsy. The biopsy method most suitable for a particular patient depends on a number of factors, including:

- whether or not an abnormality can be felt or only seen with imaging;

- how suspicious the abnormality appears on x-ray (or feels on palpation);

- the size, shape, and other distinct characteristics of the abnormality;

- the location of the abnormality in the breast and in relation to other anatomic structures;

- the number of abnormalities detected during physical examination or with x-ray imaging;

- the patient's medical history and current medications; and

- the preference of the patient, as long as an option is medically safe and appropriate.

In addition, the systems available at a given breast imaging center or surgical center may influence which method of biopsy a patient receives. For example, vacuum-assisted biopsy (brand name, Mammotome or MIBB) is currently not available at all facilities.

Many biopsy methods rely on image guidance to help the radiologist or breast surgeon precisely locate the lesion (abnormality) within the breast. Imaging may be necessary when a lesion (breast abnormality) cannot be felt during examination and is only detected on imaging studies such as mammography or ultrasound. It may also be necessary to use imaging to assure that a mass felt during examination is, indeed, the same abnormality noted on a mammogram or ultrasound.

If image guidance is required, each of the factors listed above will also be considered in terms of what type of image guidance is most appropriate for the biopsy. Biopsy methods that may require image guidance include:

- fine needle aspiration biopsy (FNA);
- core needle biopsy;
- vacuum-assisted biopsy (Mammotome or MIBB);
- large core biopsy (ABBI); and
- open surgical biopsy (excisional or incisional).

Of these methods, FNA, core needle, and vacuum-assisted biopsies are performed as percutaneous ("through the skin") procedures rather than surgical biopsies.

Though percutaneous ("through the skin") biopsy methods only provide partial information for pathologists, they are usually very accurate when performed by a skilled radiologist or surgeon who has significant experience with image guidance.

However, because percutaneous biopsies only provide samples of tissue (and not the entire lesion as a surgical biopsy does), occasionally, additional procedures may be needed for final diagnosis and treatment of a breast abnormality. This is especially true if there are faint calcifications (calcium deposits), small or low density masses, or diffuse (spread out) abnormalities. Diffuse lesions can be difficult to locate accurately in two stereotactic x-ray views.

Therefore, women should always discuss the risks and benefits of any recommended procedure with their physicians before deciding on the most suitable diagnostic option.

Digital Spot-View Mammography Improves Breast Biopsy

A recent advance in the field of mammography is digital mammography. Digital (computerized) mammography is similar to standard mammography except that breast images are obtained using a system that is equipped with a digital receptor and a computer instead of a film cassette. Digital spot view mammography is often used during breast biopsy and typically allows a faster and more accurate stereotactic biopsy. This usually results in a shorter procedure, increasing patient comfort.

With digital spot-view mammography, images are acquired digitally and displayed immediately on the system monitor. Traditional stereotactic biopsy requires a mammogram film be exposed, developed and then reviewed, significantly increasing the time before the breast biopsy can be completed. Today, the majority of facilities use digital mammography when image guidance is needed for stereotactic biopsy.

Breast Biopsy with Ultrasound Image Guidance

Fine needle aspiration (FNA), core needle biopsy, and vacuum-assisted biopsy may be performed using ultrasound (or stereotactic image guidance) if a breast lesion is easily visualized with this method.

Ultrasound is an excellent method of imaging the breasts; ultrasound guidance allows biopsy of the breast from almost any orientation.

During an ultrasound-guided biopsy, small samples of tissue are removed from the breast using a hollow core needle or vacuum-assisted biopsy device that is precisely guided to the correct location using continuous ultrasound imaging. During the procedure, the patient will lie face up on the standard ultrasound table while being modestly draped, exposing only the area of the breast undergoing biopsy. The area is identified by a preliminary ultrasound.

Breast Biopsy with Prone (Face Down) Stereotactic Image Guidance

During a prone stereotactic biopsy, the patient lies face down (prone) on a specially designed table with the breast placed through an opening in the tabletop. "Stereotactic" means that the breast biopsy path is imaged from two slightly angled directions to help guide the needle. The tabletop is raised and the radiologist and technologist perform the procedure from beneath. The patient's breast is slightly compressed and held in position throughout the procedure. Several stereotactic pairs of x-ray images are made. Small samples of tissue are then removed from the breast using a hollow core needle or vacuum-assisted biopsy device that is precisely guided to the correct location using x-ray imaging and computer coordinates.

Patients who weigh over 300 pounds are usually not appropriate candidates for biopsies that require the use of the prone table. These patients may be better candidates for upright stereotactic image guidance biopsies.

Breast Biopsy with Upright Stereotactic Image Guidance

Breast biopsy using upright stereotactic mammography requires the patient to sit upright in a chair or to lie on her side (lateral recumbent position). The breast biopsy path is imaged from two slightly angled directions to help guide the needle using an upright stereotactic mammography system. The patient's breast is slightly compressed and held in position throughout the procedure. Several stereotactic pairs of x-ray images are made. Small samples of tissue are then removed from the breast using a hollow core needle or vacuum-assisted biopsy device that is precisely guided to the correct location using x-ray imaging and computer coordinates. Upright biopsy is the best method for guiding a biopsy of the axilla or "tail" of the breast; 41% of breast cancers occur in this region.

Perhaps the most difficult part of a biopsy with upright stereotactic image guidance for many patients is the need to sit upright without moving during the biopsy. Therefore, upright stereotactic mammography may not be a viable option for some elderly, anxious, or physically impaired persons. However, upright stereotactic mammography may be an appropriate method for patients who would find it difficult to climb up onto the prone table.

Relative Cost of Different Breast Biopsy Methods

Many health insurance providers cover the cost of a breast biopsy. However, women should always check with their insurance companies before undergoing any medical procedure to determine whether the cost of the biopsy and related costs will be covered (and at what rate). Women should also check to see if special referrals are necessary, as many health maintenance plans require these prior to any specialist consultations or procedures.

The cost of a breast biopsy can range from approximately $1,000 to approximately $5,000 depending several factors, including the type of biopsy performed, the equipment used during the biopsy, whether image guidance or other additional equipment is necessary to perform the biopsy, etc. The cost of a breast biopsy typically increases as the procedure becomes more invasive. This is due to increases in associated costs of using technologically advanced equipment and forms of anesthesia. The type of facility where the biopsy is performed may also influence the cost. For example, the cost may be higher if the biopsy is performed in an outpatient suite at a hospital versus an outpatient surgical center. Fine needle aspiration (FNA) is usually the least expensive biopsy method while open surgical biopsy tends to be the most expensive.

Average Expense for Breast Biopsy

1. Fine Needle Aspiration (FNA)—least expensive

2. Core Needle

3. Vacuum-Assisted (Mammotome or MIBB)

4. Large Core (ABBI)

5. Open Surgical—most expensive

Section 18.4

Endometrial Biopsies

In this procedure, your doctor or nurse will take a tissue sample from the endometrium (the inside lining of the uterus) and have it examined.

Why Do This Test?

- The test is useful for determining the cause of heavy, prolonged, or irregular bleeding, bleeding after menopause, or bleeding associated with taking hormone replacement medications.

- It can be used to screen for endometrial cancer.

- It may be able to help determine why some women have been unable to get pregnant.

The Procedure

You will lie on an examination table with your feet in the stirrups, and your doctor or nurse will use a speculum to make the cervix more visible. You may choose to have spray anesthesia.

Your doctor or nurse will clean the cervix with antiseptic, then steady it with an instrument called a tenaculum. He or she will pass a small plastic tube into the uterus, and use gentle suction to take a small sample of the lining. A pathologist will examine it for abnormalities.

After the Test

Slight bleeding is common after this procedure, and there is a small chance of infection.

Abnormal Results

An abnormal result may indicate uterine fibroids or polyps, endometrial cancer, or other conditions.

If you are having the test because of pregnancy issues, it should indicate whether your uterine lining is suitable for implantation of a fertilized egg.

Section 18.5

Cervical Biopsies

Alternative names: Cervical punch biopsy; Biopsy—cervical punch; Biopsy of the cervix

Definition: A cervical biopsy is a test in which tissue samples are taken from the cervix and examined for disease or other problems.

How the test is performed: You will be asked to lie on your back with your feet in the stirrups. As in a regular pelvic examination, a speculum (an instrument used to hold the vaginal canal open in order to examine the interior) will be inserted into the vagina and opened slightly so that the cervix is visible.

The area is then viewed with a colposcope, a small low-power microscope used to magnify the surface of the vagina and cervix (the most accurate method). The cervix is swabbed with a vinegar solution (acetic acid), which removes the mucus to help highlight abnormal areas. The colposcope is then positioned at the opening of the vagina and the area is examined. Photographs may be taken.

An alternative method is the Schiller's test, which uses an iodine solution to stain the cervix. The stain is inserted through the speculum. The iodine solution stains the normal portions of the cervix, but does not stain abnormal tissues.

When an abnormality is located, a sample (biopsy) may be taken using a small biopsy forceps or a large needle. More than one sample may be taken. Cells from the cervical canal may be used as samples as well. This is called an endocervical curettage or biopsy (ECC) and may further help identify and locate abnormal cervical cells. When the procedure is completed, all the instruments are removed.

How to prepare for the test: There is no special preparation. Before the procedure, you should empty your bladder and bowel for your comfort. Do not douche or have sexual intercourse for 24 hours before the exam.

How the test will feel: A colposcopy is painless. The biopsy may feel like a pinch each time a tissue sample is taken and may cause some cramping with it. Any pain or cramping occurring during the biopsy may be helped by relaxing and taking a few slow deep breaths.

Some cramping may occur after the biopsy. Many women have a tendency to hold their breath during pelvic procedures in anticipation of pain. Making an effort to concentrate on slow, regular breathing will help you relax and reduce or eliminate some pain.

Why the test is performed: A cervical biopsy is usually performed when a pap smear indicates significant abnormalities, or when an abnormal area is seen on the cervix during a routine pelvic examination. The biopsy identifies the abnormality. When a positive pap smear shows minor cell changes or abnormalities, a biopsy probably will not be done immediately, unless there is a reason to believe you may be in a high-risk category. It is usually recommended that a repeat pap smear be done in six months if minor changes are detected.

Normal results: The tissue sample from the cervical biopsy will be examined by a pathologist who will report to your doctor whether the cells appear normal or abnormal.

What abnormal results mean: Abnormal results of the biopsy may indicate problems, such as abnormal tissue development or cell growth in the cervix (cervical intraepithelial neoplasia), or an invasive carcinoma (cancer).

Colposcopy may be used to keep track of precancerous abnormalities and look for recurrent abnormalities after treatment. Abnormalities that may be noted and either biopsied or monitored include any abnormal patterns in the blood vessels, whitish patches on the cervix, and areas that are inflamed, eroded, or atrophic (tissue wasting away).

Additional findings may indicate cervical polyps.

Risks: There may be some bleeding after the biopsy for up to a week. Avoid sexual intercourse, douching, or using tampons for a week to allow the cervix to heal. If bleeding is unusually heavy or lasts for longer than two weeks, or if you notice any signs of infection (fever, foul odor, or discharge), notify your health care provider.

Considerations: When the colposcopic examination or biopsy does not show why the pap smear was abnormal, a more extensive biopsy may be suggested.

Section 18.6

Colposcopy and Loop Electrosurgical Excision Procedure (LEEP)

Colposcopy

A colposcopy is a procedure that examines and, if necessary, takes a biopsy of the cervix. It is usually performed after you receive an abnormal Pap smear. It is used to identify cervical cancer or pre-cancerous conditions.

The Procedure

You will lie on an examination table with your feet in the stirrups, and your doctor or nurse will use a speculum to make the cervix more visible. He or she will then swab the cervix with acetic acid to highlight any abnormal cells. A colposcope (a microscope) will aid in examining the cervix. If your provider finds abnormal cells, he or she will use a very small instrument to remove some cells for examination.

Some women feel discomfort during a colposcopy, but your provider will use anesthetic spray to minimize any feeling. You may have cramping or slight bleeding after the procedure.

Abnormal Results

If your colposcopy indicates that you have abnormal cells, it may mean that you have:

- genital warts (HPV),
- precancerous tissue changes (cervical dysplasia), or
- cervical cancer.

Your provider will follow your biopsy with more testing as necessary to track the changes in your cervix.

Loop Electrosurgical Excision Procedure (LEEP)

LEEP is the most common procedure performed for preinvasive disease of the cervix (dysplasia), a condition that causes cells to become abnormal but not yet cancerous. Dysplasia is often first discovered if a Pap smear is abnormal, or during a colposcopy. LEEP is a quick and precise way to remove just the abnormal tissue.

The Procedure

- A LEEP procedure begins in the same way as a standard pelvic exam. You'll lie on an examination table with your feet in the stirrups, and your healthcare provider will insert a speculum into your vagina.

- You will receive some local anesthetic and a mild iodine or vinegar solution to show any abnormal cells. Your doctor or nurse will look at the cells through a magnifying device called a colposcope.

- A thin wire loop running a high-frequency electrical current will let your provider remove the abnormal cells very precisely. The loop is very thin and will seal any opened blood vessels as it goes.

- The tissue is then sent to the lab to look for cancerous cells.

Afterwards

The procedure is relatively painless, although you may experience some cramping and light bleeding.

For the next few weeks, it is a good idea to avoid the following:

- Sexual intercourse
- Tampons or douching
- Heavy lifting
- Vigorous exercise

Section 18.7

Heart Biopsies

Why is a heart biopsy done?

A heart biopsy is done to see what the cells in the heart muscle look like. The test is most often done after a heart transplant to see if the heart is being rejected by the body. It may also be done if the doctor suspects an infection in the heart, or if the heart is not pumping well for unknown reasons.

How is a heart biopsy done?

To do this test, some small pieces of the heart are removed and looked at under a microscope. To get the sample of heart cells, a doctor places a small tube into a large vein in the leg which is then passed into the heart. Some tiny pieces of the heart muscle are removed and sent to the lab where they are carefully examined.

Where is the test done?

This test may be done while a child is in the hospital or as an outpatient procedure. If your child is coming in for this test from home, be sure to come to the Pediatric Cardiology Clinic early that morning. Your child should not eat or drink anything the morning of the biopsy. If your child has had a transplant, do not give Tacrolimus or CellCept the morning of the biopsy. Bring these medications with you he or she can take them after a drug level has been drawn and the biopsy is completed. All other medicines may be taken prior to the biopsy. Your child may be given medicines to make him or her sleepy during the test. Older children sometimes prefer to have only a local anesthetic.

How long will the test take?

The biopsy takes about an hour to complete. After the test, your child will need to lie flat for two hours. A normal diet can be resumed as soon as the child is hungry.

Section 18.8

Kidney Biopsies

From "Kidney Biopsy," National Institute of Diabetes and
Digestive and Kidney Diseases, NIH Pub. No. 05-4763, January 2005.

A biopsy is a diagnostic test that involves collecting small pieces of tissue, usually through a needle, for examination under a microscope. A kidney biopsy can help find a diagnosis and determine the best course of treatment. Your doctor may recommend a kidney biopsy if you have any of the following conditions:

- Hematuria which is blood in your urine

- Proteinuria which is excessive protein in your urine

- Impaired kidney function which causes excessive waste products in your blood

A pathologist will look at the kidney tissue samples to check for unusual deposits, scarring, or infecting organisms that would explain your condition. The doctor may discover that you have a condition that can be treated and cured. If you have progressive kidney failure, the biopsy may indicate how quickly the disease is advancing. A biopsy can also help explain why a transplanted kidney is not working properly.

Talk with your doctor about what information might be obtained from the biopsy and the risks involved so that you can help make a decision about whether a biopsy is worthwhile in your case.

Preparation

You will have to sign a consent form indicating that you understand the risks involved in this procedure, although they are very slight. Discuss these risks thoroughly with your doctor before you sign the form.

Make sure your doctor is aware of all the medicines you take and any drug allergies you might have. You may be told to avoid food and fluids for eight hours before the test. Shortly before the biopsy, you will give blood and urine samples to make sure you don't have a condition that would make doing a biopsy less desirable.

Test Procedures

Kidney biopsies are usually done in a hospital. You may be fully awake with light sedation, or you may be asleep under general anesthesia. If you are awake, you will be given a local anesthetic before the needle is inserted.

You will lie on your stomach to position the kidneys near the surface of your back. If you have a transplanted kidney, you will lie on your back. The doctor will mark the entry site, clean the area, and inject a local painkiller. For a percutaneous (through the skin) biopsy, your doctor will use a locating needle and x-ray or ultrasound equipment to find the right spot and then a collecting needle to gather the tissue. You will be asked to hold your breath as the doctor inserts the biopsy needle and collects the tissue, usually for about 30 seconds or a little longer for each insertion. Do not exhale until you are told. You may feel a small "popping" sensation as the needle enters the kidney. The doctor may need three or four passes to collect the needed samples.

The entire procedure usually takes about an hour, including time to locate the kidney, clean the biopsy site, inject the local painkiller, and obtain the tissue samples.

Some patients shouldn't have a percutaneous biopsy because they are prone to bleeding problems. These patients may still undergo a kidney biopsy through an open operation in which the surgeon makes an incision and can see the kidney to obtain a biopsy. Another method is the transjugular biopsy. To obtain the tissue sample, the needle is inserted through a catheter that enters the patient's jugular vein at the neck. The needle threads down through the blood vessel to the right kidney in order to obtain the tissue from the inside without puncturing the outside skin of the kidney.

After the Test

You should lie on your back for 12 to 24 hours. During this time, your back will probably feel sore. If you have a transplanted kidney, you will lie on your stomach. You will likely stay in the hospital overnight after the procedure so that staff can check your condition. You may notice some blood in your urine for 24 hours after the test. To detect any problems, your team will monitor your blood pressure and pulse, take blood samples to measure the amount of red cells, and examine the urine that you pass. On rare occasions when bleeding does not stop on its own, it may be necessary to replace lost blood with a transfusion.

A rare complication is infection from the biopsy procedure.

Tell your doctor or nurse if you have any of these problems:

- Bloody urine more than 24 hours after the test
- Inability to urinate
- Fever
- Worsening pain in the biopsy site
- Faintness or dizziness

Getting the Results

After the biopsy, the doctor will inspect the tissue samples in the laboratory under one or more microscopes, perhaps using dyes to identify different substances that may be deposited in the tissue. It usually takes a few days to get the complete biopsy results. If your case is urgent, you may have a preliminary report within a few hours.

Section 18.9

Liver Biopsies

From "Liver Biopsy," National Institute of Diabetes and
Digestive and Kidney Diseases, NIH Pub. No 05-4731, November 2004.

In a liver biopsy, the physician examines a small piece of tissue from your liver for signs of damage or disease. A special needle is used to remove the tissue from the liver. The physician decides to do a liver biopsy after tests suggest that the liver does not work properly. For example, a blood test might show that your blood contains higher than normal levels of liver enzymes or too much iron or copper. An x-ray could suggest that the liver is swollen. Looking at liver tissue itself is the best way to determine whether the liver is healthy or what is causing it to be damaged.

Preparation

Before scheduling your biopsy, the physician will take blood samples to make sure your blood clots properly. Be sure to mention any medications you take, especially those that affect blood clotting, like blood thinners. One week before the procedure, you will have to stop taking aspirin, ibuprofen, and anticoagulants.

You must not eat or drink anything for eight hours before the biopsy, and you should plan to arrive at the hospital about an hour before the scheduled time of the procedure. Your physician will tell you whether to take your regular medications during the fasting period and may give you other special instructions.

Procedure

Liver biopsy is considered minor surgery, so it is done at the hospital. For the biopsy, you will lie on a hospital bed on your back with your right hand above your head. After marking the outline of your liver and injecting a local anesthetic to numb the area, the physician will make a small incision in your right side near your rib cage, then insert the biopsy needle and retrieve a sample of liver tissue. In some cases, the physician may use an ultrasound image of the liver to help guide the needle to a specific spot.

You will need to hold very still so that the physician does not nick the lung or gallbladder, which are close to the liver. The physician will ask you to hold your breath for five to ten seconds while he or she puts the needle in your liver. You may feel pressure and a dull pain. The entire procedure takes about 20 minutes.

Two other methods of liver biopsy are also available. For a laparoscopic biopsy, the physician inserts a special tube called a laparoscope through an incision in the abdomen. The laparoscope sends images of the liver to a monitor. The physician watches the monitor and uses instruments in the laparoscope to remove tissue samples from one or more parts of the liver. Physicians use this type of biopsy when they need tissue samples from specific parts of the liver.

Transvenous biopsy involves inserting a tube called a catheter into a vein in the neck and guiding it to the liver. The physician puts a biopsy needle into the catheter and then into the liver. Physicians use this procedure when patients have blood-clotting problems or fluid in the abdomen.

Recovery

After the biopsy, the physician will put a bandage over the incision and have you lie on your right side, pressed against a towel, for one to two hours. The nurse will monitor your vital signs and level of pain.

You will need to arrange for someone to take you home from the hospital since you will not be allowed to drive after having the sedative. You must go directly home and remain in bed (except to use the bathroom) for eight to 12 hours, depending on your physician's instructions. Also, avoid exertion for the next week so that the incision and liver can heal. You can expect a little soreness at the incision site and possibly some pain in your right shoulder. This pain is caused by irritation of the diaphragm muscle (the pain usually radiates to the shoulder) and should disappear within a few hours or days. Your physician may recommend that you take Tylenol for pain, but you must not take aspirin or ibuprofen for the first week after surgery. These medicines decrease blood clotting, which is crucial for healing.

Like any surgery, liver biopsy does have some risks, such as puncture of the lung or gallbladder, infection, bleeding, and pain, but these complications are rare.

Section 18.10

Lung Biopsies

Lung Needle Biopsy

Alternative names: Transthoracic needle aspiration; Percutaneous needle aspiration

Definition: A lung needle biopsy is a method to remove a piece of lung tissue for examination.

How the test is performed: A chest x-ray or chest computed tomography (CT) scan may be used to locate the precise spot of the biopsy. If the biopsy is done using a CT scan, you may be lying down during the exam.

A needle biopsy of the lung may also be performed during bronchoscopy or mediastinoscopy.

You sit with your arms resting forward on a table. You should try to keep still and not cough during the biopsy. The doctor will ask you to hold your breath. The skin is scrubbed and a local anesthetic is injected.

The surgeon will make a small (about 1/8-inch) cut in the skin, and will insert the biopsy needle into the abnormal tissue, tumor, or lung tissue. A small piece of tissue is removed with the needle and sent to a laboratory for examination.

When done, pressure is placed over the site. Once bleeding has stopped, a bandage is applied.

A chest x-ray is taken immediately after the biopsy.

The procedure usually takes 30–60 minutes. Laboratory analysis usually takes a few days.

How to prepare for the test: Before a needle biopsy of the lung is conducted, a chest x-ray or chest CT scan may be performed. Sometimes, you will be given a mild sedative before the biopsy. You must sign a consent form. It is important to remain as still as possible for the biopsy and to avoid coughing.

How the test will feel: A lung needle biopsy is preceded by a local injection of anesthetic, which will sting for a moment. You will feel pressure and a brief, sharp pain when the needle touches the lung.

Why the test is performed: A needle lung biopsy is performed when there is an abnormal condition that is near the surface of the lung, in the lung itself, or on the chest wall. The test is usually performed to diagnose relatively large abnormalities seen on chest x-ray or CT scan. Most often, the abnormality is not believed to be accessible by other diagnostic techniques, such as bronchoscopy.

Normal results: Normal tissues and no microbial growth, if a culture is performed, are normal.

What abnormal results mean: Bacterial, viral, or fungal lung infection; pneumonia; cancerous cells (lung cancer, mesothelioma); immune disorder.

Additional conditions under which the test may be performed: Metastatic cancer to the lung; pneumonia with lung abscess.

Risks: The risks include a collapsed lung, bleeding, and infection. A needle biopsy should not be performed if other tests show that you have any of the following:

- Bullae (enlarged alveoli associated with emphysema)
- Cysts
- Blood coagulation disorder of any type
- Severe hypoxia
- Pulmonary hypertension
- Cor pulmonale

Considerations: Signs of a collapsed lung include the following:

- Shortness of breath
- Rapid heart rate (rapid pulse)
- Blueness of the skin

If any of these occur, report them to the health care provider immediately.

Open Lung Biopsy

Alternative names: Biopsy—open lung

Definition: An open lung biopsy is surgery to remove a small piece of tissue from the lung. The sample is then examined for cancer, infection, or lung disease.

How the test is performed: An open lung biopsy is done in a hospital operating room under general anesthesia, which means you are asleep and pain-free. A tube will be placed through the mouth and into the airway that leads to the lungs.

After cleaning the skin, the surgeon makes a cut in the chest area and removes a small piece of lung tissue. The wound is closed with stitches.

A chest tube may be left in place for one to two days to prevent the lung from collapsing.

How to prepare for the test: You should tell the health care provider if you are pregnant, allergic to any medications, and if you have a bleeding problem. Be sure to tell the health care team which medications you are taking (including any herbal preparations).

You will be asked not to eat or drink for eight to 12 hours before the procedure.

How the test will feel: When you wake up after the procedure, you will feel drowsy for several hours. You may have a mild sore throat from the tube. You will feel some discomfort and pain at the incision site.

Why the test is performed: The open lung biopsy is done to evaluate lung problems seen on x-ray or CT scan.

Normal results: The lungs and lung tissue will be normal.

What abnormal results mean: Abnormal results may indicate cancer, benign tumors, lung diseases, and certain infections. The procedure may also help diagnose the following conditions:

- Acute pulmonary eosinophilia (Loeffler syndrome)

- Chronic pulmonary coccidioidomycosis
- Disseminated coccidioidomycosis
- Disseminated tuberculosis (infectious)
- Chronic pulmonary histoplasmosis
- Mesothelioma (benign-fibrous)
- Mesothelioma (malignant)
- Pneumonia with lung abscess
- Primary lung cancer
- Pulmonary aspergillosis
- Pulmonary tuberculosis
- Rheumatoid lung disease
- Sarcoidosis
- Viral pneumonia
- Wegener granulomatosis

Risks: There is a possibility of infection or an air leak into the chest. Your risk depends on whether or not you already have lung disease.

Section 18.11

Muscle Biopsies

A muscle biopsy is a surgical procedure in which one or more small pieces of muscle tissue are removed for further microscopic or biochemical examination. The procedure, often used in the diagnosis of a neuromuscular disorder, is considered "minor" surgery and is usually performed under local anesthetic.

A doctor is likely to call for a muscle biopsy after looking at preliminary blood tests, performing an electromyogram (EMG) and physical examination, and determining that the patient's symptoms indicate an underlying neuromuscular disorder. The muscle biopsy can help distinguish between muscular and neurological problems and can help pinpoint the exact neuromuscular disorder present.

Not everyone suspected of having a neuromuscular disease requires a muscle biopsy. In some cases, diagnosis can be made by symptoms and a DNA test based on a blood sample.

Open or Needle Biopsy

There are two types of muscle biopsy. The open biopsy involves the removal of one or more small pieces of muscle tissue with sharp scissors.

The neuromuscular specialist selects a muscle, usually the biceps, triceps, deltoid, or quadriceps muscle, that should yield the most information about the disease. Usually moderately affected muscles are chosen; the weakest muscles may already be too degraded for analysis. The procedure involves a two-to-three-inch incision, which is then closed with stitches and may feel sore for a few days.

In a needle biopsy, used since the 1960s, a pea-sized muscle sample is collected with a large bore needle. Although this is less invasive than the open biopsy, the doctor loses the ability to examine the muscle visually first, and the specimen collected is smaller.

Analyzing the Sample

When the muscle samples are sent to a laboratory for analysis, the technicians cut them into many thin sections for examination. Using different tests on different sections, they look at the tissue's overall appearance, chemical activities in the tissue, and the presence or absence of critical proteins. The information these tests provide helps determine exactly what disease and what form of it the person has.

Histology tests (histo means tissue) employ chemical stains to see the muscle's overall appearance and the structure of the muscle cells. This analysis can yield information about muscle degeneration and regeneration, fiber type abnormalities, mitochondrial abnormalities, scar tissue, inflammation, and other clues to specific disorders.

Histochemistry uses stains to detect chemical activities in the cells, including the actions of specific enzymes and metabolic processes. A lab that performs only histology may miss important metabolic abnormalities.

Immunohistochemistry uses antibodies to detect the presence or absence of proteins. This analysis can show whether the cells are missing dystrophin (indicating Duchenne or Becker MD), sarcoglycans (limb-girdle MD), merosin (congenital MD), or other proteins whose absence causes specific muscular dystrophies. Specific antibodies can also be used to identify the nature of inflammatory cells found in the muscle.

The lab may also use electron microscopy to get very high magnification views of the cellular structure, which can confirm structural abnormalities, like the presence of nemaline rods.

Finally, a DNA analysis can be performed on a muscle sample to detect a genetic mutation. Although a blood sample is usually adequate for a DNA test, a muscle sample may be needed to test for mitochondrial DNA mutations.

Multiple Biopsies

Yadollah Harati, a neurologist and director of the Muscle and Nerve Pathology Laboratory at Baylor College of Medicine in Houston, usually takes as many as five separate muscle samples from different regions of the muscle incision. Several are analyzed and at least one is frozen for future use. Harati believes no biopsy should be done unless the amount of tissue removed is adequate for a complete study.

Having at least three muscle samples gives the lab an adequate amount of tissue to work with. In some disorders, particularly "patchy" disorders like the inflammatory myopathies, signs of the disease may not be present in all regions of the muscles, so more samples give a better chance of accuracy.

It's important that the tissue samples be frozen promptly and properly after the biopsy and be stored carefully. If they're not handled and stored correctly, the results may be inaccurate.

Your doctor may occasionally recommend a new biopsy even though you've had one in the past, especially if you've been given a tentative diagnosis or now suspect your diagnosis was incorrect. With many new muscle-protein antibodies now available for testing biopsy samples, as well as new understanding of mitochondrial disorders and new DNA tests, a new biopsy may be desirable.

According to Harati, tissue that was frozen promptly after removal and maintained carefully is useful for many years. In autoimmune diseases, tissue changes over time in your body may necessitate a new biopsy for the most accurate diagnosis.

Getting Results

The analysis of a muscle biopsy sample is a very tedious and labor-intensive process in which many sections of the muscle must be cut, many different types of procedures performed, and the results carefully analyzed. Harati's lab usually performs a few basic histology tests immediately after the biopsy and then, based on these results, determines what further tests should be made.

His lab typically makes an initial report on the day of the biopsy and a full report in two to three weeks.

Section 18.12

Skin Biopsies

This information is reprinted with the permission from DermNet, the website of the New Zealand Dermatological Society. Visit www.dermnet .org.nz for patient information on numerous skin conditions and their treatment. © 2007 New Zealand Dermatological Society.

A skin biopsy is when your dermatologist removes a piece of skin and sends it to a pathology laboratory where a histopathologist looks at it under the microscope.

Why Do You Need to Have a Skin Biopsy?

Skin biopsies are performed to help with the diagnosis of your skin condition. Sometimes, different skin conditions can look similar to the naked eye so additional information is required. This is obtained by looking at the structure of the skin under the microscope after the cells have been stained with special colored dyes.

There are two situations in which this usually occurs:

- To distinguish between different types of rashes or skin lesions. Your dermatologist maybe considering a number of possible diagnoses, and the skin biopsy provides additional information in this process.

- The dermatologist suspects you have a skin cancer. A biopsy is taken to confirm that the skin cancer is present. The biopsy may also give information on the type of skin cancer, which may determine the best treatment.

What Is Involved in Having a Skin Biopsy?

Your dermatologist will explain to you why the skin biopsy is needed and the particular procedure involved.

Shortly before the skin biopsy, you will be given a small injection of local anesthetic to make the area numb. This usually stings momentarily but the skin quickly becomes numb.

The dermatologist will perform the skin biopsy. You may feel a pushing sensation in the area where the skin biopsy is being performed but there should not be any pain. You should tell the doctor if the procedure is painful during the biopsy.

You may have stitches depending on the type of skin biopsy. Your dermatologist will tell you when to get them removed.

A dressing will usually be applied to the site of the biopsy. This should be left in place for the first 24 hours. After that you can remove the dressing.

Your dermatologist will arrange to tell you the result of the biopsy. It usually takes about one week for the doctor to obtain the result from the pathology laboratory, but can sometimes take longer if special stains are required. There will be a small scar left after the skin biopsy site has healed.

Punch Biopsy

Punch biopsies are quick, convenient and usually only produce a small wound. They allow the pathologist to get a full thickness view of the skin. More than one punch biopsy may be required depending on the condition being investigated.

The punch biopsy blade takes a small round core of tissue ranging from 2 mm to 6 mm in diameter although 3 to 4 mm is the usual size.

Sometimes a stitch will be required or, if the wound is small, it may heal adequately without a stitch.

Shave Biopsy

A shave biopsy may be used if the skin lesion is suspected to only affect the top layers of the skin (epidermis and dermis).

The dermatologist will take a very superficial slice of skin from the area affected with a scalpel, Dermablade or razor blade. There are usually no stitches required after a shave biopsy but there will be a small scab that should heal in one to two weeks depending on the skin lesion involved.

Incisional Biopsy

Incisional biopsies are used when a larger piece of skin is needed to make a correct diagnosis. The dermatologist will cut out a piece of skin with a scalpel blade. Stitches are usually required after an incisional biopsy.

Section 18.13

Thyroid Biopsies

A fine needle aspiration (FNA) biopsy or thyroid biopsy, is usually carried out to determine the nature of the cells in a thyroid nodule. The biopsy is done with a small needle, and local anesthesia is not generally required. Your physician should be advised if you have any medical conditions that increase your risk of bleeding, or if you are taking drugs that may increase your chances of bleeding during the biopsy, such as aspirin, other non-steroidal agents, anti-platelet agents, or blood thinners such as Coumadin or warfarin.

Most studies have shown that the greater number of separate needle aspirations done at the time of the biopsy, the greater yield and ultimate accuracy of the biopsy procedure. Hence it is common practice for several attempts to be made in the course of the biopsy procedure, or for the needle to be inserted into a few different locations within the thyroid nodule.

Firm pressure applied locally to the biopsy site for about five minutes is usually sufficient to stop any bleeding that may develop following the biopsy. Some minor degree of discomfort in the neck, perhaps soreness or occasionally ear pain, may be noticeable for one to three days after the biopsy, but the majority of patients do not experience these complaints after thyroid biopsy.

Patients should be aware that thyroid biopsies may frequently not be diagnostic, and there are limitations to the success and utility of the biopsy procedure. These limitations include the local anatomy of the patients' neck, the skill of the person carrying out the biopsy, and the experience of the cytopathologist examining the biopsy material. Furthermore, it is often not possible for even a superb experienced pathologist to make a determination of benign versus malignant thyroid cells, even if an excellent biopsy is obtained, depending on the nature of the underlying thyroid pathology.

Most patients are surprised to learn that a biopsy may not always give 100% accurate results. Although good centers will end up with informative and accurate results about 80–90% of the time a biopsy is done, certain types of nodules showing lots of follicular cells or Hurthle cells result in an inability to make an accurate preoperative diagnosis. Given the limitations of the test, it is not uncommon for a patient to have more than one biopsy in the first year of assessment, depending on the size of the nodule, the clinical appearance of the nodule, and the judgment of the physician.

It is important to remember that all diagnostic procedures, including thyroid fine needle aspiration biopsies, have their limitations. For a representative overview of the sensitivity and specificity and predictive value of biopsy results from several centers. In some centers, the reported results using ultrasound guided (FNAB) biopsies are very accurate when correlated with the final surgical diagnosis. In contrast, even academic teaching centers report less than optimal accuracy of thyroid biopsies when correlated with the final diagnosis after surgical removal of the thyroid gland.

Furthermore, analysis of ultrasound guided biopsies at a Harvard teaching hospital demonstrated that only 63% of biopsies done under ultrasound yielded sufficient cells for accurate initial assessment. Nevertheless, there is evidence that biopsies done under ultrasound guidance yield more accurate results than biopsies done by a physician without the use of ultrasound. Comparison of palpation-guided fine-needle aspiration biopsy to ultrasound-guided fine-needle aspiration biopsy in the evaluation of thyroid nodules.

There are ongoing research studies examining whether newer molecular techniques can improve the diagnostic accuracy of the thyroid biopsy. Some studies have shown that a combination of gene expression profiles can improve the ability of scientists to distinguish benign versus malignant follicular tumors, but these studies are still experimental and not widely available.

Nodules that are partly cystic may yield only cyst fluid and degenerating cells, with little in the way of informative thyroid cells for a pathologist to review. Alternatively, despite several reasonable attempts, only blood cells and inflammatory cells may be obtained, precluding a definitive cytology interpretation. Thyroid adenomas that are benign and follicular thyroid cancers may look the same following a thyroid biopsy to even the most experienced cytopathologist, and sometimes the only way to make a definitive diagnosis in these cases is to remove the nodule surgically.

Depending on the size of the nodule, the anatomical location, the local anatomy, and skill of the individual physician, a nodule may be biopsied in the office, or under ultrasound guidance. Ultrasound-guided biopsies may be particularly valuable for small nodules that are difficult to access, or for nodules that are partly cystic, where biopsy of the solid component is desired.

Chapter 19

Throat Culture

A child's throat can be sore for many reasons. If due to an infection, the most common cause is a virus. In most cases, the soreness goes away as the infection does and almost never leads to further problems. But in some cases, sore throats are caused by a more serious bacterial infection from germs known as group A streptococci, or strep. These germs cause strep throat, an infection that commonly affects school-age children.

It's important to find out whether strep is the cause of a sore throat because prompt treatment can decrease symptoms and reduce the risk of complications such as rheumatic fever (which can cause heart damage). To determine this, doctors usually perform either a strep screen or throat culture.

How is a strep screen or throat culture done?

In a strep screen, the doctor or medical assistant wipes the back of the throat with a long cotton swab. This tickles the back of the throat, and can cause a child to gag. While a strep screen can be uncomfortable for a few seconds, it should not be painful. It may help to tell your child exactly that—the test will tickle and feel a little uncomfortable, but will be over very quickly, especially if your child stays still.

In a laboratory, the swab is placed in a test tube with a chemical mix that extracts part of the strep germ (the antigen) from the swab. This extract is then combined with antibodies, which attach to the strep antigen if it is present. A third substance is added to the tube that detects the antigen-antibody combination. If this combination is present, a color change is seen. This means that strep was present in the initial sample from the throat swab. The specimen for a throat culture is taken in the same way, but the fluid from the swab is put into a culture dish in which the bacteria from the specimen must be grown for two to three days before strep germs, if present, can be identified.

A positive strep screen or throat culture means the child has strep throat and would benefit from taking antibiotics to kill the strep germs.

How long does it take to get the results?

A rapid strep screen can offer results in minutes, whereas a throat culture takes two to three days. Waiting for results will still leave enough time to treat the strep infection and avoid potentially serious, preventable complications. Sometimes, depending on the severity of your child's symptoms and other specific circumstances, your doctor may recommend beginning antibiotic treatment while waiting for the culture results.

If the rapid strep screen is negative, a throat culture is done as well because the rapid test can miss some cases of strep throat. Often, the doctor will take both samples at once, in case the culture is needed. That way, your child only feels uncomfortable once. If the throat culture results are negative for strep, antibiotic treatment can be avoided or stopped. This reduces the risk of your child experiencing an allergic reaction or other side effects from unnecessary antibiotic treatment. A negative throat culture means that a virus is probably the cause of your child's sore throat. Talk to your doctor if you have any other questions or concerns.

Chapter 20

Lumbar Puncture (Spinal Tap)

Alternative names: Spinal tap; Ventricular puncture; Lumbar puncture; Cisternal puncture; Cerebral spinal fluid culture

Definition: Cerebral spinal fluid (CSF) collection is a test to look at the fluid that surrounds the brain and spinal cord. Cerebral spinal fluid acts like a cushion, protecting the brain and spine from injury. The fluid is normally clear. The test is also used to measure pressure in the spinal fluid.

How the test is performed: There are different ways to get a sample of spinal fluid. Lumbar puncture, commonly called a spinal tap, is the most common method. The test is usually performed in the following manner:

- The patient must lay on his or her side, with the knees pulled up toward the chest, and the chin tucked downward. Sometimes the test is done with the person sitting up, but bent over.

- After the back is cleaned, the health care provider will inject a local numbing medicine (anesthetic) into the lower spine.

- A spinal needle is inserted, usually into the lower back area.

- Once the needle is properly positioned, spinal fluid pressure is measured, and fluid is collected.

"Cerebral Spinal Fluid (CSF) Collection," © 2008 A.D.A.M., Inc. Reprinted with permission.

- The needle is removed, the area is cleaned, and a bandage is placed over the needle site. The patient is often asked to lie down for a short time after the test.

Occasionally, special x-rays are used to help guide the needle into the proper position. This is called fluoroscopy.

Lumbar puncture with fluid collection may also be part of other procedures, particularly a myelogram (x-ray or CT scan after dye has been inserted into the CSF).

Alternative methods of CSF collection are rarely used, but may be necessary in the event of a back deformity or infection.

Cisternal puncture uses a needle placed below the occipital bone (back of the skull). It can be dangerous because it is so close to the brain stem.

Ventricular puncture is even rarer, but may be recommended in persons with possible brain herniation. This test is usually done in the operating room. A hole is drilled in the skull, and a needle is inserted directly into one of brain's ventricles.

How to prepare for the test: The patient (or guardian) must give the health care team permission to do the test.

How the test will feel: The position may be uncomfortable, but it is extremely important that the patient stays in the bended position to avoid moving the needle and possibly injuring the spinal cord.

The anesthetic will sting or burn when first injected. There will be a hard pressure sensation when the needle is inserted, and there is usually some brief pain when the needle goes through the tissue surrounding the spinal cord. This pain should stop in a few seconds.

Overall, discomfort is minimal to moderate. The entire procedure usually takes about 30 minutes, but it may take longer. The actual pressure measurements and fluid collection only take a few minutes.

Why the test is performed: This test is done to measure pressures within the cerebrospinal fluid and to collect a sample of the fluid for further testing. CSF can be used to diagnose certain neurologic disorders, particularly infections (such as meningitis) and brain or spinal cord damage.

Normal results: Normal values vary from lab to lab but typically range as follows:

- Pressure: 50–180 mm H20

- Appearance: clear, colorless
- CSF total protein: 15–45 mg/100 mL
- Gamma globulin: 3–12% of the total protein
- CSF glucose: 50–80 mg/100 mL (or approximately 2/3 of blood sugar level)
- CSF cell count: 0–5 white blood cells, no red blood cells
- Chloride: 110–125 mEq per liter

Note: mg/mL = milligrams per milliliter; mEq/L = milliequivalent per liter

What abnormal results mean: If the CSF looks cloudy, it could mean there is an infection or a build up of white blood cells or protein.

If the CSF looks bloody or red, it may be a sign of bleeding or spinal cord obstruction. If it is brown, orange, or yellow, it may be a sign of increased CSF protein or previous bleeding (more than three days ago).

Increased CSF pressure may be due to increased intracranial pressure (pressure within the skull). Decreased CSF pressure may be due to spinal cord tumor, shock, fainting, or diabetic coma.

Increased protein may be due to blood in the CSF, diabetes, polyneuritis, tumor, injury, or any inflammatory or infectious condition. Decreased protein is a sign of rapid CSF production.

Increased CSF gamma globulin levels may be due to diseases such as multiple sclerosis, neurosyphilis, or Guillain-Barré syndrome.

Increased CSF glucose is a sign of high blood sugar. Decreased CSF glucose may be due to hypoglycemia (low blood sugar), bacterial or fungal infection (such as meningitis), tuberculosis, or certain types of meningitis.

Increased white blood cells in the CSF may be a sign of meningitis, acute infection, beginning of a chronic illness, tumor, abscess, stroke, or demyelinating disease (such as multiple sclerosis).

Red blood cells in the CSF sample may be a sign of bleeding into the spinal fluid or the result of a traumatic lumbar puncture.

Additional conditions under which the test may be performed:

- Chronic inflammatory polyneuropathy
- Dementia due to metabolic causes
- Encephalitis

- Epilepsy
- Febrile seizure (children)
- Generalized tonic-clonic seizure
- Hydrocephalus
- Inhalation anthrax
- Normal pressure hydrocephalus (NPH)
- Pituitary tumor
- Reye syndrome

Risks: Risks of lumbar puncture include the following:

- Hypersensitivity (allergic) reaction to the anesthetic
- Discomfort during the test
- Headache after the test
- Bleeding into the spinal canal

There is an increased risk of bleeding in persons who take blood thinners.

Brain herniation may occur if this test is done on a person with a mass in the brain (such as a tumor or abscess). This can result in brain damage or death. This test is not done if an exam or test reveals signs of a brain mass.

Damage to the nerves in the spinal cord may occur, particularly if the person moves during the test.

Cisternal puncture or ventricular puncture carry additional risks of brain damage and bleeding within the brain.

Considerations: This test should not be performed on people who may have increased intracranial pressure.

References

Nathan, BR. Cerebrospinal Fluid and Intracranial Pressure. In: Goetz, CG, ed. *Textbook of Clinical Neurology*, 2nd ed. Philadelphia, Pa: WB Saunders Company; 2003:511–524.

Chapter 21

Urinalysis

At A Glance

Why get tested?

To screen for metabolic and kidney disorders and for urinary tract infections.

When to get tested?

During a routine physical or when you have symptoms of a urinary tract infection, such as abdominal pain, back pain, frequent or painful urination, or blood in the urine; as part of a pregnancy checkup, a hospital admission, or a pre-surgical work-up.

Sample required?

One to two ounces of urine; first morning sample is most valuable.

The Test Sample

What is being tested?

A urinalysis is a group of tests that detect and semi-quantitatively measure various compounds that are eliminated in the urine, including the byproducts of normal and abnormal metabolism as well as cells, including bacteria, and cellular fragments. Urine is produced by the kidneys, located on either side of the spine at the bottom of the ribcage. The kidneys filter wastes and metabolic byproducts out of the blood, help regulate the amount of water in the body, and conserve proteins, electrolytes, and other compounds that the body can reuse. Anything that is not needed is excreted in the urine and travels from the kidneys to the bladder, through the urethra, and out of the body. Urine is generally yellow and relatively clear, but every time someone urinates, the color, quantity, concentration, and content of the urine will be slightly different because of varying constituents.

Many disorders can be diagnosed in their early stages by detecting abnormalities in the urine. These include increased concentrations of constituents that are not usually found in significant quantities in the urine, such as: glucose, protein, bilirubin, red blood cells, white blood cells, crystals, and bacteria. They may be present because there are elevated concentrations of the substance in the blood and the body is trying to decrease blood levels by "dumping" them in the urine, because kidney disease has made the kidneys less effective at filtering, or in the case of bacteria, due to an infection.

A complete urinalysis consists of three distinct testing phases:

1. Physical examination, which evaluates the urine's color, clarity, and concentration.

2. Chemical examination, which tests chemically for nine substances that provide valuable information about health and disease.

3. Microscopic examination, which identifies and counts the type of cells, casts, crystals, and other components (bacteria, mucus) that can be present in urine.

Usually, a routine urinalysis consists of the physical and the chemical examinations. These two phases can be completed in just a few minutes in the laboratory or doctor's office. A microscopic examination is then performed if there is an abnormal finding on the physical or chemical examination, or if the doctor specifically orders it.

How is the sample collected for testing?

Urine for a urinalysis can be collected at any time. The first morning sample is the most valuable because it is more concentrated and more likely to yield abnormal results. Because of the potential to contaminate urine with bacteria and cells from the surrounding skin during collection (particularly in women), it is important to first clean the genitalia. Women should spread the labia of the vagina and clean from front to back; men should wipe the tip of the penis. As you start to urinate, let some urine fall into the toilet, then collect one to two ounces of urine in the container provided, then void the rest into the toilet. This type of collection is called a midstream collection or a clean catch.

A urine sample will only be useful for a urinalysis if it is collected as a clean catch and taken to the doctor's office or laboratory for processing within a short period of time. If it will be longer than an hour between collection and transport time, then the urine should be refrigerated.

NOTE: If undergoing medical tests makes you or someone you care for anxious, embarrassed, or even difficult to manage, you might consider reading one or more of the following articles: "Coping with Test Pain, Discomfort, and Anxiety," "Tips on Blood Testing," "Tips to Help Children through Their Medical Tests," and "Tips to Help the Elderly through Their Medical Tests" which can be found online at http://www .labtestsonline.org/understanding/testtips.

Is any test preparation needed to ensure the quality of the sample?

No test preparation is needed.

The Test

How is it used?

The urinalysis is used as a screening and/or diagnostic tool because it can help detect substances or cellular material in the urine associated with different metabolic and kidney disorders. It is ordered widely and routinely to detect any abnormalities that should be followed up on. Often, substances such as protein or glucose will begin to appear in the urine before patients are aware that they may have a problem. It is used to detect urinary tract infections (UTI) and other disorders of the urinary tract. In patients with acute or chronic conditions, such as kidney disease, the urinalysis may be ordered at intervals as a rapid method to help monitor organ function, status, and response to treatment.

When is it ordered?

A routine urinalysis may be done when you are admitted to the hospital. It may also be part of a wellness exam, a new pregnancy evaluation, or a work-up for a planned surgery. A urinalysis will most likely be performed if you see your health care provider complaining of abdominal pain, back pain, painful or frequent urination, or blood in the urine, symptoms of a UTI. This test can also be useful in monitoring whether a condition is getting better or worse.

What does the test result mean?

NOTE: A standard reference range is not available for this test. Because reference values are dependent on many factors, including patient age, gender, sample population, and test method, numeric test results have different meanings in different labs. Your lab report should include the specific reference range for your test. Lab Tests Online strongly recommends that you discuss your test results with your doctor.

Urinalysis results can have many interpretations. They are a red flag, a warning that something may be wrong and should be evaluated further. Generally, the greater the concentration of the abnormal substance (such as greatly increased amounts of glucose, protein, or red blood cells), the more likely it will be that there is a problem that needs to be addressed. But the results do not tell the doctor exactly what the cause of the finding is or whether it is a temporary or chronic condition. A normal urinalysis also does not guarantee that there is no illness. Some people will not release elevated amounts of a substance early in a disease process and some will release them sporadically during the day (which means they may be missed by a single urine sample). In very dilute urine, small quantities of chemicals may be undetectable.

Is there anything else I should know?

The urinalysis is a set of screening tests that can provide a general overview of a person's health. Your doctor must correlate the urinalysis results with your health complaints and clinical findings and search for the causes of abnormal findings with other targeted tests (such as a comprehensive metabolic panel (CMP), complete blood count (CBC), or urine culture (to look for a urinary tract infection).

Common Questions

How long does it take to get results for urinalysis?

This depends on the laboratory and the equipment used. Usually, once the specimen is in the laboratory, the test takes approximately 30 minutes or less to complete.

Is the time of day a factor when collecting a urine sample?

Because this is a general screening test, time is usually not important, although a first morning void is usually preferred. However, if your doctor is looking for a specific finding, he may ask that you collect a sample at a specific time. For example, if he is looking for the excretion of glucose, it's better to collect a specimen after a meal. If he is looking for low levels of protein, it's better to collect a concentrated specimen, such as a first morning specimen.

Are there home test kits available?

Kits to perform a urinalysis are not available because the test requires special equipment and technical skills. However, some commercial testing strips can be purchased at a pharmacy to perform part of the chemical examination, such as urine pH, urine glucose, and urine ketones.

Chapter 22

Stool Tests

Chapter Contents

243

Section 22.1

Fecal Occult Blood Test

The fecal occult blood test is one of a variety of colorectal cancer screening tests. When doctors test for fecal occult blood, they are testing for the presence of microscopic or invisible blood in the stool, or feces. Fecal occult blood can be a sign of a problem in your digestive system, such as a growth, or polyp, or cancer in the colon or rectum. If microscopic blood is detected, it is important for your doctor to determine the source of bleeding to properly diagnose and treat the problem.

What causes blood to appear in stool?

Blood may appear in the stool because of one or more of the following conditions:

- Benign (non-cancerous) or malignant (cancerous) growths or polyps of the colon
- Hemorrhoids (swollen blood vessels near the anus and lower rectum that can rupture, causing bleeding)
- Anal fissures (splits or cracks in the lining of the anal opening)
- Intestinal infections that cause inflammation
- Ulcers
- Ulcerative colitis
- Crohn disease
- Diverticular disease, caused by outpouchings of the colon wall
- Abnormalities of the blood vessels in the large intestine

Gastrointestinal bleeding may be microscopic (occult blood), or may be easily seen as red blood, or black tar-like bowel movements, called melena.

How do I take a fecal occult blood test?

The fecal occult blood test requires the collection of three stool samples. The stool samples should be taken one day apart, because colon cancers may bleed from time to time, rather than consistently.

You can purchase fecal occult blood test kits at the pharmacy to perform the test at home, or your doctor may give you the home test during one of your appointments. These tests provide specific instructions, and most offer a toll-free number to call if you have questions.

The stool samples are collected in a clean container and evaluated by detecting color changes on a test card or by sending the samples, in a special container and envelope, directly to the doctor's office for analysis. Your doctor may examine the samples with a microscope or with chemical tests.

How should I prepare for a fecal occult blood test?

The test results are largely affected by how you prepare for the test, so it is important to follow the instructions carefully.

Do not perform the test if you have:

- Diarrhea
- Colitis
- Constipation
- Diverticulitis
- Ulcers
- Severe throat irritation
- Hemorrhoid flare-ups
- Your period

Because certain foods can alter the test results, a special diet is often recommended for 48 to 72 hours before the test.

The following foods should not be eaten 48 to 72 hours before taking the test:

- Beets
- Broccoli
- Cantaloupe
- Carrots
- Cauliflower
- Cucumbers
- Fish
- Grapefruit
- Horseradish
- Mushrooms
- Poultry
- Radishes

- Red meat (especially meat that is cooked rare)
- Turnips
- Vitamin C-enriched foods or beverages

Your doctor will go over your medicines with you before the test, since you may need to stop taking certain medicines 48 hours before the test.

How often do I need to do this test?

To allow for the early detection and prevention of colorectal cancer, the fecal occult blood test is recommended yearly for everyone starting at age 50.

What do the test results mean?

A positive fecal occult blood test means that blood has been found in the stool. Your doctor will have to determine the source of the bleeding, either by doing a colonoscopy (an examination of the entire colon) or by doing an upper endoscopy (an examination to determine if the bleeding is coming from the stomach or small intestine).

A negative test result means that no blood was found in the stool sample during the testing period. You should continue to follow your doctor's recommendations for regular cancer screening.

Section 22.2

Fecal Culture

Definition: A fecal culture is a laboratory test to isolate and identify organisms in the feces that may cause gastrointestinal symptoms and disease. Normally, many organisms are present in the feces, but some can act as pathogens (disease-causing organisms).

Some bacteria cause symptoms directly and others cause symptoms through toxins they produce.

How the test is performed: For adults and children, there are many ways to collect the samples. You can catch the stool on plastic wrap that is loosely placed over the toilet bowl and held in place by the toilet seat. Then, put the sample in a clean container. One test kit supplies a special toilet tissue that you use to collect the sample, then put the sample in a clean container.

For infants and young children in diapers, line the diaper with plastic wrap. If the plastic wrap is positioned properly, isolating the stool from any urine output, mixing of urine and stool can be prevented for a better sample.

A sample of the specimen is placed in culture media to encourage the growth of microorganisms. The culture is observed for growth at regular intervals in the laboratory. When growth is observed, the organisms are identified. Further tests to determine sensitivity of the organisms to antimicrobial therapy may also be carried out.

How to prepare for the test: A collection container will be provided for the stool specimen. Return the sample to the laboratory as soon as possible. The specimen should not include toilet tissue or urine.

How the test will feel: There is no discomfort.

Why the test is performed: The test is performed when gastrointestinal distress is present and an infection is suspected as a cause of the distress. It may be performed if severe, persistent, or recurrent diarrhea of unknown cause is present.

It may also be performed when long-term antibiotic therapy has been used, to see if bacteria that don't usually live in the intestine such as *Clostridium difficile* are now in the intestine.

Normal results: Normal fecal organisms are present.

What abnormal results mean: Abnormal results may indicate an intestinal infection.

Risks: There are no risks.

Considerations: Often other stool tests such as gram stain of stool, stool ova and parasites exam, and fecal smear are done in addition to the culture.

Section 22.3

Stool Clostridium Difficile

"Stool C. Difficile Toxin,"
© 2008 A.D.A.M., Inc. Reprinted with permission.

Definition: The stool *C. difficile* toxin test detects harmful substances produced by the bacteria *Clostridium difficile* (*C. difficile*) in a stool sample. This bacteria is a common cause of diarrhea after antibiotic use.

How the test is performed: A sample of a stool is submitted for laboratory analysis. There are several laboratory methods used to detect *C. difficile* toxin in the stool specimen.

Today, an enzyme immunoassay (EIA) is most often used to detect substances produced by the bacteria. The EIA is faster that previous culture tests, simpler to perform, and results are available in about an hour. However, it is slightly less sensitive than previous methods. Several stool samples may be needed to obtain an accurate result.

How to prepare for the test: There are many ways to collect the samples. You can catch the stool on plastic wrap that is loosely placed over the toilet bowl and held in place by the toilet seat. Then put the sample in a clean container. One test kit supplies a special toilet tissue that you use to collect the sample. After collecting the sample, you put it in a clean container.

Do not mix urine, water, or toilet tissue with the sample.

For children wearing diapers, you can line the diaper with plastic wrap. If the plastic wrap is positioned properly, mixing of urine and stool can be prevented for a better sample.

How the test will feel: There is no discomfort.

Why the test is performed: The test may be done when your doctor suspects that diarrhea is the result of recent antibiotic use. Antibiotics alter the bacterial flora in the colon ("helpful bacteria"), and this sometimes results in excessive growth of *C. difficile* and its toxins. Diarrhea caused by *C. difficile* following antibiotic use occurs frequently in hospitalized patients.

Normal results: No *C. difficile* toxin is detected. (Note: Normal value ranges may vary slightly among different laboratories. Talk to your doctor about the meaning of your specific test results.)

What abnormal results mean: Abnormal results mean that *C. difficile* toxins are likely present in the stool and are causing diarrhea.

Risks: There are no risks associated with testing for *C. difficile* toxin.

Considerations: Since the test for *C. difficile* toxin is not 100% sensitive, several stool samples may be needed to detect it.

Section 22.4

Stool Ova and Parasites

"Stool Ova and Parasites Exam,"
© 2008 A.D.A.M., Inc. Reprinted with permission.

Definition: Stool ova and parasites exam is an analysis of stool to check for the presence of a parasite or worm-like infection of the intestine. Ova refers to the egg stage of a parasite's life cycle. Some parasites are single-cell organisms such as amoeba, Giardia, and trichomonas, while others have a worm-like appearance.

How the test is performed: For adults and children, there are many ways to collect the samples. You can catch the stool on plastic wrap that is loosely placed over the toilet bowl and held in place by the toilet seat. Then, put the sample in a clean container. One test kit supplies a special toilet tissue that you use to collect the sample, then put the sample in a clean container.

For infants and young children in diapers, line the diaper with plastic wrap. If the plastic wrap is positioned properly, isolating the stool from any urine output, mixing of urine and stool can be prevented for a better sample.

A small smear of stool is placed on a microscope slide and examined.

How to prepare for the test: You will be given a specimen container for the stool sample. Do not mix urine or toilet tissue in with the stool specimen.

How the test will feel: There is no discomfort.

Why the test is performed: The test is performed if a parasitic infestation is suspected, for prolonged diarrhea of unknown cause, or other intestinal symptoms.

Normal results: The presence of normal bacteria and other microorganism in the stool is normal.

What abnormal results mean: Parasites or eggs are present in the stool indicating parasitic infestation.

Risks: There are no risks.

Chapter 23

Genetic Testing

Chapter Contents

Section 23.1

What You Should Know about Genetic Testing

Excerpted from "Genetic Testing," *Genetics Home
Reference: Your Guide to Understanding Genetic Conditions*,
National Library of Medicine, January 2008.

What is genetic testing?

Genetic testing is a type of medical test that identifies changes in
chromosomes, genes, or proteins. Most of the time, testing is used to
find changes that are associated with inherited disorders. The results
of a genetic test can confirm or rule out a suspected genetic condition
or help determine a person's chance of developing or passing on a
genetic disorder. Several hundred genetic tests are currently in use,
and more are being developed.

Genetic testing is voluntary. Because testing has both benefits and
limitations, the decision about whether to be tested is a personal and
complex one. A genetic counselor can help by providing information
about the pros and cons of the test and discussing the social and emotional aspects of testing.

What are the types of genetic tests?

Genetic testing can provide information about a person's genes and
chromosomes. Available types of testing include the following:

Newborn screening: Newborn screening is used just after birth to
identify genetic disorders that can be treated early in life. Millions of
babies are tested each year in the United States. All states currently test
infants for phenylketonuria (a genetic disorder that causes mental retardation if left untreated) and congenital hypothyroidism (a disorder
of the thyroid gland). Most states also test for other genetic disorders.

Diagnostic testing: Diagnostic testing is used to identify or rule
out a specific genetic or chromosomal condition. In many cases, genetic
testing is used to confirm a diagnosis when a particular condition is
suspected based on physical signs and symptoms. Diagnostic testing

can be performed before birth or at any time during a person's life, but is not available for all genes or all genetic conditions. The results of a diagnostic test can influence a person's choices about health care and the management of the disorder.

Carrier testing: Carrier testing is used to identify people who carry one copy of a gene mutation that, when present in two copies, causes a genetic disorder. This type of testing is offered to individuals who have a family history of a genetic disorder and to people in certain ethnic groups with an increased risk of specific genetic conditions. If both parents are tested, the test can provide information about a couple's risk of having a child with a genetic condition.

Prenatal testing: Prenatal testing is used to detect changes in a fetus's genes or chromosomes before birth. This type of testing is offered during pregnancy if there is an increased risk that the baby will have a genetic or chromosomal disorder. In some cases, prenatal testing can lessen a couple's uncertainty or help them make decisions about a pregnancy. It cannot identify all possible inherited disorders and birth defects, however.

Preimplantation testing: Preimplantation testing, also called preimplantation genetic diagnosis (PGD), is a specialized technique that can reduce the risk of having a child with a particular genetic or chromosomal disorder. It is used to detect genetic changes in embryos that were created using assisted reproductive techniques such as in-vitro fertilization. In-vitro fertilization involves removing egg cells from a woman's ovaries and fertilizing them with sperm cells outside the body. To perform preimplantation testing, a small number of cells are taken from these embryos and tested for certain genetic changes. Only embryos without these changes are implanted in the uterus to initiate a pregnancy.

Predictive and presymptomatic testing: Predictive and presymptomatic types of testing are used to detect gene mutations associated with disorders that appear after birth, often later in life. These tests can be helpful to people who have a family member with a genetic disorder, but who have no features of the disorder themselves at the time of testing. Predictive testing can identify mutations that increase a person's risk of developing disorders with a genetic basis, such as certain types of cancer. Presymptomatic testing can determine whether a person will develop a genetic disorder, such as hemochromatosis (an iron overload disorder), before any signs or symptoms appear. The results of predictive and presymptomatic testing can provide information about a person's risk of developing a specific disorder and help with making decisions about medical care.

Forensic testing: Forensic testing uses DNA sequences to identify an individual for legal purposes. Unlike the tests described above, forensic testing is not used to detect gene mutations associated with disease. This type of testing can identify crime or catastrophe victims, rule out or implicate a crime suspect, or establish biological relationships between people (for example, paternity).

How is genetic testing done?

Once a person decides to proceed with genetic testing, a medical geneticist, primary care doctor, specialist, or nurse practitioner can order the test. Genetic testing is often done as part of a genetic consultation.

Genetic tests are performed on a sample of blood, hair, skin, amniotic fluid (the fluid that surrounds a fetus during pregnancy), or other tissue. For example, a procedure called a buccal smear uses a small brush or cotton swab to collect a sample of cells from the inside surface of the cheek. The sample is sent to a laboratory where technicians look for specific changes in chromosomes, DNA, or proteins, depending on the suspected disorder. The laboratory reports the test results in writing to a person's doctor or genetic counselor.

Newborn screening tests are done on a small blood sample, which is taken by pricking the baby's heel. Unlike other types of genetic testing, a parent will usually only receive the result if it is positive. If the test result is positive, additional testing is needed to determine whether the baby has a genetic disorder.

Before a person has a genetic test, it is important that he or she understands the testing procedure, the benefits and limitations of the test, and the possible consequences of the test results. The process of educating a person about the test and obtaining permission is called informed consent.

What is direct-to-consumer genetic testing?

Traditionally, genetic tests have been available only through healthcare providers such as physicians, nurse practitioners, and genetic counselors. Healthcare providers order the appropriate test from a laboratory, collect and send the samples, and interpret the test results. Direct-to-consumer genetic testing refers to genetic tests that are marketed directly to consumers via television, print advertisements, or the internet. This form of testing, which is also known as at-home genetic testing, provides access to a person's genetic information without necessarily involving a doctor or insurance company in the process.

If a consumer chooses to purchase a genetic test directly, the test kit is mailed to the consumer instead of being ordered through a doctor's office. The test typically involves collecting a DNA sample at home, often by swabbing the inside of the cheek, and mailing the sample back to the laboratory. In some cases, the person must visit a health clinic to have blood drawn. Consumers are notified of their results by mail or over the telephone, or the results are posted online. In some cases, a genetic counselor or other healthcare provider is available to explain the results and answer questions. The price for this type of at-home genetic testing ranges from several hundred dollars to more than a thousand dollars.

The growing market for direct-to-consumer genetic testing may promote awareness of genetic diseases, allow consumers to take a more proactive role in their health care, and offer a means for people to learn about their ancestral origins. At-home genetic tests, however, have significant risks and limitations. Consumers are vulnerable to being misled by the results of unproven or invalid tests. Without guidance from a healthcare provider, they may make important decisions about treatment or prevention based on inaccurate, incomplete, or misunderstood information about their health. Consumers may also experience an invasion of genetic privacy if testing companies use their genetic information in an unauthorized way.

Genetic testing provides only one piece of information about a person's health—other genetic and environmental factors, lifestyle choices, and family medical history also affect a person's risk of developing many disorders. These factors are discussed during a consultation with a doctor or genetic counselor, but in many cases are not addressed by at-home genetic tests. More research is needed to fully understand the benefits and limitations of direct-to-consumer genetic testing.

What do the results of genetic tests mean?

The results of genetic tests are not always straightforward, which often makes them challenging to interpret and explain. Therefore, it is important for patients and their families to ask questions about the potential meaning of genetic test results both before and after the test is performed. When interpreting test results, healthcare professionals consider a person's medical history, family history, and the type of genetic test that was done.

A positive test result means that the laboratory found a change in a particular gene, chromosome, or protein of interest. Depending on the purpose of the test, this result may confirm a diagnosis, indicate that a person is a carrier of a particular genetic mutation, identify an increased risk of developing a disease (such as cancer) in the future, or suggest a need for further testing. Because family members have some genetic material in common, a positive test result may also have implications for certain blood relatives of the person undergoing testing. It is important to note that a positive result of a predictive or presymptomatic genetic test usually cannot establish the exact risk of developing a disorder. Also, health professionals typically cannot use a positive test result to predict the course or severity of a condition.

A negative test result means that the laboratory did not find a change in the gene, chromosome, or protein under consideration. This result can indicate that a person is not affected by a particular disorder, is not a carrier of a specific genetic mutation, or does not have an increased risk of developing a certain disease. It is possible, however, that the test missed a disease-causing genetic alteration because many tests cannot detect all genetic changes that can cause a particular disorder. Further testing may be required to confirm a negative result.

In some cases, a negative result might not give any useful information. This type of result is called uninformative, indeterminate, inconclusive, or ambiguous. Uninformative test results sometimes occur because everyone has common, natural variations in their DNA, called polymorphisms, which do not affect health. If a genetic test finds a change in DNA that has not been associated with a disorder in other people, it can be difficult to tell whether it is a natural polymorphism or a disease-causing mutation. An uninformative result cannot confirm or rule out a specific diagnosis, and it cannot indicate whether a person has an increased risk of developing a disorder. In some cases, testing other affected and unaffected family members can help clarify this type of result.

What is the cost of genetic testing, and how long does it take to get the results?

The cost of genetic testing can range from under $100 to more than $2,000, depending on the nature and complexity of the test. The cost increases if more than one test is necessary or if multiple family members must be tested to obtain a meaningful result. For newborn screening, costs vary by state. Some states cover part of the total cost, but most charge a fee of $15 to $60 per infant.

From the date that a sample is taken, it may take a few weeks to several months to receive the test results. Results for prenatal testing are usually available more quickly because time is an important consideration in making decisions about a pregnancy. The doctor or genetic counselor who orders a particular test can provide specific information about the cost and time frame associated with that test.

Will health insurance cover the costs of genetic testing?

In many cases, health insurance plans will cover the costs of genetic testing when it is recommended by a person's doctor. Health insurance providers have different policies about which tests are covered, however. A person interested in submitting the costs of testing may wish to contact his or her insurance company beforehand to ask about coverage.

Some people may choose not to use their insurance to pay for testing because the results of a genetic test can affect a person's health insurance coverage. Instead, they may opt to pay out-of-pocket for the test. People considering genetic testing may want to find out more about their state's privacy protection laws before they ask their insurance company to cover the costs.

What are the benefits of genetic testing?

Genetic testing has potential benefits whether the results are positive or negative for a gene mutation. Test results can provide a sense of relief from uncertainty and help people make informed decisions about managing their health care. For example, a negative result can eliminate the need for unnecessary checkups and screening tests in some cases. A positive result can direct a person toward available prevention, monitoring, and treatment options. Some test results can also help people make decisions about having children. Newborn screening can identify genetic disorders early in life so treatment can be started as early as possible.

What are the risks and limitations of genetic testing?

The physical risks associated with most genetic tests are very small, particularly for those tests that require only a blood sample or buccal smear (a procedure that samples cells from the inside surface of the cheek). The procedures used for prenatal testing carry a small but real risk of losing the pregnancy (miscarriage) because they require a sample of amniotic fluid or tissue from around the fetus.

Many of the risks associated with genetic testing involve the emotional, social, or financial consequences of the test results. People may feel angry, depressed, anxious, or guilty about their results. In some cases, genetic testing creates tension within a family because the results can reveal information about other family members in addition to the person who is tested. The possibility of genetic discrimination in employment or insurance is also a concern.

Genetic testing can provide only limited information about an inherited condition. The test often can't determine if a person will show symptoms of a disorder, how severe the symptoms will be, or whether the disorder will progress over time. Another major limitation is the lack of treatment strategies for many genetic disorders once they are diagnosed.

A genetics professional can explain in detail the benefits, risks, and limitations of a particular test. It is important that any person who is considering genetic testing understand and weigh these factors before making a decision.

What is genetic discrimination?

Genetic discrimination occurs when people are treated differently by their employer or insurance company because they have a gene mutation that causes or increases the risk of an inherited disorder. People who undergo genetic testing may be at risk for genetic discrimination.

The results of a genetic test are normally included in a person's medical records. When a person applies for life, disability, or health insurance, the insurance company may ask to look at these records before making a decision about coverage. An employer may also have the right to look at an employee's medical records. As a result, genetic test results could affect a person's insurance coverage or employment. People making decisions about genetic testing should be aware that when test results are placed in their medical records, the results might not be kept private.

Fear of discrimination is a common concern among people considering genetic testing. Several laws at the federal and state levels help protect people against genetic discrimination; however, genetic testing is a fast-growing field and these laws don't cover every situation.

How does genetic testing in a research setting differ from clinical genetic testing?

The main differences between clinical genetic testing and research testing are the purpose of the test and who receives the results. The goals of research testing include finding unknown genes, learning how genes work, and advancing our understanding of genetic conditions. The results of testing done as part of a research study are usually not available to patients or their healthcare providers. Clinical testing, on the other hand, is done to find out about an inherited disorder in an individual patient or family. People receive the results of a clinical test and can use them to help them make decisions about medical care or reproductive issues.

It is important for people considering genetic testing to know whether the test is available on a clinical or research basis. Clinical and research testing both involve a process of informed consent in which patients learn about the testing procedure, the risks and benefits of the test, and the potential consequences of testing.

Section 23.2

Points to Consider about Genetic Services

GeneTests: Medical Genetics Information Resource (database online). Educational Materials: About Genetic Services. Copyright © University of Washington, Seattle. 1993-2008. Available at http://www.genetests.org. Accessed January 2, 2008.

Clinically applicable genetic tests may be used for:

- diagnostic testing,
- predictive testing,
- carrier testing,
- prenatal testing,
- preimplantation testing, or
- newborn screening.

Research tests generally do not give clinically applicable results. Research testing is discussed further in the next section.

Diagnostic testing: Diagnostic testing is used to confirm or rule out a known or suspected genetic disorder in a symptomatic individual. Points to consider:

- DNA testing may yield diagnostic information at a lower cost and with less risk than other procedures.

- Diagnostic testing is appropriate in symptomatic individuals of any age.

- Confirming a diagnosis may alter medical management for the individual.

- Diagnostic testing of an individual may have reproductive or psychosocial implications for other family members as well.

- Establishing a diagnosis may require more than one type of genetic test.

- DNA testing may not always be the best way to establish a clinical diagnosis.

Predictive testing: Predictive testing is offered to asymptomatic individuals with a family history of a genetic disorder. Predictive testing is of two types: presymptomatic (eventual development of symptoms is certain when the gene mutation is present, for example, Huntington disease) and predispositional (eventual development of symptoms is likely but not certain when the gene mutation is present, for example, breast cancer). Points to consider:

- Predictive testing is medically indicated if early diagnosis allows interventions which reduce morbidity or mortality.

- Even in the absence of medical indications, predictive testing can influence life planning decisions.

- Because predictive testing can have psychological ramifications, careful patient assessment, counseling, and follow-up are important.

- Many laboratories will not proceed with predictive testing without proof of informed consent and genetic counseling.

- Identification of the specific gene mutation in an affected relative or establishment of linkage within the family should precede predictive testing.

- Predictive testing of asymptomatic children at risk for adult onset disorders is strongly discouraged when no medical intervention is available (American College of Medical Genetics, ACMG, Policy Statement).

Carrier testing: Carrier testing is performed to identify individuals who have a gene mutation for a disorder inherited in an autosomal recessive or X-linked recessive manner. Carriers usually do not themselves have symptoms related to the gene mutation. Carrier testing is offered to individuals who have family members with a genetic condition, family members of an identified carrier, and individuals in ethnic or racial groups known to have a higher carrier rate for a particular condition. Points to consider:

- Identifying carriers allows reproductive choices.

- Genetic counseling and education should accompany carrier testing because of the potential for personal and social concerns.

- Molecular genetic testing of an affected family member may be required to determine the disease-causing mutation(s) present in the family.

- In some situations, DNA testing may not be the primary way of determining carrier status.

- Carrier testing can improve risk assessment for members of racial and ethnic groups more likely to be carriers for certain genetic conditions.

Prenatal testing: Prenatal testing is performed during a pregnancy to assess the health status of a fetus. Prenatal diagnostic tests are offered when there is an increased risk of having a child with a genetic condition due to maternal age, family history, ethnicity, or suggestive multiple marker screen or fetal ultrasound examination. Routine prenatal diagnostic test procedures are amniocentesis and chorionic villus sampling (CVS). More specialized procedures include placental biopsy, periumbilical blood sampling (PUBS), and fetoscopy with fetal skin biopsy. Points to consider:

- A laboratory that performs the disease-specific test of interest must be identified before any prenatal diagnostic test procedure is offered.

- All prenatal diagnostic test procedures have an associated risk to the fetus and the pregnancy; therefore, informed consent is required, most often in conjunction with genetic counseling.

- In most cases, before prenatal diagnosis using molecular genetic testing can be offered, specific gene mutation(s) must be identified in an affected relative or carrier parent(s).

- Prenatal testing for adult-onset conditions is controversial. Individuals seeking prenatal diagnosis for these conditions should be referred to a professional trained in genetic counseling for a complete discussion of the issues (ACMG Policy Statement).

Preimplantation testing (preimplantation genetic diagnosis): Preimplantation testing is performed on early embryos resulting from in vitro fertilization in order to decrease the chance of a particular genetic condition occurring in the fetus. It is generally offered to couples with a high chance of having a child with a serious disorder. Preimplantation testing provides an alternative to prenatal diagnosis and termination of affected pregnancies. Points to consider:

- Preimplantation testing is only performed at a few centers and is only available for a limited number of disorders.

- Preimplantation testing is not possible in some cases due to difficulty in obtaining eggs or early embryos and problems with DNA analysis procedures.

- Due to possible errors in preimplantation diagnosis, traditional prenatal diagnostic methods are recommended to monitor these pregnancies.

- The cost of preimplantation testing is very high and is usually not covered by insurance.

Newborn screening: Newborn screening identifies individuals who have an increased chance of having a specific genetic disorder so that treatment can be started as soon as possible. Points to consider:

- Newborn screening programs are usually legally mandated and vary from state to state.

- Newborn screening is performed routinely at birth, unless specifically refused by the parents in writing.

- Screening tests are not designed to be diagnostic, but to identify individuals who may be candidates for further diagnostic tests.

- Many parents do not realize that newborn screening has been done (or which tests were included), even if they signed a consent form when their child was born.

- Education is necessary with positive screening results in order to avoid misunderstandings, anxiety, and discrimination.

Section 23.3

Points to Consider when Ordering Genetic Testing

GeneTests: Medical Genetics Information Resource (database online). Educational Materials: Ordering Genetic Testing. Copyright © University of Washington, Seattle. 1993-2008. Available at http://www.genetests.org. Accessed January 2, 2008.

Genetic tests may be ordered by a medical geneticist or genetic counselor as part of a genetic consultation, or they may be ordered by a primary or specialty care provider. Considerations when ordering a genetic test include the following:

- Choosing a laboratory
- Pretest counseling and informed consent
- Sample logistics and supporting documentation
- Test result interpretation and follow-up

Choosing a Laboratory

GeneTests (www.genetests.org) was created to simplify the search for genetic testing laboratories, which may be difficult to locate. For many diseases, there may be only one laboratory providing genetic testing. U.S. patents have been issued covering diagnostic testing for some genetic disorders. A given laboratory may or may not be the exclusive licensee to such a patent. If there is a choice of laboratories, the following factors should be considered:

Laboratory personnel: Genetics laboratory personnel have two major roles: processing patient samples (technologists), and interfacing with referring clinicians regarding their patients (clinical consultants).

Lab personnel, who are usually certified in their specialty, may include lab directors, supervisors, technologists, and genetic counselors.

Compatibility: The test offered by the laboratory must match the specific clinical need.

- Clinical testing gives a result which can be used in patient care; research testing usually does not. If only research testing is available, the patient or family may choose to defer testing until a clinical test is available.

- The test methodology must be suited to the testing purpose (for example, Prader-Willi syndrome can be diagnosed with methylation testing, but other tests are required for recurrence risk counseling).

- Some diseases are caused by mutations in more than one gene. It is important to be sure that the lab selected is testing the appropriate gene(s).

- Different kinds of DNA tests are available. The laboratory selected should offer what is most appropriate for a specific clinical situation. For instance:

  - A specific gene mutation (for example, if the familial mutation has been identified)

  - A panel of mutations (for example, the Ashkenazi Jewish BRCA1 panel of three mutations)

  - The complete gene sequence

Reliability: Direct contact with the laboratory is needed to assess the laboratory's experience and qualifications.

- Does the laboratory have any other certification? (Laboratories with clinical listings in GeneTests have Clinical Laboratory Improvement Amendments, CLIA, certification.)

- Is the laboratory associated with a reputable company or university?

- Is the laboratory director board-certified?

- Is the laboratory's work published in the medical literature?

- What is the laboratory's experience with the specific test being ordered?

Ease of communication:

- What professionals are on staff to help assess the appropriateness of testing, determine the best testing paradigm for the family, and interpret test results?

- Does the laboratory have information on tests offered and logistics of sample collection and shipping easily available by phone, fax, or internet?

- What information is contained in the test result report (for example, raw data, interpretation, references, sensitivity, and specificity information)?

Geographical location:

- Some states have restrictions on insurance coverage or, as is the case in New York, additional regulatory restrictions.

- Samples shipped outside of the U.S. must go through Customs, which requires that hazard identification and a statement of value accompany the sample. Language barriers and time zones can also be an issue.

Turn-around time: Time from sample receipt to test result report may vary.

- Clinical laboratories generally have similar turn-around times for tests performed using the same methodology.

- A shorter turn-around time is advantageous only when it can be determined that quality control and thoroughness are not compromised.

- Test results for pregnancy management (prenatal diagnosis) are considered urgent due to restrictions on options late in pregnancy. Pregnancy dating should be included with all prenatal samples.

- The laboratory should be notified in advance of any sample that is "stat" (rush), as the sample processing may be different.

Cost: May vary from less than $100 to more than $2000 based on several factors.

- Test methodology. Low complexity tests (for example, single gene mutation) are less expensive than high complexity tests (for example, full gene sequencing).

- Laboratory testing strategy. Some labs test for a large number of mutations all at once; other labs test in stepwise fashion, beginning with the most common mutations.

- Number of individuals tested. Several family members may need to be tested to obtain a meaningful test result.

- Contractural agreements. Hospitals, insurers, and laboratories negotiate contracts to set the price of testing and amount of reimbursement.

- Specimen handling. Some cell types require culturing or other special handling before testing.

- Additional services. Genetic consultation or counseling is usually recommended and sometimes required before genetic testing is performed. These fees should be considered in the total cost.

Pretest Counseling and Informed Consent

If genetic testing is clinically available and useful for a particular patient, the patient needs to understand why it is being offered and its implications for medical management and psychosocial well-being. If a competent patient (or parent/guardian) agrees to the proposed genetic test after full disclosure, this constitutes informed consent. Informed consent may be verbal or written. Some laboratories require written documentation of informed consent.

Pretest counseling includes:

- assessing the patient's risk perception, expectations and support systems.

- explaining the implications of testing vs. not testing for medical management and reproductive options.

- describing the methods used to obtain specimens and associated risks.

- reviewing test accuracy (sensitivity and specificity).

- estimating the chance that the test will be positive based on available information (for example, family history, clinical symptoms).

- discussing any out-of-pocket costs to the patient.

- establishing a plan for conveying test results. Depending on the circumstances, results may be given:

- in person,
- by phone, with or without a follow-up appointment,
- by mail (negative results only), or
- only when positive (for example, newborn screening).

Results should be revealed only to the individual tested, or his/her parent or guardian, unless explicit permission has been granted to share results.

Additional issues relevant in some testing situations:

- Need to clarify biological relationships (parentage, zygosity) for linkage studies.
- Potential discrimination in employment, insurability or educational opportunities, especially in predictive testing. (Some states have State Genetics Laws in place prohibiting genetic discrimination).
- Results from research testing are not generally available for patient care.

Sample Logistics and Supporting Documentation

Contact the lab directly to ask the following questions:

What are the sample requirements?

- Are samples from other family members needed?
- What specimen type is needed?
- Does the specimen need to be cultured before shipping?
- What is the requested amount of specimen? Will less be accepted in hard-to-draw situations?
- What information should be included on the label?

What supporting documentation is needed?

- Does the lab have a specific requisition form?
- What clinical history should be included?
- Are medical records or test results on family members needed?
- Is family history needed for test interpretation? A pedigree is an efficient way to show family relationships.

- Is ethnicity relevant to test interpretation?
- If crossing international borders, are hazard labels and customs paperwork included?

How should the sample be transported?

- What is the correct delivery address?
- When is delivery accepted?
- Should the sample be frozen, refrigerated or at room temperature during shipping?
- Is there a courier to the lab, or is there a taxicab, mail, or overnight shipping required?

Table 23.1. For Positive Test Results

If the test purpose was...	The interpretation is...	And follow-up includes genetic counseling[1] and...
Diagnostic testing	Clinical diagnosis is confirmed	Medical management and treatment
Predictive testing	The likelihood of showing disease symptoms is increased	Counseling for life planning; Medical management if available
Carrier testing	The patient is a carrier	Testing offered to partner; Prenatal testing offered if indicated
Prenatal testing	A fetus is diagnosed with a specific condition	Pregnancy treatment/management or termination
Newborn screening	Disease in a newborn is suggested;	Confirmatory testing; if positive, medical management and treatment
	Carrier status in a newborn may be identified	Carrier testing offered to parents

1. Genetic Counseling includes discussion of expected course of the disorder; possible interventions; underlying cause; risks to family members; reproductive options; support.

Test Result Interpretation and Follow-Up

Test results are provided in writing by the laboratory to the referring clinician. The details of the lab report vary by lab, but may include:

- raw data;
- clinical interpretation of test result;
- sensitivity and specificity information; and
- references.

The clinician explains the meaning of the test result to the patient and to other family members as needed. Test results and follow-up

Table 23.2. For Negative Test Results

If the test purpose was...	The interpretation is...	And follow-up may include...
Diagnostic testing	Clinical symptoms are unexplained	Further testing and/or follow-up genetic consultation
Predictive testing	The likelihood of showing symptoms is decreased	Counseling for survivor guilt and long-range life planning; No high-risk surveillance needed
Carrier testing	High likelihood that the individual is not a carrier; Low risk of having a child affected with the condition in question	Testing offered to other family members if indicated
Prenatal testing	If fetus was symptomatic (for example, by ultrasound findings), clinical symptoms remain unexplained and may need further investigation. If fetus was not symptomatic, the chance of the condition tested for is very small.	If fetus was symptomatic, further testing and/or pregnancy management. If fetus was not symptomatic, no follow-up.
Newborn screening	The newborn is not expected to have the condition tested for	No follow-up

should be documented in the medical record and a copy made available to the patient. For many conditions, educational materials may be available from patient support organizations.

Parent support and information:

- The Genetic Alliance (www.geneticalliance.org)
- Family Village (www.familyvillage.wisc.org)
- Family Voices (www.familyvoices.org)
- Kansas University Medical Center (www.kumc.edu/gec/support)
- March of Dimes (www.modimes.org)

Section 23.4

Genetic Testing for Breast and Ovarian Cancer Risk

National Cancer Institute (www.cancer.gov), September 2005.

Breast cancer is the second most common form of cancer and the second leading cause of cancer deaths for American women. Each year, more than 210,000 women in the United States learn that they have breast cancer.

Some kinds of cancer, such as breast and ovarian cancer, seem to run in families. There is a test that may tell some people if they are at risk for breast, ovarian, and other cancers. Before getting tested, though, there are many factors you should consider.

This section will give you an overview of testing for breast and ovarian cancer risk. This information may also apply to risk of other cancers. It describes the advantages and disadvantages of this kind of testing. It also gives basic medical terms to help as you talk with your doctor or other health care professionals trained in genetics.

Who is at higher risk of breast and ovarian cancer?

A woman with a significant family history of breast and/or ovarian cancer has a higher risk of getting these cancers. You have a significant family history if:

- you have two or more close family members who have had breast and/or ovarian cancer, and/or
- the breast cancer in the family members has been found before the age of 50.

Talk with your doctor or other health care professional trained in genetics about your family history. He or she can help you know if you have a significant family history of breast and/or ovarian cancer. This information may help you learn about your cancer risk and help you decide if genetic testing is right for you.

About family history: A close family member can be your mother, father, sister, brother, grandparent (on your mother's or father's side), mother's sister and/or brother, or father's sister and/or brother.

Having a family history of cancer does not mean you are going to get cancer. Many things, such as family history and age, may increase a person's chance (or risk) of getting cancer. But family history alone is not the only reason people get cancer. Scientists do not know all the reasons why people get cancer.

How do genes affect breast and ovarian cancer risk?

Genes are nature's blueprints for every living thing. Most genes come in pairs: one set of genes is passed down (or inherited) from your mother and the other set from your father. Genes determine how your body will function and grow, as well as the color of your hair and eyes.

Sometimes genes do not function properly because there is a mistake in them. If a gene has a mistake, it is said to be mutated or altered. When a gene with a mistake is passed along in family members, it is called an inherited altered gene. All people have altered forms of some genes. Certain altered genes can increase your risk of illnesses such as cancer. Gene alterations have been found in many families with a history of breast cancer. Some women in these families have also had ovarian cancer.

These alterations are most often found in genes named BRCA1 and BRCA2 (Breast Cancer Gene 1 and Breast Cancer Gene 2). Both men and women have BRCA1 and BRCA2 genes, so alterations in these genes can be passed down from either the mother or the father. More genes like these may be discovered in the future.

Does every woman with an inherited altered BRCA gene get cancer?

A woman with a BRCA1 or BRCA2 alteration is at higher risk for developing breast, ovarian, and other cancers than a woman without an alteration. However, not every woman who has an altered BRCA1 or BRCA2 gene will get cancer, because genes are not the only factor that affects cancer risk.

Most cases of breast cancer do not involve altered genes that are inherited. At most, about one in 10 breast cancer cases can be explained by inherited alterations in BRCA1 and 2 genes.

What about men with an inherited altered BRCA gene?

Although breast cancer in men is rare, men with altered BRCA1 and BRCA2 genes have higher rates of breast cancer than men without an altered gene. Men with an altered BRCA1 or 2 gene may also have a slightly higher risk of other cancers. Even if a man never develops cancer, he can pass the altered gene to his sons and daughters.

What is genetic testing for inherited cancer risk?

Genetic testing is a process that looks for inherited genetic alterations that may increase your risk of certain cancers. This type of testing may show whether the risk in a family is passed through their genes.

Although the lab test itself is quite complex, only a blood sample is needed. For breast and ovarian cancer risk, the testing involves looking for altered genes such as BRCA1 and BRCA2. Finding an altered gene can take several weeks. So your test results may not be ready right away.

The price of testing varies and, in some cases, may not be covered by health insurance. Ask your doctor or other health professionals for more information on genetic testing, privacy issues, and insurance coverage.

What should I think about before getting tested?

- The limits of the test
- The advantages and disadvantages of the test
- Would knowing this information cause me to make changes in my medical care?

What are the limits of the test?

Testing for breast and ovarian cancer risk will not give you a simple "yes" or "no" answer. If a gene alteration is found, this will tell that you have an increased risk of getting cancer, but it will not tell if or when cancer will develop. If an alteration is not found, it still is no guarantee that cancer won't develop.

What are the advantages and disadvantages of testing?

Genetic testing can affect relationships with family members. Think about who in your family might want to know your test results, and who you'd like to tell.

If you are thinking about being tested, you should decide what the advantages and disadvantages of testing are for you. What is right for one person is not always right for another.

Having a genetic test may help you achieve these advantages:

- Make medical and lifestyle choices
- Clarify your cancer risk
- Decide whether or not to have risk-reducing surgery
- Give other family members useful information (if you choose to share your results)
- May explain why you or other family members have developed cancer

The disadvantages to testing include the following:

- There is no guarantee that your test results will remain private
- Although rare, you may face discrimination for health, life, disability, and other insurance
- You may find it harder to cope with your cancer risk when you know your test results
- If you find that you do not have an inherited altered gene, you may think that you have no chance of getting cancer. People who are found not to have an inherited cancer gene can still get cancer.

What is informed consent?

If you are thinking about genetic testing, you should be informed, both verbally and in writing, about the risks of getting tested, as well as what the test can and cannot tell you. You can decide if testing is or is not right for you. You may also choose to delay the decision if this is not the best time for you to be tested.

What can I do if I find out that I have an inherited altered gene?

You can make choices that help lower your risk of getting cancer or help find cancer early. You do not need to be tested to consider these options.

- **Increased monitoring:** You may choose to be watched more closely for any sign of cancer. This can include more frequent breast and pelvic exams, mammograms, breast MRI, breast self-exams, ultrasound of the ovaries and breasts, and blood tests.

- **Risk-reducing surgery:** Called prophylactic surgery, this is when women choose to have healthy ovaries and/or breasts removed to reduce their chance of getting cancer. You may want to talk with your doctor and other health care professionals to learn more about this.

Who can I call?

A person who is considering genetic testing should talk with a professional trained in genetics before deciding whether to be tested. For more information on genetic testing or for a referral to centers that have health care professionals trained in genetics, call the National Cancer Institute's Cancer Information Service toll-free at 800-4-CANCER (800-422-6237), or visit online at http://www.cancer.gov. The Cancer Information Service can also provide information about clinical trials, other research studies, and current risk management information.

What are the main questions I should ask?

If you are thinking about genetic testing, be sure to talk with your doctor, nurse, genetic counselor, or other health professionals, and take some time to answer these questions together. You may want to get more than one opinion.

- What are the chances that an inherited gene alteration is involved in the cancer in me or my family?

- What are my chances of having an inherited altered gene?

- Besides having altered genes, what are my other risk factors for breast and ovarian cancer?

- Are all genetic tests the same? How much does the test cost? How long will it take to get my results?

- What are the possible results of the test?

- What would a positive result mean for me?

- What would a negative result mean for me?

- How might a positive test result affect my health, life, and disability insurance options?

- How might a positive test result affect my employment?

- Do I want to ask my insurance company to pay for my test?

- Where will my test results be placed/recorded? Who will have access to them?

- Would knowing this information cause me to make changes in my medical care?

- What are my reasons for wanting to be tested?

- What type of cancer screening is recommended if I don't get tested?

Other questions to think about and discuss with your family:

- What effect will the test results have on me and my relationship with my family members if I have an inherited altered gene? If I don't have an altered gene?

- Should I share my test results with my spouse or partner? Parents? Children? Friends? Others? How will they react to the news, which may also affect them?

- Are my children ready to learn new information that may one day affect their own health?

Section 23.5

Genetic Discrimination in Health Insurance

National Human Genome Research Institute (www.genome.gov), November 2007. Concluding information about the passage of the Genetic Information Nondiscrimination Act (GINA) in May 2008 was added by the editor.

What is the issue?

More than a decade of research on the human genome has yielded a wealth of information. Scientists have mapped and sequenced the genome, identified individual genes or sets of genes that are associated with diseases ranging from Alzheimer disease to diabetes and certain forms of cancer, and developed genetic tests to determine an individual's predisposition for some of these diseases. Developments and discoveries like these—and others likely to come in the years ahead—offer hope that many deadly illnesses can be diagnosed, treated and perhaps even cured both earlier and with better results than is now possible.

By learning more about their genetic makeup and susceptibility to certain diseases, people now have more choices, and potentially more control, when dealing with their health and future. Genetic information may lead people to ask their physicians to screen them regularly for certain diseases, to take preventive measures earlier in life, or even to rethink their reproductive plans and choices.

But genetic information can also be misused. It can be used to discriminate against people in health insurance and employment. People known to carry a gene that increases their likelihood of developing cancer, for example, may get turned down for health insurance. Without health insurance, it may be impossible for some people to get treatment for a disease that could be fatal. This may lead some people to decide against genetic testing for fear of what the results might show, and who might find out about them. It also could lead some people to decline participation in biomedical research such as studies of gene mutations associated with certain diseases that examine the history of families prone to those maladies.

Each of us probably has half a dozen or more genetic mutations that place us at risk for some disease. That does not mean that we will develop the disease, only that we are more likely to get it than people who do not have the same genetic mutations we do. As our knowledge of the human genome increases, more and more people will likely be identified as carriers of mutations associated with a greater risk of certain diseases. That means that virtually all people are potential victims of genetic discrimination in health insurance.

What are the public concerns?

As a result, Americans have become concerned about the possible misuse of genetic information, especially in health insurance and employment. A *Time magazine*/Cable News Network (CNN) poll, published in June 2000, found that 75 percent of those surveyed would not want their insurance company to have information about their genetic code. A 1998 survey released by the National Center for Genome Resources (NCGR) found that 85 percent of those polled think employers should not have access to information about their employees' genetic conditions, risks, or predispositions.

People have reason to be concerned. Employer-sponsored health insurance plans in the private sector cover more than half of all Americans. Numerous reports in the news media and from expert groups have already uncovered instances where people were denied health insurance or coverage for particular conditions based on genetic information. In one case, a young boy, who had inherited an altered gene from his mother making him susceptible to a potentially fatal heart condition, was denied coverage by a health insurer when the boy's father lost his job and group coverage, and then tried to buy new insurance.

In 1993, the Ethical, Legal, and Social Implications (ELSI) Working Group of the Human Genome Project issued a report titled "Genetic Information and Health Insurance". The report recommended that people be eligible for health insurance no matter what is known about their past, present, or future health status. Two years later, the ELSI Working Group and the National Action Plan on Breast Cancer (NAPBC) jointly developed guidelines to assist federal and state agencies in preventing genetic discrimination in health insurance.

Further, the ELSI Working Group and NAPBC recommended that health insurers be prohibited from using genetic information or an individual's request for genetic services to deny or limit health insurance coverage, establish differential rates or have access to an individual's genetic information without that individual's written authorization. Written authorization, the groups said, should be required for each separate disclosure and should specify the recipient of the disclosed information.

Next, the National Human Genome Research Institute (NHGRI) and the United States Department of Energy, acting through the ELSI Working Group, cosponsored a series of workshops in the mid-1990s on genetic discrimination in health insurance and the workplace. The findings and recommendations of the workshop participants were published in *Science: (Genetic Information and the Workplace: Legislative Approaches and Policy Challenges* [sciencemag.org]) magazine, the monthly journal of the American Association for the Advancement of Science.

What are the legislative protections?

Those recommendations, and earlier ones issued by the ELSI Working Group and NAPBC led, in part, to new legislation and policies at both the federal and state levels. The Health Insurance Portability and Accountability Act (HIPAA) of 1996 provided the first federal protections against genetic discrimination in health insurance. The act prohibited health insurers from excluding individuals from group coverage due to past or present medical problems, including genetic predisposition to certain diseases. It limited exclusions from group plans for preexisting conditions to 12 months and prohibited such exclusions for people who had been covered previously for that condition for 12 months or more. And the law specifically stated that genetic information in the absence of a current diagnosis of illness did not constitute a preexisting condition.

On the other hand, HIPAA did not prohibit health insurers from charging a higher rate to individuals based on their genetic makeup, prevent insurers from collecting genetic information, or limit the disclosure of genetic information about individuals to insurers. Nor did it prevent insurers from requiring applicants to undergo genetic testing.

The next step in addressing the issue of genetic discrimination was taken by President Bill Clinton. The President had earlier supported proposed legislation that would have banned all health plans—group or individual—from denying coverage or raising premiums on the basis of genetic information. When the legislation failed to pass Congress, President Clinton issued an executive order (Executive Order 13145 to Prohibit Discrimination in Federal Employment Based on

Genetic Information) in February 2000 prohibiting agencies of the federal government from obtaining genetic information about their employees or job applicants and from using genetic information in hiring and promotion decisions. In announcing the order, President Clinton said, "We must not allow advances in genetics to become the basis of discrimination against any individual or any group. We must never allow these discoveries to change the basic belief upon which our government, our society, and our system of ethics is founded—that all of us are created equal, entitled to equal treatment under the law."

Both before and since that Executive Order, a number of bills were introduced into Congress to further deal with genetic discrimination in health insurance and employment. Nine bills were introduced in the 106th Congress (1999–2001) and four in the 107th Congress (2001–03). In 2005, the Senate passed S.306, but the comparable house bill, H.R.1227 did not reach a vote. Meanwhile, 41 states have enacted legislation related to genetic discrimination in health insurance and 31 states have adopted laws regarding genetic discrimination in the workplace. The state laws regarding health insurance conform to HIPAA.

On April 25, 2007, the Genetic Information Nondiscrimination Act (GINA) of 2007, H.R. 493 [thomas.loc.gov], was passed in the U.S. House of Representatives, by a vote of 420-3.

The Senate approved a version of GINA in April 2008; it was subsequently approved by the House on May 1, 2008 and signed into law on May 21, 2008.

Part Four

Imaging Tests

Chapter 24

Radiography (X-Rays)

Chapter Contents

Section 24.1

What You Should Know about X-Rays

Who's Taking Your X-Ray?

More than 300 million medical imaging procedures are performed in the United States each year. Some are as familiar as dental x-rays and others are as complex as magnetic resonance brain images. Chances are, if you've had a chest x-ray, an annual mammogram or a CT scan, a radiologic technologist performed your examination.

Radiologic technologists use knowledge of physics, radiation protection, human anatomy, and a mastery of highly technical equipment to create medical images. They work closely with radiologists, who are physicians trained to interpret the images. Medical imaging examinations often are the first tool doctors use to diagnose illness so that treatment can begin.

Certified technologists are known as registered technologists and can use the credentials R.T. after their names. Radiologic technologists may specialize in a wide range of areas. Technologists show that they are competent to perform these examinations by passing additional certification tests. These radiologic technologists have additional credentials after the R.T.

Why It Matters That a Qualified R.T. Performs Your Exam

The one thing medical imaging procedures have in common is that they must be accurate and precise. An image is only as good as the person who takes it; a treatment is only as effective as the individual who administers it. How can you be sure that your radiologic exam or procedure is being performed by a qualified, competent professional? Just ask.

When you meet the person who will perform your examination, ask if he or she is certified by a national agency or licensed by the state. In addition to asking about qualifications, you should ask questions about the procedure you're scheduled to receive. A competent radiologic technologist will be able to explain the procedure in detail, help you prepare for it and tell you what to expect.

Some Common Radiologic Exams and Procedure

Diagnostic x-ray (radiography): During a radiographic examination, x-rays pass through a patient's body and are recorded on film, video, or computer, producing anatomical images. Diagnosing pneumonia, assessing broken bones, or determining the cause of intestinal bleeding are just a few of the many uses of radiographs. Health professionals who perform these examinations are known as radiographers and have the credential (R) after R.T.

Mammography: Mammograms are low-dose x-ray examinations of the breast that can be used to detect a small breast tumor years before it can be felt. Mammographers are specially trained professionals whose certification is indicated by an (M).

Computed tomography: CT technologists use a rotating x-ray unit and computers to create cross-sectional images of patient anatomy. CT images are especially useful to diagnose diseases of the brain, abdomen and pelvis. Technologists who have passed the CT certification exam are identified by the credential (CT).

Magnetic resonance imaging: This imaging method uses strong magnetic fields, radiofrequency pulses, and computers to produce detailed, cross-sectional images of the body. Knee injuries, herniated disks, and rotator cuff tears are some of the conditions imaged using MR. Certification for magnetic resonance is indicated by (MR).

Cardiovascular-interventional technology: These procedures use radiologic imaging to guide catheters, balloons, stents, and other tools through the body to diagnose and treat disease without open surgery. For example, blocked arteries often are treated using interventional radiology. Technologists who assist interventional radiologists in these procedures have the additional credential (CV).

Nuclear medicine: Nuclear medicine technologists use trace amounts of radioactive materials to gather information about how organs function. Special equipment detects the gamma rays emitted by radiopharmaceuticals and creates images of the body part being studied. Nuclear medicine exams can be used to study illnesses such as thyroid disorders and heart disease. Technologists who have passed a nuclear medicine certification exam may use the credential (N) after R.T. or the designation certified nuclear medicine technologist (CNMT).

Shields and Safety

Have you ever wondered why the person taking your x-ray sometimes partially covers you with a heavy lead apron? And why that person leaves the room or steps behind a barrier before he or she takes your film? Perhaps not, but for the certified radiologic technologist who performs your diagnostic imaging examination, it's a matter of safety and quality patient care.

Natural and Artificial Radiation

Radiation is a frightening word to many people, but humans are exposed to different forms of radiation every day. Sources of radiation include cosmic rays from the sun, radioactive elements in the earth's crust, and even radioactive elements in our bodies. Natural sources contribute approximately 82% of the annual radiation dose to the U.S. public.

Medical uses of radiation, such as x-rays and nuclear medicine procedures, represent most of the exposure to artificial or man-made radiation. Each year, the average American is exposed to about three millisieverts (mSv) of naturally occurring background radiation from his or her environment. By comparison, a typical dental x-ray exposes a patient to approximately 0.06 mSv, a chest x-ray delivers 0.08 mSv and a mammogram delivers about 1.0 mSv.

Are X-Rays Safe?

X-rays are a form of ionizing radiation. When this type of radiation passes through living cells, ions are formed that react with other atoms in the cell, causing damage. With low doses of radiation, cells repair the damage quickly. Although we have no direct evidence that small doses of radiation are harmful, the medical community operates under the assumption that any exposure, no matter how small, carries some potential for biological damage.

Any potential risk associated with radiation exposure should be balanced against the potential benefits of the examination. For example, early detection of breast cancer far outweighs the very small risk associated with radiation exposure from a mammogram.

Radiation Protection

Radiation protection includes those practices and devices that limit exposure to ionizing radiation. Qualified radiologic technologists are educated in radiation safety and protection and use techniques to minimize dose and exposure. That's why it's important to ensure that your medical imaging examination is performed by a radiologic technologist who is nationally certified or licensed by the state. In addition, new techniques and equipment are continually being developed to decrease the total amount of radiation received by the patient.

Certain organs are radiosensitive, which means they are more sensitive to the effects of radiation exposure than other parts of the body. Those organs, including the thyroid gland and the male and female reproductive organs, usually are shielded when they are in the path of the x-ray beam. Shields commonly are made of lead strips or materials saturated with lead, which block the x-rays. Because a developing fetus also is radiosensitive, pregnant women should seek a physician's advice before undergoing an x-ray examination. If you must remain in the room with a child or other family member during an exam, ask about shielding for yourself.

Radiation protection extends to medical imaging professionals as well. Although the radiation dose for each examination is relatively small, the total dose to medical professionals can add up over time. Many state and federal regulations strictly limit the total dose that people working with radiation can receive. Before the radiologic technologist makes an exposure, he or she will move to a shielded control booth or behind a protective barrier. Lead aprons protect technologists who must remain in the examination room with the patient.

If you have questions or concerns about radiation safety, ask a certified radiologic technologist.

Pregnancy and X-Ray Safety

Are you pregnant or is there a chance that you might be pregnant? This may seem like a personal question, but if you are a woman of child-bearing age, it's one of the things the radiologic technologist will ask before performing an x-ray examination. Radiologic technologists are skilled medical professionals who have received specialized education in the areas of radiation protection, patient care and radiation safety. Their job is to produce the best quality diagnostic image while minimizing your exposure to the x-rays. This is of particular concern if you are pregnant or if you might be pregnant.

Why Is This Question Important?

Because the cells of the developing baby are rapidly dividing and growing into specialized organs and tissue, the unborn child is more sensitive to the effects of radiation exposure than an adult. The same is true for other things such as alcohol, certain drugs, and infection.

Many x-ray examinations, such as imaging the arms, legs, head, and chest, don't involve exposing your reproductive organs or unborn baby to the direct x-ray beam. In these cases, lead shielding can be used to block any scattered radiation.

X-ray examinations of your abdominal area, such as the stomach, lower back, pelvis, and kidneys, are more of a concern because they expose the developing fetus to the direct x-ray beam.

Scientists disagree about the exact amount of risk to the unborn child from the radiation used in x-ray examinations, but it's believed to be small. Yet, even small risks should not be taken if they're unnecessary.

The benefits of diagnostic x-ray exams often outweigh the risks. In some cases, the risk of not having the information provided by the exam may be greater than the risk from the radiation.

Protecting Yourself and Your Unborn Child

Once you let the radiologic technologist know whether you are pregnant or you might be pregnant, several different things may happen. For example, if you have been trying to get pregnant or you have any symptoms of pregnancy such as nausea, vomiting, or breast tenderness, the exam may be delayed until a pregnancy test is performed. The technologist may ask you the date of your last regular menstrual period.

If you are pregnant and scheduled to have an examination that does not involve the abdominal area, the radiologic technologist will use lead shielding to protect your reproductive organs and the developing baby.

If you are pregnant and must have an abdominal-area x-ray exam, your procedure may be delayed while the radiologist consults with the physician who ordered the exam. Radiologists are physicians who specialize in the interpretation of medical images, and along with radiologic technologists, they make sure that the procedure is necessary and is performed properly.

Don't be alarmed if you had an x-ray examination before you knew you were pregnant. Remember that the risk is considered very small. However, if you are worried about the radiation exposure your baby may have received, you can discuss your concerns with your physician.

Sometimes a mother is asked to hold her child during an x-ray examination. If you are pregnant or if there is the possibility that you are pregnant, another person should take your place. Even if you are not pregnant, you should ask for a lead apron to protect your reproductive organs during the procedure.

Remember that radiologic technologists are committed to safety and quality patient care. If you have concerns about pregnancy and radiation safety, ask a radiologic technologist before your x-ray examination.

Section 24.2

Chest X-Rays

What is chest radiography?

Chest x-ray is the most commonly performed diagnostic x-ray examination. Approximately half of all x-rays obtained in medical institutions are chest x-rays. A chest x-ray is usually done for the evaluation of lungs, heart, and chest wall. Pneumonia, heart failure, emphysema, lung cancer, and other medical conditions can be diagnosed or suspected on a chest x-ray. Traditionally, chest x-rays have been taken prior to employment, prior to surgery, or during immigration. These "routine" chest x-rays are being reevaluated because of inadequate evidence for their usefulness, and many insurance companies no longer pay for these "routine" x-rays obtained in absence of specific signs, symptoms, or medical conditions.

What are some common uses of the procedure?

Chest x-ray is typically performed as the first imaging test for symptoms of shortness of breath, a bad or persistent cough, chest pain, chest injury, or fever. Individuals with known or suspected medical conditions such as congestive heart failure or cancer may have chest x-rays to follow their response to treatment, or to determine changes that would require a change in their medical management.

How should I prepare for the procedure?

This procedure requires no special preparation. Women should always inform their doctor or x-ray technologist if there is any possibility that they are pregnant.

What does the equipment look like?

The most common radiography equipment used for chest x-rays consists of a box-like apparatus containing the recording material such as film, against which the individual places their chest, and the apparatus containing the x-ray tube, usually positioned about six feet away. In some instances, the radiography equipment consists of a large, flat table with a drawer that holds an x-ray film cassette into which a film is placed. With this arrangement, the x-ray tube is suspended above the table.

How does the procedure work?

Radiography involves exposing a part of the body to a small dose of radiation to produce an image of the internal organs. When x-rays penetrate the body, they are absorbed in varying amounts by different parts of the anatomy. The ribs and spine, for example, absorb much of the radiation and appear white or light gray on the image. Lung tissue absorbs little radiation and appears dark on the image. Depending upon the type of image recording medium, chest x-rays can be maintained as hard copy film for filing, or more commonly, as filmless digital images that are archived electronically. Digital images can also be transferred for storage onto CD-ROM. Stored images may be used to compare with later images if illness develops. Indeed, historical comparison films are often very important in the decision process as to whether a finding is clinically important or not.

How is the procedure performed?

Patients must remove their clothing, including undergarments that may contain metal. Most medical centers will give the patient a loose-fitting gown to wear. Patients will also be asked to remove all metallic jewelry that may interfere with the x-rays. Normally, a frontal, or posteroanterior view is obtained, in which the patient stands with the chest pressed to the photographic plate, with hands on hips and elbows pushed in front in a somewhat exaggerated position. The technologist will ask the patient to be still and to take a deep breath and hold it. Breath-holding after a deep breath reduces the possibility of a blurred image, and also enhances the quality of the x-ray image, since abnormalities in air-filled lungs are easier to see than in deflated lungs. Next, the technologist walks into a cubicle or small room to activate the radiographic equipment, which sends a beam of x-rays from the x-ray source behind the patient, through the patient's chest, to the recording medium (film or digital cassette). Some newer equipment is designed to accommodate patients who cannot stand for chest x-rays.

The technologist may need to take additional views to properly see all parts of the chest, or may take a side view, or lateral view, of the chest. S/he will remove the exposed film and place a new, unexposed film in its place (or, with digital imaging, exchanges or refreshes the digital receptor). For a lateral view, the patient stands sideways to the photographic plate with arms elevated, and the process is repeated. Views from other angles may be obtained if the radiologist needs to evaluate additional areas of the chest. Finally, a chest x-ray may be repeated within days or months to evaluate for any changes. These repeated, sequential examinations are called serial chest x-rays.

When the chest x-rays are completed you will be asked to wait until the technologist checks the images for motion and makes sure that the entire chest is included. Ultimately, a radiologist will interpret the chest x-ray images using a lighted view box to review films or using a computer and monitor to review digital images.

What will I experience during the procedure?

This is a painless procedure. The primary discomfort may come from the coldness of the recording plate. Individuals with arthritis or injuries to the chest wall, shoulders, or arms may have discomfort trying to maintain position for the chest x-ray. In these circumstances, the technologist will assist you in finding a position that still ensures diagnostic image quality.

Who interprets the results and how do I get them?

A radiologist, who is a physician specifically trained to supervise and interpret radiology examinations, will analyze the images and send a signed report with his or her interpretation to your primary care physician or other health care provider, who will inform you of your test results. New communications technology also allows for confidential distribution of diagnostic reports and digital images over the internet at many facilities.

Section 24.3

Bone X-Rays

What is bone radiography?

Radiography, known to most people as x-ray, is the oldest and most frequently used form of medical imaging. For nearly a century, diagnostic images have been created by passing small, highly controlled amounts of radiation through the human body, capturing the resulting shadows and reflections on a photographic plate.

X-ray imaging is the fastest and easiest way for a physician to view and assess broken bones, cracked skulls, and injured backbones.

At least two films are taken of a bone, and often three films if the problem is around a joint (knee, elbow, or wrist). X-rays also play a key role in orthopedic surgery and the treatment of sports injuries. X-ray is useful in detecting more advanced forms of cancer in bones. Very early cancer findings require other methods.

Radiologists have developed alternative imaging methods that do not rely on radiation, such as ultrasound and magnetic resonance imaging (MRI). However, because x-ray was the first imaging modality, many people (and medical imaging professionals) continue to use the term "radiology" to include all types of imaging. Strictly speaking, though, radiology refers to the use of x-rays.

One century ago, Wilhelm Konrad Roentgen discovered the x-ray (called that because X meant they didn't know what it was) which began the use of energy to visualize medical problems in patients. X-rays themselves (a form of energy) are not visible with the eye. Another method or material must be used to convert the information to a visible or useable form. X-rays typically use film or TV screens to make the structures penetrated by x-rays visible.

X-rays are used in a variety of ways to make regular pictures, angiograms (study of blood vessels), or CT scans. Other forms of energy such as ultrasound magnetic waves, and isotopes are used to also make pictures.

What are some common uses of the procedure?

Probably the most common use of bone radiographs is to assist the physician in identifying and treating fractures. X-ray images of the skull, spine, joints, and extremities are performed every minute of every day in hospital emergency rooms, sports medicine centers, orthopedic clinics, and physician offices. Images of the injury can show even very fine hairline fractures or chips, while images produced after treatment ensure that a fracture has been properly aligned and stabilized for healing. Bone x-rays are an essential tool in orthopedic surgery, such as spinal repair, joint replacements, or fracture reductions. X-ray images can be used to diagnose and monitor the progression of degenerative diseases such as arthritis. They also play an important role in the detection and diagnosis of cancer, although usually computed tomography (CT) or MRI is better at defining the extent and the nature of a suspected cancer. On regular x-rays severe osteoporosis is visible, but bone density determination detects early loss of bone density. Bone density determination is usually done on special equipment.

How should I prepare for the procedure?

There is no special preparation required for most bone radiographs. Once you arrive, you may be asked to change into a gown before your examination. You will also be asked to remove jewelry, eyeglasses, and any metal objects that could obscure the images, since those show up on x-rays and may block the bones. Women should always inform their doctor or x-ray technologist if there is any possibility that they are pregnant.

What does the equipment look like?

Radiography equipment consists of a large, flat table with a drawer that holds an x-ray film cassette into which a film is placed. Suspended above the table is an apparatus that holds the x-ray tube which can be moved over the body to direct the x-ray.

How does the procedure work?

Radiography involves exposing a part of the body to a small dose of radiation to produce an image of the internal organs. When x-rays penetrate the body, they are absorbed in varying amounts by different part of the anatomy. Ribs, for example, will absorb much of the radiation and, therefore, appear white or light gray on the image. Soft tissue such as the liver or lungs will appear darker because it absorbs less radiation. Broken bones or malignancies in the bone can usually be detected with radiography.

The images may be placed on film or may be stored electronically on PACS (picture archiving and communication systems). Films are usually stored in a film jacket in the radiology department or in the doctor's office for approximately seven years (unless the patient is a child, then until age 21). Images may be digitally acquired or may be digitized from analog images and can be stored on PACS.

How is the procedure performed?

The technologist positions the patient on the examination table, places a flat holder (cassette) under the table in the area of the body to be imaged. Sandbags or pillows may help the patient hold the proper position. Then the technologist goes to a small adjacent room and asks the patient to hold very still without breathing for a few seconds. The radiographic equipment is activated, sending a beam of x-rays through the body to expose the film. The technologist then re-positions the patient for another view, and the process is repeated.

When the x-rays are completed you will be asked to wait until the technologist checks the images for adequate exposure and motion.

What will I experience during the procedure?

In most cases, x-ray imaging is painless and the only discomfort results from the coldness of the plate. Sometimes, to get a clear image of an injury such as a possible fracture, you may be asked to hold an uncomfortable position for a short time. Any movement could blur the image and make it necessary to repeat the procedure to get a useful, clear picture.

Who interprets the results and how do I get them?

A radiologist, who is a physician experienced in bone x-ray and other radiology examinations, will analyze the images and send a signed report with his or her interpretation to your primary care or referring physician, who will inform you on your test results.

Chapter 25

Contrast Radiography

Chapter Contents

Section 25.1

Contrast Agents

Although bones show up clearly on x-ray images, some other organs and tissues do not. Contrast agents, also known as contrast media, often are used during medical imaging examinations to highlight specific parts of the body and make them easier to see. Contrast agents can be used with many types of imaging examinations, including x-ray exams, computed tomography (CT) scans, and magnetic resonance imaging (MRI).

Contrast agents are administered in different ways: Some are given as a drink, others are injected or delivered through an intravenous line or an enema. After the examination, some contrast agents are harmlessly absorbed by the body; others are excreted through the urine or bowel movements. Contrast agents are not dyes; they do not permanently discolor internal organs. Instead, they temporarily change the way x-rays or other imaging tools interact with your body.

If the exam your physician requested for you requires a contrast agent, a radiologic technologist will explain how it is used before the exam begins. Radiologic technologists are skilled health professionals who have specialized education in the safe use of contrast agents as well as in radiation protection, radiographic positioning, and procedures. The technologist will answer any questions you have about the examination or the contrast agent.

Some contrast agents carry a small risk of allergic reaction, so it is important to tell the radiologic technologist who will perform your examination if you have any type of allergy. Also, if you notice any unusual or uncomfortable symptoms during the examination, be sure to tell the technologist. It is his or her job to make you as comfortable as possible while obtaining the best image possible.

One of the most commonly used contrast agents is barium sulfate. Barium blocks the passage of x-rays, so barium-filled organs stand out better on x-ray exams. For an examination of the esophagus or stomach, patients are asked to drink a mixture of barium sulfate and water, sometimes with vanilla or fruit flavoring added. This mixture usually is thick and white.

For an examination of the rectum or colon, barium is administered rectally through an enema tube. After the exam is finished, you can go to the bathroom and expel the barium. It is a good idea to increase your fluid intake after the exam to help remove the contrast from your body. Your bowel movements may be white for a few days.

Contrast agents containing iodine are used to image the gallbladder, urinary tract, blood vessels, spleen, liver, and bile duct. Iodine contrast agents are clear liquids and usually are injected. Patients who are allergic to iodine should not receive this type of contrast agent. Be sure to tell the technologist which medications you are taking and your current medical conditions before the exam begins. Some conditions and medications make the use of iodine contrast agents riskier.

You may notice side effects associated with the use of iodine-containing contrast agents. These include a feeling of warmth or flushing, a metallic taste in the mouth, light headedness, nausea, itching, and hives. Usually, these symptoms are mild and disappear quickly. However, it is a good idea to tell the radiologic technologist if you experience any of them. In extremely rare instances, these side effects can be serious. The technologist will monitor you carefully for signs of side effects.

Section 25.2

Angiograms

"Coronary Angiography,"
National Heart Lung and Blood Institute, March 2007.

What is coronary angiography?

Coronary angiography is a test that uses dye and special x-rays to show the inside of your coronary arteries. The coronary arteries supply blood and oxygen to your heart.

A material called plaque can build up on the inside walls of the coronary arteries and cause them to narrow. When this happens, it's called coronary artery disease (CAD). CAD can prevent enough blood from flowing to your heart and can lead to angina (chest discomfort or pain) and heart attack. Coronary angiography shows if you have CAD.

Most of the time, the coronary arteries can't be seen on an x-ray. During coronary angiography, a special dye is injected into the bloodstream to make the coronary arteries show up on an x-ray.

To deliver the dye to your coronary arteries, a procedure called cardiac catheterization is used. A long, thin, flexible tube called a catheter is put into a blood vessel in your arm, groin (upper thigh), or neck. The tube is then threaded into your coronary arteries, and the dye is injected into your bloodstream. Special x-rays are taken while the dye is flowing through the coronary arteries.

Cardiologists (doctors who specialize in heart problems) usually perform cardiac catheterizations in a hospital. You're awake during cardiac catheterization. The procedure usually causes little to no pain, although you may feel some soreness in the blood vessel where your doctor put the catheter.

Cardiac catheterization rarely causes serious complications.

Who needs coronary angiography?

Coronary angiography is a test for coronary artery disease (CAD). Your may need coronary angiography if you have signs or symptoms of CAD. These include the following:

- Angina: This is unexplained pain or pressure in your chest. This chest discomfort may only happen when you're active.

- Sudden cardiac arrest: This is when your heart suddenly and unexpectedly stops beating.

- Results from an EKG (electrocardiogram), exercise stress test, or other test that suggest you have heart disease.

You also may need coronary angiography on an emergency basis if you're having a heart attack. This test combined with a procedure called angioplasty can open the blocked artery causing the heart attack and prevent further damage to your heart.

Coronary angiography also can help your doctor decide how to treat CAD after a heart attack. This is especially true if the heart attack caused major damage to your heart, or if you're still having chest pain.

What should I expect before coronary angiography?

Before having coronary angiography, discuss the following with your doctor:

- The test and how to prepare for it

- Any medicines you're taking, and whether you should stop taking them before the test

- Whether you have diabetes, kidney disease, or other conditions that may require taking extra steps during or after the test to avoid complications

Your doctor will tell you exactly which procedures will be performed. For example, your doctor may recommend angioplasty if the angiography shows a blocked artery. You will have the opportunity to ask questions about the procedure, and you will be asked to provide written informed consent to have the procedures done.

It may not be safe to drive right after having cardiac catheterization. If your doctor says you can go home the same day as the test, you should arrange for a ride home from the hospital. You may have to stay overnight for this test.

What should I expect during coronary angiography?

During coronary angiography, you're kept on your back and awake. That way, you can follow your doctor's instructions during the test.

299

You'll be given medicine to help you relax. This medicine may make you sleepy.

Your doctor will numb the area where the small plastic tube (catheter) will enter the blood vessel through a small cut in the arm, groin (upper thigh), or neck. The doctor then threads the catheter through the vessel up to the opening of the coronary arteries. Special x-ray movies are taken of the catheter as it's moved up into the heart. The movies help your doctor see where to position the tip of the catheter.

Your doctor will put a special dye in the catheter when it reaches the correct spot. This dye will flow through your coronary arteries and make them show up on an x-ray. This x-ray is called an angiogram. If the angiogram reveals blocked arteries, your doctor may use angioplasty to restore blood flow to your heart.

After your doctor completes the angiography, or the angiography and angioplasty, he or she will remove the catheter from your body. The opening left in the blood vessel will then be closed up and bandaged. A small sandbag or other type of weight may be put on top of the bandage to apply pressure. This will help prevent major bleeding from the site.

What should I expect after coronary angiography?

After coronary angiography, you will be moved to a special care area, where you will rest and be monitored for several hours or overnight. During this time, your movement will be limited to avoid bleeding from the site where the catheter was inserted. While you recover in this area, nurses will check your heart rate and blood pressure regularly and see if there is any bleeding from the tube insertion site.

A small bruise may develop on your arm, groin (upper thigh), or neck at the site where the catheter was inserted. That area may feel sore or tender for about a week. Be sure to let your doctor know if you develop problems such as a constant or large amount of blood at the site that can't be stopped with a small bandage, or unusual pain, swelling, redness, or other signs of infection at or near the insertion site.

Talk to your doctor about whether you should avoid certain activities, such as heavy lifting, for a short time after the procedure.

What are the risks of coronary angiography?

Coronary angiography is a common medical test that rarely causes serious problems. But complications can include problems such as the following:

- Bleeding, infection, and pain in the arm, groin (upper thigh), or neck where the catheter was inserted

- Damage to blood vessels. This is a very rare complication caused by the catheter scraping or poking a hole in a blood vessel as it is threaded up to the heart.

- An allergic reaction to the dye used.

Other less common complications of the test include the following:

- An arrhythmia (irregular heartbeat), which often goes away on its own, but may need treatment if it persists;

- Damage to the kidneys caused by the dye used

- Blood clots that can trigger strokes, heart attacks, or other serious problems

- Low blood pressure

- A buildup of blood or fluid in the sac that surrounds the heart. This fluid can prevent the heart from beating properly

As with any procedure involving the heart, complications can sometimes, although rarely, be fatal. The risk of complications with coronary angiography is higher if you have diabetes or kidney disease, or if you're 75 years old or older. The risk for complications also is greater in women and in people having coronary angiography on an emergency basis.

Section 25.3

Intravenous Pyelograms

What is an intravenous pyelogram (IVP)?

An intravenous pyelogram (IVP) is an x-ray examination of the
kidneys, ureters, and urinary bladder. Most people are familiar with
x-ray images, which produce a still picture of the body's interior by
passing small, highly controlled amounts of radiation through the
body, and capturing the resulting shadows and reflections on film. An
IVP study uses a contrast material to enhance the x-ray images. The
contrast material is injected into the patient's system, and its progress
through the urinary tract is then recorded on a series of quickly captured images. The exam enables the radiologist to review the anatomy
and the function of the kidneys and urinary tract.

What are some common uses of the procedure?

A radiologist can use an IVP study to find the cause of a wide variety of disorders, including frequent urination, blood in the urine, or
pain in the side or lower back. The IVP exam can enable the radiologist to detect problems within your urinary tract resulting from kidney stones; enlarged prostate; internal injuries after an accident or
trauma; tumors in the kidney, ureters, or urinary bladder; and other
changes.

How should I prepare for the procedure?

You should tell your doctor about any allergies you have to foods
or medications, as well as any recent illnesses or other medical conditions. If you are diabetic, make sure your doctor is aware of your
condition and the medications you take. Women should always inform
their doctor or x-ray technologist if there is any possibility that they
are pregnant. Your doctor will give you detailed instructions on how
to prepare for your IVP study. You will likely be instructed not to eat

or drink after midnight the night before your exam. You may also be asked to take a mild laxative (in either pill or liquid form) the evening before the procedure. Follow your doctor's instructions. Once you arrive at the imaging center, you may be asked to change into a gown before your examination. You will also be asked to remove jewelry, eyeglasses, or any metal objects that could obscure the images. Underwear with metallic components should also be removed.

What does the equipment look like?

The equipment used for most IVP examinations consists of a large, flat table. Suspended above the table is an apparatus containing the x-ray tube. The apparatus moves on a jointed "arm" so that it can be properly positioned.

How does the procedure work?

Different tissues, such as bone, blood vessels, and muscles and other soft tissues, absorb x-ray radiation at different rates. When a special film plate is exposed to the absorbed x-rays, an image of the inside of the body is captured.

An IVP study requires the use of a contrast material to help tissues show more clearly on the x-ray film. As the contrast material moves into and through the kidneys, ureters, and urinary bladder, the technologist captures a series of images that track its progress. By reviewing these images, a radiologist can then assess abnormalities in the urinary system, as well as how quickly and efficiently the patient's system is able to handle waste.

How is the procedure performed?

Before introducing the contrast material, the radiologist or technologist will ask whether the patient has any allergies and whether the patient has a history of diabetes, asthma, a heart condition, kidney problems, or thyroid conditions. These conditions may indicate a higher risk of reaction to the contrast material, or potential problems eliminating the material from the patient's system after the exam. You may also be asked if you have had any prior surgery on the urinary system.

An IVP examination is usually done on an outpatient basis. The patient is positioned on the table, and a contrast material is injected, usually in a vein in the patient's arm. Images are taken both before and after the injection of the contrast material. As the contrast material is processed by the kidneys, a series of images is captured to determine the actual size of the kidneys and to show the collecting system as it begins to empty. Some kidneys don't empty at the same rate and delayed films from thirty minutes to three or four hours may be requested. However, a typical IVP study usually takes about an hour.

What will I experience during the procedure?

Aside from the minor sting from the injection of contrast material, an IVP causes no pain. When the contrast material is injected, some people report feeling a flush of heat and, sometimes, a metallic taste in the mouth. These common side effects usually disappear within a minute or two and are no cause for alarm. Some people experience a mild itching sensation. If it persists or is accompanied by hives, the itch can be treated easily with medication. In rare cases, a patient may become short of breath or experience swelling in the throat or other parts of the body. These can be indications of a more serious reaction to the contrast material that should be treated promptly, so tell the radiologist or technologist immediately if you experience these symptoms.

During the imaging process, you may be asked to turn from side to side and to hold several different positions, to enable the radiologist to capture views from several angles. Near the end of the exam, you may be asked to empty your bladder so that an additional film can be taken of your urinary bladder as it empties.

The contrast material used for IVP studies will not discolor your urine or cause any discomfort when you urinate. If you experience such symptoms after your IVP exam, they are likely to indicate some other problem. Let your doctor know right away.

Who interprets the results and how do I get them?

A radiologist, who is a physician experienced in IVP and other radiology examinations, will analyze the images and send a signed report with his or her interpretation to the patient's primary care physician. The patient receives IVP results from the referring physician who ordered the test results. New technology also allows for distribution of diagnostic reports and referral images over the internet at many facilities.

Section 25.4

Cystograms

A cystogram is an x-ray examination of the urinary bladder, which is located in the lower pelvic area. A cystogram can show the bladder's position and shape, and the exam often is used to diagnose a condition called reflux. Reflux occurs when urine in the bladder moves back up the ureters, the tubes that transport urine from the kidneys to the bladder. This condition can cause repeated urinary tract infections. A cystogram may be performed after a patient has experienced a pelvic injury to ensure that the bladder has not torn. Cystograms also are used to detect polyps or tumors in the bladder.

Patient Preparation

Before your examination, a radiographer will explain the procedure to you and answer any questions you might have. A radiographer, also known as a radiologic technologist, is a skilled medical professional who has specialized education in the areas of radiation protection, patient care and radiographic positioning and procedures.

If you are a woman of childbearing age, the radiographer will ask the date of your last menstrual period and if there is any possibility you are pregnant. Next, the radiographer will ask if you have any allergies. It is important to list all allergies to food and medicine, as well as to let the radiographer know if you have a history of hay fever or asthma. Some allergies may indicate a possible reaction to the contrast agent that will be used during the examination.

You will be asked to put on a hospital gown and then the radiographer will direct you to the restroom and ask you to completely empty your bladder.

During the Examination

You will be positioned on your back on the x-ray table, with your knees flexed. Your pubic area will be washed, and then the radiographer or a radiology nurse will gently insert a small, flexible catheter into your ure-thra, the duct from which you urinate. Skin tape may be used to hold the catheter to your inner thigh.

Next, a radiologist (a physician who specializes in the diagnostic interpretation of medical images) or an urologist (a physician who specializes in conditions of the urinary system) will slowly fill your bladder with a contrast agent. The contrast agent is a substance that helps make organs easier to see on radiographs and is administered through the catheter. You will feel pressure and fullness in your blad-der and will have an urge to urinate.

After your bladder is full, the physician will take radiographs us-ing fluoroscopy. A fluoroscope is an x-ray unit attached to a television screen. You will be asked to lie on your side or to turn slightly from side to side while the physician watches your bladder on the TV screen. The radiographer also may take a few additional x-ray images.

Following this portion of the exam, the catheter will be removed, and you will be allowed to use the restroom. In addition to being sticky, the contrast agent that you expel is clear and odorless, so it will not be visible to you. After you return to the x-ray room, an additional x-ray image will be taken. This final radiograph will show whether any contrast agent stays in your bladder following urination. Any remain-ing contrast will be expelled the next time you urinate.

Voiding Cystourethrogram

Voiding cystourethrograms follow the same routine as cystograms with one difference. Toward the end of the examination, when the urinary catheter is removed, you will be asked to urinate into a spe-cial urinal. Radiographs will be taken while you urinate. These im-ages will show the size and shape of the bladder when it is under stress caused by urination.

Post-Examination Information

Your radiographs will be reviewed by the radiologist, and your personal physician will receive a report of the findings. Your physi-cian then will advise you of the results and discuss what further pro-cedures, if any, are needed.

Section 25.5

Upper and Lower GI Series

"Upper GI Series," National Digestive Diseases Information
Clearinghouse (NDDIC), NIH Pub. No. 05-4335, November 2004; and
"Lower GI Series," NDDIC, NIH Pub. No. 05-4334, November 2004.

Upper GI Series

The upper gastrointestinal (GI) series uses x-rays to diagnose problems in the esophagus, stomach, and duodenum (first part of the small intestine). It may also be used to examine the small intestine. The upper GI series can show a blockage, abnormal growth, ulcer, or a problem with the way an organ is working.

During the procedure, you will drink barium, a thick, white, milkshake-like liquid. Barium coats the inside lining of the esophagus, stomach, and duodenum, and makes them show up more clearly on x-rays. The radiologist can also see ulcers, scar tissue, abnormal growths, hernias, or areas where something is blocking the normal path of food through the digestive system. Using a machine called a fluoroscope, the radiologist is also able to watch your digestive system work as the barium moves through it. This part of the procedure shows any problems in how the digestive system functions, for example, whether the muscles that control swallowing are working properly. As the barium moves into the small intestine, the radiologist can take x-rays of it as well.

An upper GI series takes one to two hours. X-rays of the small intestine may take three to five hours. It is not uncomfortable. The barium may cause constipation and white-colored stool for a few days after the procedure.

Preparation

Your stomach and small intestine must be empty for the procedure to be accurate, so the night before you will not be able to eat or drink anything after midnight. Your physician may give you other specific instructions.

Lower GI Series

A lower gastrointestinal (GI) series uses x-rays to diagnose problems in the large intestine, which includes the colon and rectum. The lower GI series may show problems like abnormal growths, ulcers, polyps, diverticula, and colon cancer.

Before taking x-rays of your colon and rectum, the radiologist will put a thick liquid called barium into your colon. This is why a lower GI series is sometimes called a barium enema. The barium coats the lining of the colon and rectum and makes these organs, and any signs of disease in them, show up more clearly on x-rays. It also helps the radiologist see the size and shape of the colon and rectum.

You may be uncomfortable during the lower GI series. The barium will cause fullness and pressure in your abdomen and will make you feel the urge to have a bowel movement. However, that rarely happens because the tube used to inject the barium has a balloon on the end of it that prevents the liquid from coming back out.

You may be asked to change positions while x-rays are taken. Different positions give different views of the colon. After the radiologist is finished taking x-rays, you will be able to go to the bathroom. The radiologist may also take an x-ray of the empty colon afterwards.

A lower GI series takes about one to two hours. The barium may cause constipation and make your stool turn gray or white for a few days after the procedure.

Preparation

Your colon must be empty for the procedure to be accurate. To prepare for the procedure you will have to restrict your diet for a few days beforehand. For example, you might be able to drink only liquids and eat only nonsugar, nondairy foods for two days before the procedure; only clear liquids the day before; and nothing after midnight the night before. A liquid diet means fat-free bouillon or broth, gelatin, strained fruit juice, water, plain coffee, plain tea, or diet soda. To make sure your colon is empty, you will be given a laxative or an enema before the procedure. Your physician may give you other special instructions.

Section 25.6

Barium Enemas

The barium enema examination demonstrates your large bowel (colon). This examination is performed when patients have a change in bowel habits, experience abdominal pain or rectal bleeding, or if your doctor suspects you may have diverticulitis or polyps.

Patient Preparation

For the barium enema examination to be successful, your intestines must be completely empty. Typically, you will be asked to follow a restricted diet for two days prior to the examination. This may include a soft diet or a liquid diet. You also will be required to take a laxative the evening before the examination, and you also may be asked not to eat or drink anything after midnight the night before the exam. Your doctor will give you specific instructions, which you should follow closely. Any residue in your lower digestive tract will show up on the x-rays and could be mistaken for an abnormality in the colon or rectum.

Before your examination, a radiographer will explain the procedure to you and answer any questions you might have. A radiographer, also known as a radiologic technologist, is a skilled medical professional who has received specialized education in the areas of anatomy, radiation protection, patient care, radiation exposure, radiographic positioning, and radiographic procedures. As part of his or her duties, the radiographer will determine the amount of radiation necessary to produce a diagnostically useful image.

Prior to performing your barium enema examination, the radiographer will give you a hospital gown to wear. This gown has no metal snaps on it, because metal can interfere with the accuracy of the image. It is important that everything underneath this gown be removed, including jewelry and underwear.

If you are a woman of childbearing age, the radiographer will ask if there is any possibility you are pregnant. Because this examination exposes the pelvic area to radiation, it is important that you tell the radiographer the date of your last menstrual period and whether there is a chance that you may be pregnant.

During the Examination

Inside the x-ray room, you will be asked to lie down on a tilting table attached to a fluoroscope, which is an x-ray unit combined with a television screen. The radiographer will take an x-ray of your abdomen to make sure that your intestines are clean. Next, the radiographer will insert a lubricated enema tip into your rectum. A radiologist will come into the room and begin the examination. Liquid barium will begin to flow through the enema tip, a little at a time. Barium is a special compound that allows radiographic visualization of the gastrointestinal tract. It coats the walls of your lower digestive tract, casting shadows that can be recorded on x-ray film. The radiologist will watch the television screen to observe the flow of barium, and films will be taken throughout the process.

As the barium is being delivered, the radiologist will ask you to turn from side to side. This allows the barium to coat the walls of your colon. If you feel uncomfortable or are not able to turn over, you should tell the radiographer or radiologist. Their goal is to make you as comfortable as possible and at the same time perform a successful examination.

After the barium has been administered, the radiographer will take a series of x-rays of your large intestine. You will be asked to hold your breath and remain still during the exposure. It also is important that you try to hold in the enema. Once the films are complete, the radiographer will show you to the toilet facilities so you can expel the barium. After you have expelled the barium, the radiographer may take another x-ray to assess whether any barium remains.

In some cases, the radiologist may introduce air along with the barium solution. This examination is called a high-density, double-contrast, or air-contrast barium enema examination. The air will be inserted through the same enema tip as the barium. During the procedure, you may experience cramping or a sensation of being bloated. It is important that you try not to expel the air or the barium. Because barium used in this procedure is thick, it clings to the walls of the colon rather than filling the colon itself. The air is used to expand the walls of the colon and allow the radiographer and radiologist to get more detailed images.

Once the examination is complete, the radiographer will process your x-ray films and determine whether they are technically acceptable. The films then will be given to a radiologist to interpret. Radiologists are physicians who specialize in the diagnostic interpretation of medical images.

Post-Examination Information

After your radiographs have been reviewed by a radiologist, your personal physician will receive a report of the findings. Your physician then will advise you of the results and discuss what further procedures, if any, are needed.

The barium will make your stools white for a few days. This is normal. If you experience constipation following the examination, tell your doctor. He or she may advise you to take a laxative. You also should increase your water consumption in the days following the examination.

The radiation that you are exposed to during this examination, like the radiation produced during any other x-ray procedure, passes through you immediately. You are not "radioactive," and it is not necessary to take any special precautions following your examination.

Please remember that the material presented here is for informational purposes only. If you have specific questions about a medical imaging procedure, contact your physician or the radiology department of the institution where your test will be performed.

Section 25.7

Hysterosalpingograms

What is a hysterosalpingogram (HSG)?

A hysterosalpingogram or HSG is an x-ray procedure performed to determine whether the fallopian tubes are open and to see if the shape of the uterine cavity is normal. An HSG is an outpatient procedure that takes less than one half-hour to perform. It is usually done after menses have ended, but before ovulation, to prevent interference with an early pregnancy.

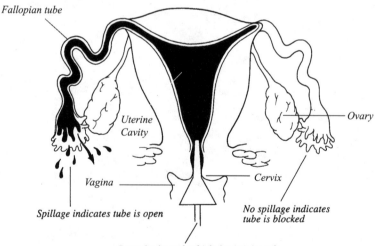

Fallopian tube

Uterine Cavity

Ovary

Vagina

Cervix

Spillage indicates tube is open

No spillage indicates tube is blocked

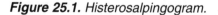

Cannula through which dye is injected

Figure 25.1. Histerosalpingogram.

How is a hysterosalpingogram done?

A patient is positioned under a fluoroscope (a real-time x-ray imager) on a table. The gynecologist or radiologist then examines her uterus and places a speculum in her vagina. Her cervix is cleaned, and a device (cannula) is placed into the opening of the cervix. The physician then gently fills the uterus with a liquid containing iodine (contrast) through the cannula. The contrast then enters the tubes, outlines the length of the tubes, and spills out their ends if they are open. Any abnormalities in the uterine cavity or fallopian tubes will be visible on a monitor. The HSG is not designed to evaluate the ovaries or diagnose endometriosis. Frequently, side views of the uterus and tubes are obtained by having the patient change her position on the table. After the HSG, a patient can immediately resume normal activities, although some physicians ask that the woman refrain from intercourse for a few days.

Is it uncomfortable?

An HSG usually causes mild or moderate uterine cramping for about five minutes; however, some women may experience cramps for several hours. The symptoms can be greatly reduced by taking medications used for menstrual cramps.

Does a hysterosalpingogram enhance fertility?

It is controversial whether this procedure enhances fertility. Some studies indicate a slight increase in fertility lasting about three months after a normal HSG. Most physicians perform the HSG only for diagnostic reasons.

What are the risks and complications of HSG?

An HSG is considered a very safe procedure. However, there is a set of recognized complications, some serious, which occur less than 1% of the time.

- **Infection:** The most common serious problem with HSG is pelvic infection. This usually occurs in the presence of previous tubal disease. In rare cases, infection can damage the fallopian tubes or necessitate their removal. A woman should call her doctor if she experiences increasing pain or a fever within one to two days of the HSG.

- **Fainting:** Rarely, the patient may get light-headed during or shortly after the procedure.

- **Radiation exposure:** Radiation exposure from a HSG is very low, less than a kidney or bowel study, and there have been no demonstrated ill effects from this radiation, even if conception occurs later the same month. The HSG should not be done if pregnancy is suspected.

- **Iodine allergy:** Rarely, a patient may have an allergy to the iodine contrast used in an HSG. A patient should inform her doctor if she is allergic to iodine, intravenous contrast dyes, or seafood. Patients who are allergic to iodine may have a sonohysterogram performed instead of HSG since that procedure uses non-iodine containing fluids. Sonohysterograms provide good detail concerning the uterine cavity, but limited information about the fallopian tubes. If a patient experiences a rash, itching, or swelling after the procedure, she should contact her doctor.

- **Spotting:** Spotting commonly occurs for one to two days after the HSG. Unless instructed otherwise, a patient should notify her doctor if she experiences heavy bleeding after the HSG.

Section 25.8

Arthrograms

An arthrogram is an exam of a joint using contrast material and x-rays to view the soft tissue and joint structures. This section will tell you about how the exam works, how to prepare for the exam, how the exam is performed, what to expect during the exam, and how to get your results.

What is an arthrogram?

An arthrogram is an x-ray exam of a joint after the injection of a dye-like contrast material and/or air to outline the soft tissue and joint structures on the pictures.

How does the exam work?

Joint fluid is removed and replaced with injected contrast material or air—sometimes both. A series of pictures are taken before the joint tissue absorbs the contrast material. Sometimes the radiologist will take more x-rays while pushing and pulling on your joint.

How should I prepare for the exam?

- No special steps are needed before an arthrogram.
- Food and fluid intake do not need to be restricted.
- A technologist may ask you to change into a gown.
- You may need to remove your jewelry if it will affect the exam.

How is the procedure performed?

1. In the x-ray exam room, you will be placed on a table.
2. Simple x-ray pictures of your joint are taken to compare with the arthrograms.

3. The skin around your joint is washed with antiseptic, and a local anesthetic may be injected into the area around the joint.

4. A needle is then placed into the joint space. The radiologist will use a syringe to drain the joint fluid, which may be sent to a lab for review.

5. The syringe is replaced with one containing contrast material. If the fluoroscopic exam shows correct needle placement, the contrast material and air are injected into the joint space.

6. After the injection, the needle is removed and the site is rubbed with a sterile sponge and may be sealed to prevent air from escaping.

7. You will be asked to move the joint to more evenly dispense the contrast material. Still pictures are then taken with the joint in a range of positions.

8. The exam usually takes 45 to 60 minutes.

What will I feel during the exam?

- After you are given an anesthetic to numb the area, you may not feel anything during the exam.

- At first, you may feel a slight pinprick and burning as the anesthesia is injected into the joint.

- You may also feel a fullness as the joint is filled, and you may feel and hear gurgling as the joint is moved.

Who interprets the results and how do I get them?

A radiologist trained to interpret arthrograms will review the pictures and send a report to your doctor, who will give you your test results.

The radiologist will not discuss the results with you. Based on the findings, you and your primary care doctor will decide the next step, such as treatment for a problem, as needed.

Section 25.9

Myelograms

Myelography is an x-ray examination of the structures within your
spinal column. The examination can show conditions such as spinal
tumors, spinal cord swelling, and herniated (slipped) disks.

Patient Preparation

Before the exam, a radiographer will explain the procedure and
answer any questions you might have. A radiographer, also known as
a radiologic technologist, is a skilled medical professional who has
received specialized education in radiation protection, patient care,
and radiographic positioning and procedures.

If you are a woman of childbearing age, the radiographer will ask
if you could be pregnant. It is important to tell the radiographer if
you have any allergies to food or medicine, or a history of hay fever
or asthma. Allergies may indicate a possible reaction to the contrast
agent that is used during the exam.

During the Examination

Before your spine can be imaged, a contrast agent is injected into
the space around your spinal cord. A contrast agent is a substance
that makes it easier to see parts of your body that are not normally
visible on a radiograph. A physician first injects a local anesthetic
to numb the area before inserting a spinal needle. This will sting
slightly.

You will be positioned in one of three ways:

- Lying on your side with knees pulled up to the chest and chest
curled forward.

- Lying face down on the table with large pillows under your
stomach.

317

- Sitting on the edge of the table, leaning forward, and grasping your ankles.

Each of these positions opens the spaces between your vertebrae to allow a needle to be inserted. Once the needle is in place, the physician removes a small amount of fluid from your spinal canal. It will be sent to a laboratory for analysis. The physician then slowly injects the contrast agent through the needle.

While the contrast is administered, a fluoroscope, which combines an x-ray unit with a television screen, is used to take images of your spine. As the contrast agent fills the space around your spinal cord, the radiographer and radiologist watch the TV screen to observe any problems or defects. The room lights will be dimmed so they can see the images more clearly.

After the contrast is administered, the needle is removed, and the radiographer positions you on the x-ray table, stomach down. A brace will be placed against your shoulders to support you as the table is tipped slowly. You will never be alone in the room, and the radiographer and radiologist will monitor you closely. If you experience any discomfort, tell them immediately.

As the table is tipped gently toward your head or feet, the radiologist will take images of your back. He or she may ask you to turn slightly onto one hip and then the other. You will be asked to hold your breath as the images are taken. Next, the radiographer will place a film cassette against the side of your abdomen and take a radiograph of your back.

Post-Examination Information

Once the exam is complete, the radiographer processes your x-ray films, determines if they are technically acceptable and decides whether additional images are needed. Follow-up films may be taken at this time. A radiologist will interpret the final films, and your personal physician will receive a report of the findings.

You may be asked to wait in the radiology department for about an hour so that caregivers can ensure that you recover fully. Before you leave, the radiographer will give you a set of instructions. It is important to follow these instructions to avoid a headache or other side effects. Any remaining contrast is absorbed by your body.

Chapter 26

Mammography

What is a screening mammogram?

A screening mammogram is an x-ray of the breast used to detect breast changes in women who have no signs or symptoms of breast cancer. It usually involves two x-rays of each breast. Mammograms make it possible to detect tumors that cannot be felt. Mammograms can also find microcalcifications (tiny deposits of calcium in the breast) that sometimes indicate the presence of breast cancer.

How are screening and diagnostic mammograms different?

A diagnostic mammogram is an x-ray of the breast that is used to check for breast cancer after a lump or other sign or symptom of breast cancer has been found. Signs of breast cancer may include pain, skin thickening, nipple discharge, or a change in breast size or shape. A diagnostic mammogram also may be used to evaluate changes found during a screening mammogram, or to view breast tissue when it is difficult to obtain a screening mammogram because of special circumstances, such as the presence of breast implants. A diagnostic mammogram takes longer than a screening mammogram because it involves more x-rays in order to obtain views of the breast from several angles. The technician may magnify a suspicious area to produce a detailed picture that can help the doctor make an accurate diagnosis.

Excerpted from "Screening Mammograms: Questions and Answers," National Cancer Institute (www.cancer.gov), September 2007.

When does the National Cancer Institute (NCI) recommend that women have screening mammograms?

- Women age 40 and older should have mammograms every one to two years.

- Women who are at higher than average risk of breast cancer should talk with their health care providers about whether to have mammograms before age 40 and how often to have them.

What are the factors that place a woman at increased risk of breast cancer?

The risk of breast cancer increases gradually as a woman gets older. However, the risk of developing breast cancer is not the same for all women. Research has shown that the following factors increase a woman's chance of developing this disease:

- **Personal history of breast cancer:** Women who have had breast cancer are more likely to develop a second breast cancer.

- **Family history:** A woman's chance of developing breast cancer increases if her mother, sister, and/or daughter have a history of breast cancer (especially if they were diagnosed before age 50).

- **Certain breast changes on biopsy:** A diagnosis of atypical hyperplasia (a noncancerous condition in which cells have abnormal features and are increased in number) or lobular carcinoma in situ (LCIS) (abnormal cells found in the lobules of the breast) increases a woman's risk of breast cancer. Women who have had two or more breast biopsies for other benign conditions also have an increased chance of developing breast cancer. This increased risk is due to the condition that led to the biopsy, and not to the biopsy itself.

- **Genetic alterations (changes):** Specific alterations in certain genes (BRCA1, BRCA2, and others) increase the risk of breast cancer. These alterations are rare; they are estimated to account for no more than 10 percent of all breast cancers.

- **Reproductive and menstrual history:** Women who began having periods before age 12 or went through menopause after age 55 are at an increased risk of developing breast cancer. Women who have their first child after age 30 or who never have a child are at an increased risk of developing breast cancer.

- **Long-term use of menopausal hormone therapy:** Women who use combination estrogen-progestin menopausal hormone therapy for more than five years have an increased chance of developing breast cancer.

- **Breast density:** Breasts appear dense on a mammogram if they contain many glands and ligaments (called dense tissue), and do not have much fatty tissue. Because breast cancers tend to develop in the dense tissue of the breast (not in the fatty tissue), those older women whose mammograms show more dense tissue are at an increased risk of breast cancer. Abnormalities in dense breasts can be more difficult to detect on a mammogram.

- **Radiation therapy ("x-ray therapy"):** Women who had radiation therapy to the chest (including the breasts) before age 30 are at an increased risk of developing breast cancer throughout their lives. This includes women treated for Hodgkin lymphoma. Studies show that the younger a woman was when she received her treatment, the higher her risk of developing breast cancer later in life.

- **DES (diethylstilbestrol):** The drug DES was given to some pregnant women in the United States between 1940 and 1971. (It is no longer given to pregnant women.) Women who took DES during pregnancy may have a slightly increased risk of breast cancer. The possible effects on their daughters are under study.

- **Body weight:** Studies have found that the chance of getting breast cancer after menopause is higher in women who are overweight or obese.

- **Physical activity level:** Women who are physically inactive throughout life may have an increased risk of breast cancer. Being active may help reduce risk by preventing weight gain and obesity.

- **Alcohol:** Studies suggest that the more alcohol a woman drinks, the greater her risk of breast cancer.

What is the best method of detecting breast cancer as early as possible?

Getting a high-quality mammogram and having a clinical breast exam (an exam done by a health care provider) on a regular basis are the most effective ways to detect breast cancer early. Like any test, mammograms have both benefits and limitations. For example, some cancers cannot be detected by a mammogram, but may be found by breast examination.

Checking one's own breasts for lumps or other unusual changes is called breast self-exam (BSE). Studies so far have not shown that BSE alone reduces the number of deaths from breast cancer. BSE should not take the place of routine clinical breast exams and mammograms.

What are the benefits of screening mammograms?

Several large studies conducted around the world show that breast cancer screening with mammograms reduces the number of deaths from breast cancer for women ages 40 to 69, especially those over age 50. Studies conducted to date have not shown a benefit from regular screening mammograms, or from a baseline screening mammogram (a mammogram used for comparison), in women under age 40.

What are some of the limitations of screening mammograms?

- Finding cancer does not always mean saving lives
- False negatives
- False positives

What is the Breast Imaging Reporting and Database System (BI-RADS®)?

The American College of Radiology (ACR) has established a uniform way for radiologists to report mammogram findings. The system, called BI-RADS, includes seven standardized categories, or levels. Each BI-RADS category has a follow-up plan associated with it to help radiologists and other physicians appropriately manage a patient's care (see Table 26.1).

Further information on BI-RADS is available on the ACR website at http://www.acr.org on the internet or by calling the ACR at 800-227-5463 (800-ACR-LINE).

What happens if mammography leads to the detection of ductal carcinoma in situ (DCIS)?

Over the past 30 years, improvements in mammography have made it possible to detect a higher number of tissue abnormalities called DCIS.

DCIS is abnormal cells that are confined to the milk ducts of the breast. The cells have not invaded the surrounding breast tissue. DCIS usually does not cause a lump, so it cannot be detected during a clinical breast exam or BSE. However, mammography is able to detect 80 percent of DCIS cases. Some of these cases later become invasive cancers.

It is not possible to predict which cases of DCIS will progress to invasive cancer. Therefore, DCIS usually is removed surgically. Until recently, DCIS was often treated with a mastectomy, but breast-conserving therapy (breast-sparing surgery plus radiation therapy) is now standard practice for many women with DCIS. Tamoxifen may also be used. Women who have been diagnosed with DCIS should talk with their doctor to make an informed decision about treatment.

How much does a mammogram cost?

Screening mammograms generally cost between $50 and $150. Most states now have laws requiring health insurance companies to reimburse all or part of the cost of screening mammograms. Insurance companies and health care providers can supply details.

All women age 40 and older with Medicare can get a screening mammogram each year. Medicare will also pay for one baseline mammogram

Table 26.1. Breast Imaging Reporting and Database System (BI-RADS)

Category	Assessment	Follow-up
0	Need additional imaging evaluation	Additional imaging needed before a category can be assigned
1	Negative	Continue annual screening mammography (for women over age 40)
2	Benign (noncancerous) finding	Continue annual screening mammography (for women over age 40)
3	Probably benign	Receive a 6-month follow-up mammogram
4	Suspicious abnormality	May require biopsy
5	Highly suggestive of malignancy (cancer)	Requires biopsy
6	Known biopsy—proven malignancy (cancer)	Biopsy confirms presence of cancer before treatment begins

for a woman between the ages of 35 and 39. There is no deductible requirement for this benefit, but Medicare beneficiaries have to pay 20 percent of the Medicare-approved amount. Information about Medicare coverage is available at http://www.medicare.gov on the internet, or through the Medicare Hotline at 800-633-4227 (800-MEDICARE). For the hearing impaired, the telephone number is 877-486-2048.

Some state and local health programs and employers provide mammograms free or at low cost. For example, the Centers for Disease Control and Prevention (CDC) coordinates the National Breast and Cervical Cancer Early Detection Program. This program provides screening services, including clinical breast exams and mammograms, to low-income women throughout the United States and in several U.S. territories. Contact information for local programs is available on the CDC's website at http://apps.nccd.cdc.gov/cancercontacts/nbccedp/contacts.asp on the internet, or by calling the CDC at 800-CDC-INFO (800-232-4636). Information on low-cost or free mammography screening programs is also available through the NCI's Cancer Information Service (CIS) at 800-4-CANCER (800-422-6237).

Where can women get high-quality mammograms?

Women can get high quality mammograms in breast clinics, hospital radiology departments, mobile vans, private radiology offices, and doctors' offices.

The Mammography Quality Standards Act (MQSA) is a federal law designed to ensure that mammograms are safe and reliable. Through the MQSA, all mammography facilities in the United States must meet stringent quality standards, be accredited by the Food and Drug Administration (FDA), and be inspected annually. The FDA ensures that mammography facilities across the country meet MQSA standards. These standards apply to the following people at the mammography facility:

- The technologist who takes the mammogram

- The radiologist who interprets the mammogram

- The medical physicist who tests the mammography equipment

Women can ask their doctors or staff at the mammography facility about FDA certification before making an appointment. All mammography facilities are required to display their FDA certificate. Women should look for the MQSA certificate at the mammography facility and check its expiration date. MQSA regulations also require mammography facilities to give patients an easy-to-read report on the results of their mammogram.

Information about local FDA-certified mammography facilities is available through the CIS at 800-4-CANCER (800-422-6237). Also, a list of these facilities is on the FDA's website at http://www.fda.gov/cdrh/mammography/certified.html on the internet.

What should women with breast implants do about screening mammograms?

Women with breast implants should continue to have mammograms. (A woman who had an implant following breast cancer surgery should ask her doctor whether a mammogram of the reconstructed breast is necessary.) It is important to inform the mammography facility about breast implants when scheduling a mammogram. The technician and radiologist must be experienced in x-raying patients with breast implants. Implants can hide some breast tissue, making it more difficult for the radiologist to detect an abnormality on the mammogram. If the technologist performing the procedure is aware a woman has breast implants, steps can be taken to make sure that as much breast tissue as possible can be seen on the mammogram.

What is digital mammography? How is it different from conventional (film) mammography?

Both digital and conventional mammography use x-ray radiation to produce an image of the breast; however, conventional mammography stores the image directly on film, whereas digital mammography takes an electronic image of the breast and stores it directly in a computer. This allows the recorded data to be enhanced, magnified, or manipulated for further evaluation. The difference between conventional mammography and digital mammography is like the difference between a traditional film camera and a new digital camera. Aside from the difference in how the image is recorded and stored, there is no other difference between the two.

In January 2000, the FDA approved the first digital mammography system. In September 2005, preliminary results from a large clinical trial (research study) of digital vs. film mammography were published. These findings show no difference between digital and film mammograms in detecting breast cancer for the general population of women in the trial. However, those women with dense breasts who are pre- or perimenopausal (women who had a last menstrual period within 12 months of their mammograms) or who are younger than age 50 may benefit from having a digital rather than a film mammogram.

Digital mammography allows a radiologist to electronically adjust, store, and retrieve digital images. These features may offer the following advantages over conventional mammography:

- Long-distance consultations with other mammography specialists may be easier.

- Subtle differences between normal and abnormal tissues may be easily noted.

- The number of follow-up procedures needed may be fewer.

- Fewer repeat images may be needed, reducing exposure to radiation.

Digital mammography can be done only in facilities that are certified to practice conventional mammography and have received FDA approval to offer digital mammography. The procedure for having a mammogram with a digital system is the same as with conventional mammography.

What other technologies are being developed for breast cancer screening?

The NCI is supporting the development of several new technologies to detect breast tumors. This research ranges from methods being developed in research labs to those that have reached clinical trials. Efforts to improve conventional mammography include digital mammography, magnetic resonance imaging (MRI), and positron emission tomography (PET scanning).

In addition to imaging technologies, NCI-supported scientists are exploring methods to detect markers (genetic traits) of breast cancer in blood, urine, or nipple aspirates (fluid from the breast) that may serve as early warning signals for breast cancer.

Chapter 27

Sonography
(Ultrasound Exams)

Chapter Contents

Section 27.1

Ultrasound: An Introduction

Ultrasound imaging—also known as sonography—uses sound waves to produce images of organs, vessels, and tissues in the body. During an ultrasound examination, a small, hand-held transducer is placed in contact with the patient's body. It emits inaudible, high-frequency sound waves that pass through the body, sending back "echoes" as they bounce off organs, vessel walls, and tissues. Special computer equipment then converts these echoes into an image.

Ultrasound imaging has many applications. It is ideal for imaging the heart and the blood vessels. It can evaluate heart wall, chamber, and valve motion, as well as blood flow within the heart and blood vessels. It may be used to detect breast cysts or gallstones and to examine the prostate and to examine the liver, kidneys, pancreas, spleen, colon, and urinary bladder for tumors, inflammation, stones, or cysts. The use of ultrasound is expanding into the field of sports medicine as an effective way to detect ligament, tendon, and nerve injuries. Ultrasound also can be used to guide needle placement for biopsies, and to guide the drainage of cysts or fluid collections in the abdomen or chest that occur with some illnesses.

Because ultrasound uses sound waves instead of radiation to create images, it is a safe form of fetal imaging. It is used in obstetrics to assess fetal well-being, determine fetal position, diagnose multiple gestations (twins, triplets, etc.), determine a delivery date, and rule out ectopic pregnancy. If the fetus is old enough and positioned correctly, a baby's sex also can be determined. Ultrasound also plays a significant role in the evaluation and treatment of infertility.

In addition to its diagnostic imaging capabilities, ultrasound also is sometimes used in therapeutic applications to help treat soft tissue injuries. The discussion contained here, however, is confined to medical imaging.

Patient Preparation

Depending upon the body part being examined, you may be advised to drink water before your ultrasound examination, because sound waves travel more easily through fluid. You also may be advised to avoid drinking carbonated beverages before the examination because the air bubbles may interfere with the image.

You should wear comfortable clothing on the day of your examination. You may or may not be asked to put on a hospital gown, depending upon the procedure.

Before the exam begins, a sonographer will explain the procedure to you, ask questions about your health, ask why your physician requested the exam, and answer any questions you might have. A sonographer is a skilled medical professional who has received specialized education in the areas of anatomy, patient care, imaging techniques and ultrasound procedures.

During the Examination

Total examination time can range from less than 30 minutes to more than an hour, depending upon the part of the body being examined.

The sonographer will position you on the examination table and apply a special lotion to your skin directly above the area being studied. The lotion is odorless, harmless, and water-soluble. It acts as a conductor, making it easier for sound waves to travel into the underlying anatomy. After the lotion is applied, the sonographer will move a device called a transducer over the lotion-covered skin. The transducer sends out sound waves and receives echoes. These echoes are relayed to a computer for processing and displayed on a monitor as a picture for the sonographer to view. Selected pictures will be saved on paper, film, videotape, or in a computerized format to be reviewed by the supervising physician.

During the procedure, you will feel light pressure from the transducer being moved over your skin. The sonographer may ask you to change the position of your body or to hold your breath for a few seconds so that certain images can be obtained.

When the exam is complete, your ultrasound scans will be given to a radiologist—a physician who specializes in the diagnostic interpretation of medical images. Other physicians who may obtain additional training and read ultrasound exams include obstetricians, gynecologists, cardiologists, vascular surgeons, oncologists, and urologists.

Other Types of Ultrasound Procedures

Echocardiography uses ultrasound to take "moving pictures" of the heart. During an echocardiography examination, you will be hooked up to an electrocardiogram unit (ECG) that monitors the timing of events in the heart. The ECG leads will be attached to your chest with small adhesive patches and wires. The sonographer will spread gel on your chest and then move the ultrasound transducer over your chest wall or upper abdomen to obtain images of your heart. To evaluate the heart's response to stress, you might also be asked to perform a series of exercises that elevate your heart rate. Another echocardiography examination will be performed while your heart rate is elevated.

Doppler ultrasound is a special application of ultrasound that detects moving objects, such as blood flow. With Doppler ultrasound, physicians can examine the amount, direction, and speed of blood flowing to the brain or coursing through the heart, vessels, or other organs.

Although the ultrasound transducer usually is placed on the outside of the body, on the surface of the skin, a few examinations require that the transducer be placed inside the body to obtain the highest quality images. Some types of gynecological and obstetric examinations, for example, require that the transducer be placed inside the vagina. These examinations, called endovaginal or transvaginal procedures, use a special type of transducer designed for maximum image quality and minimum patient discomfort.

During a transesophageal echocardiogram, the transducer is threaded down a patient's throat into his or her esophagus. Placement of the transducer in the esophagus permits the sonographer to obtain clear images of specific areas of the heart.

A rectal transducer is used for ultrasound examinations of the prostate. This procedure may be used to acquire a tissue sample (biopsy) from areas of the prostate.

Post-Examination Information

After your ultrasound images have been reviewed by a radiologist, your personal physician will receive a report of the findings. Your physician then will advise you of the results and discuss what further procedures, if any, are needed.

There are no known side effects or after effects from ultrasound imaging, and it is not necessary to take any special precautions following your examination.

Please remember that the material presented here is for informational purposes only. If you have specific questions about a medical imaging procedure, contact your physician or the radiology department of the institution where your test will be performed.

Section 27.2

Obstetric Ultrasound

What is obstetric ultrasound imaging?

Ultrasound (US) imaging, also called ultrasound scanning or sonography, is a method of obtaining images of internal organs by sending high-frequency sound waves into the body. The soundwave echoes are recorded and displayed as a real-time visual image. No ionizing radiation (x-ray) is involved in ultrasound imaging. Obstetric ultrasound refers to the specialized use of sound waves to visualize and thus determine the condition of a pregnant woman and her embryo or fetus.

General Electric Medical System's new ultrasound technology that displays clinical images of the human body, allowing physicians and patients to see revolutionary "4D images," is now available at Rose Hill Imaging Services.

The fourth-dimension is real-time motion added to three-dimensional images. This technology dramatically expands diagnostic capabilities, therapy planning and ultrasound-guided minimally invasive diagnostic procedures such as biopsies.

Widely recognized for its clinical use in obstetrics and gynecology, 4D ultrasound with real-time motion is a new, powerful tool that can aid physicians studying the baby's motion, behavior, the baby's surface anatomy, and problems related to a woman's uterus and ovaries.

What are some common uses of the procedure?

Obstetric ultrasound should be performed only when clinically indicated. Some indications may be:

- to establish the presence of a living embryo/fetus;
- to estimate fetal age;
- to diagnose congenital abnormalities;
- to evaluate the position of the fetus;
- to evaluate the position of the placenta;
- to determine if there are multiple pregnancies.

How should I prepare for the procedure?

You should wear a loose fitting two-piece outfit for the examination. Only the lower abdominal area needs to be exposed during this procedure; consequently, a two-piece outfit will prevent you from having to readjust or remove all of your clothing.

If an ultrasound is required early in your pregnancy, you may be required to have a full bladder for the procedure. Air interferes with soundwaves, so if your bladder is distended, the air-filled bowel is pushed out of the way and an image of the uterus and embryo or fetus is obtained. About an hour and a half before the procedure, you should empty your bladder. You may be instructed to drink up to six glasses of water and avoid urinating until the procedure is completed. A full bladder is usually not necessary in the later stages of pregnancy.

What does the equipment look like?

The equipment consists of a transducer and a monitoring system. The transducer is a small hand-held device that resembles a microphone. The radiologist or sonographer spreads a lubricating gel on the area being examined and then presses this device firmly against the skin.

The ultrasound image is immediately visible on a nearby screen that looks much like a computer or television monitor. The radiologist or sonographer watches this screen during an examination and captures representative images for storage. Often, the patient is able to see it as well.

How does the procedure work?

Ultrasound imaging is based on the same principles involved in the sonar used by bats, ships at sea, and anglers with fish detectors. As a controlled sound bounces against objects, its echoing waves can be used to identify how far away the object is, how large it is, its shape and its internal consistency (fluid, solid, or mixed).

The ultrasound transducer functions as both a loudspeaker (to create the sounds) and a microphone (to record them). For obstetric ultrasound, when the transducer is pressed against the skin, it directs a stream of inaudible, high-frequency sound waves into the lower abdomen. As the sound waves echo from the embryo or fetus and surrounding structures in the uterus, the sensitive microphone in the transducer records tiny changes in the sound's pitch and direction. These signature waves are instantly measured and displayed by a computer, which in turn creates a real-time picture on the monitor.

The live images of the examination can be recorded on videotape. In addition, still frames of the moving picture are usually "frozen" to capture a series of images.

Doppler ultrasonography is the application of diagnostic ultrasound used to detect moving blood cells or other moving structures and measure their direction and speed of movement. The Doppler effect is used to evaluate movement by measuring changes in frequency of the echoes reflected from moving structures.

The movement of the embryo or fetus and fetal heart can be seen as an ongoing ultrasound "movie." Most ultrasound devices also have an audio component that processes the echoes produced by blood flowing through the fetal heart, blood vessels, and umbilical cord. This sound can be made audible to human ears and has been described by patients as a "whooshing noise."

How is the procedure performed?

You will be asked to lie on your back or side. You will also be asked to expose your lower abdominal area. The sonographer or radiologist then spreads a warm water-soluble gel over your lower abdomen. This gel allows better transmission of the sound waves by making it easier to move the transducer over your abdomen and by sending the sound beam directly into the body without the interference from even a tiny amount of air on the skin. The transducer emits high-frequency sound waves as the sonographer or radiologist moves it over your abdomen. The transducer also detects the echoes that bounce off anatomic structures as reflections.

Sometimes the radiologist determines that a transvaginal scan will need to be performed. Instead of a transducer being moved over your abdomen, the high-frequency waves will be emitted by a probe (transvaginal transducer) placed in the vagina. This technique often provides improved, more detailed images of the uterus and ovaries. It is especially useful in early pregnancy. With this approach the urinary bladder needs to be empty. Only two to three inches of the transducer are inserted into the vagina. The rest of the probe is a handle for use by the operator.

What will I experience during the procedure?

This is a painless procedure. There may be varying degrees of discomfort from pressure as the sonographer or radiologist guides the transducer over your abdomen, especially if you are required to have a full bladder. At times the sonographer may have to press more firmly to get closer to the embryo or fetus to better visualize the structure. This discomfort is temporary. Also, you may dislike the feeling of the water-soluble gel applied to your abdomen. With transvaginal scanning, there may be minimal discomfort as the probe is moved in the vagina.

Who interprets the results and how do I get them?

A radiologist, who is a physician experienced in obstetric ultrasound and other radiology examinations, will analyze the images and send a signed report with his or her interpretation to the patient's personal physician. The patient receives ultrasound results from the referring physician who ordered the test. New technology also allows for distribution of diagnostic reports and referral images over the internet at many facilities.

Section 27.3

Pelvic Ultrasound

What is pelvic ultrasound imaging?

Ultrasound (US) or sonography involves the sending of sound waves into the body. Those sound waves are reflected off the internal organs. The reflections are then recorded by special instruments that subsequently create an image of anatomic parts. No ionizing radiation (x-ray) is involved in ultrasound imaging.

For women, pelvic ultrasound is most often used to examine the uterus and ovaries and, during pregnancy, to monitor the health and development of the embryo or fetus. In males, a pelvic ultrasound usually focuses on the bladder and the prostate gland. Ultrasound images are captured in real-time, so they can show movement of internal tissues and organs, such as the flow of blood in arteries and veins.

What are some common uses of the procedure?

Millions of expectant parents have seen the first "picture" of their unborn child thanks to pelvic ultrasound examinations of the uterus and fetus. However, monitoring of fetal development is not the only reason for a pelvic ultrasound exam.

For females, ultrasound examinations can help determine the causes of pelvic pain, abnormal bleeding, or other menstrual problems. Ultrasound images can also help to identify palpable masses such as ovarian cysts and uterine fibroid growths, as well as ovarian or uterine cancers. Sonohysterography (saline infusion sonography) is a relatively new procedure in which sterile saline is injected into the uterus while a transvaginal sonogram is performed. The purpose is to distend the uterine cavity (endometrial cavity) to look for polyps, fibroids, or cancer, especially in patients with abnormal uterine bleeding. Other indications include evaluation of the uterine cavity looking for uterine anomalies (abnormal formations since birth) or scars. The saline outlines the lesion and allows for easy visualization and measurement.

For males, pelvic ultrasound is a valuable tool for evaluating the prostate, as well as for evaluating the tubes that carry semen.

In both sexes, a pelvic ultrasound exam can help to identify tumors and other disorders in the urinary bladder. Because ultrasound provides real time images, it can also be used to guide procedures, such as needle biopsies, in which a needle is used to sample cells from an abnormal area for laboratory testing.

How should I prepare for the procedure?

You should wear comfortable, loose-fitting clothing for your ultrasound exam. Other preparation depends on the type of examination you will have. For some scans, your doctor may instruct you not to eat or drink for as many as 12 hours before your appointment. You may be asked to drink up to six glasses of water two hours prior to your exam, so that your bladder is full when the scan begins. A full bladder helps with visualization of the uterus, ovaries, and bladder wall.

What does the equipment look like?

The equipment consists of a transducer and a monitoring system. The transducer is a small, hand-held device that resembles a microphone. The radiologist or sonographer spreads a lubricating gel on the patient's lower abdomen, where the uterus and ovaries are located, and then presses this device firmly against the skin.

Transvaginal ultrasound uses a wand like device that is lubricated and inserted into the vaginal canal.

The ultrasound image is immediately visible on a nearby screen that looks much like a computer or television monitor. The radiologist or sonographer watches this screen during an examination and captures representative images for storage. Often, the patient is able to see it as well.

How does the procedure work?

Ultrasound imaging is based on the same principles as the sonar used by bats, ships at sea, and anglers with fish detectors. As a controlled sound wave bounces against objects, its echoing waves can be used to identify how far away the object is, how large it is, its shape and its internal consistency (fluid, solid or mixed).

The ultrasound transducer functions as both a loudspeaker (to transmit the sounds) and a microphone (to record them). When the transducer is pressed against the skin, it directs a stream of inaudible, high-frequency sound waves into the body. As the sound waves echo back from the body's fluids and tissues, the sensitive microphone in the transducer records the strength and character of the reflected waves—with Doppler ultrasound the microphone captures and records tiny changes in the sound wave's pitch and direction. These signature waves are instantly measured and displayed by a computer, which in turn creates a real-time picture on the monitor.

The live images of the examination can be recorded on videotape or on a disc. In addition, still frames of the moving picture are usually "frozen" to capture a series of images.

How is the procedure performed?

There are three methods of performing pelvic ultrasound: abdominal (transabdominal), vaginal (transvaginal, endovaginal) in women, and rectal (transrectal) in men. The same principles of high-frequency sound apply in each technique.

For the transabdominal approach, the patient has a full urinary bladder and is positioned on an examination table. A clear gel is applied to the lower abdomen to help the transducer make secure contact with the skin. The sound waves produced by the transducer cannot penetrate air, so the gel helps to eliminate air pockets between the transducer and the skin. The sonographer then presses the transducer firmly against the skin and sweeps it back and forth to image the pelvic organs. Doppler sonography can be performed through the same transducer.

Transvaginal ultrasound involves the insertion of the transducer into the vagina after the patient empties her bladder and is performed very much like a gynecologic exam. The tip of the transducer is smaller than the standard speculum used when performing a Pap test. A protective cover is placed over the transducer, lubricated with a small amount of gel, and then inserted into the vagina. Only two to three inches of the transducer end are inserted into the vagina. The images are obtained from different orientations to get the best views of the uterus and ovaries. Doppler sonography can be performed through the transvaginal transducer, which is the same transducer used during sonohysterography. Below is an example of a transvaginal transducer (probe). Transvaginal ultrasound is usually performed with the patient lying on her back. In some cases she may bring her knees toward her chest with her legs spread—stirrups may be used as is common during a Pap smear or internal exam.

The prostate gland is located directly in front of the rectum, so the ultrasound exam is performed transrectally. A protective cover is placed over the transducer, lubricated, and then placed into the rectum so the sound need only travel a short distance. The images are obtained from different orientations to get the best view of the prostate gland. Ultrasound of the prostate is most often performed with the patient lying with his left side down on the table and with his knees bent up slightly.

Each method has its advantages. The transabdominal approach offers an expanded view of the entire pelvis, showing where one internal structure is in relation to another. Since the transducer is brought closer to the area being examined in the transvaginal and transrectal approaches, improved visualization may be achieved. Thus, it can be helpful in locating the embryonic heartbeat in an early pregnancy, evaluating the uterine texture, or measuring a cyst in an ovary. Your physician or radiologist will decide whether one or a combination of approaches is best for your particular case.

When the examination is complete, the patient may be asked to dress and wait while the ultrasound images are reviewed, either on film or on a monitor. Often, though, the sonographer or radiologist is able to review the ultrasound images in real time as they are acquired, and the patient can be released immediately.

Section 27.4

Abdominal Ultrasound

What is abdominal ultrasound imaging?

Ultrasound of the abdomen uses sound waves to obtain pictures inside of the abdomen. The organs examined most often include the liver, gallbladder, biliary system, spleen, pancreas, kidneys, and bladder. Ultrasound can also check the blood vessels in the abdomen.

How does the exam work?

Ultrasound sends sound waves into the body using a transducer, a hand-held device that sends and receives sound waves. After gel is applied to the skin, the sonographer (technologist) presses the transducer against the skin to obtain pictures, which then appear on a screen. As the sound waves echo from the body's fluids and tissues, a picture is created showing the tissues that are being studied.

How should I prepare for the exam?

- If the gallbladder or biliary system will be studied, you must fast for at least eight hours before your exam. This results in the highest accuracy in checking for biliary disease. When you eat, the gallbladder normally contracts to help digest your food. If you haven't fasted, the gallbladder may look abnormal. Clear liquids are fine, as long as there is no fat or sugar. Black coffee, tea, and water are fine.

- For ultrasound of the other abdominal organs, no preparation is needed.

- Wear loose-fitting, comfortable clothing.

How is the exam performed?

1. You will lie on an exam table, with your clothing moved away from your abdomen.

2. A warm gel is applied to your abdomen to help the transducer make contact with your skin.

3. The sonographer then presses the transducer against your skin and moves it around to obtain all the pictures.

4. The radiologist may obtain more pictures after the sonographer is done.

What will I feel during the exam?

- Ultrasound of the abdomen is fast, painless, and easy.

- You will feel the sonographer apply warm gel to your abdomen, and press the transducer against your skin.

- The transducer will be moved over your skin until all the pictures are obtained.

339

- You may be asked to roll on either side, or change your position.

- There is little or no discomfort with the exam, which usually takes less than 45 minutes.

Who interprets the results of the exam and how do I get them?

The radiologist who specializes in ultrasound will review the pictures and send the report to your referring doctor. You will receive your results from the doctor who ordered the test. The radiologist may discuss early findings with you when your exam is over.

Section 27.5

Heart Ultrasound (Echocardiography)

Reprinted with permission from "Frequently Asked Questions about Heart Ultrasound (Echocardiography)," "The Most Common Heart Ultrasound: Transthoracic Echocardiogram," and "Pediatric and Fetal Ultrasound," © 2007 American Society of Echocardiography. For more information, visit http://www.seemyheart.org.

Frequently Asked Questions about Heart Ultrasound (Echocardiography)

Why should you be concerned?

- Every year, about 1.2 million Americans will have a coronary attack. About 494,000 will die and many could be avoided.

- Cardiovascular diseases, including CHD and stroke, remain the number one cause of death in the United States, killing more than 953,000 Americans each year.

- Stroke is the third leading cause of death in the U.S. and a leading cause of death worldwide.

- Cardiovascular disease claims more women's lives than the next six causes of death combined—about 500,000 women's lives a year.

- Worldwide, about one in 150 babies are born with cardiac defects.

Heart ultrasound (echocardiography) can be very helpful to:

- Evaluate a heart murmur;
- Diagnose and determine the extent of valve conditions;
- Determine the presence of abnormalities in the structure of the heart;
- Measure the size and thickness of the heart and its chambers;
- Assess the motion of the chamber walls and the extent of damage to the heart muscle after a heart attack;
- Assess how different parts of the heart are functioning in patients with chronic heart disease;
- Determine if fluid is collecting around the heart (congestive heart problems);
- Identify the presence of tumors in the heart;
- Assess for and monitor congenital defects;
- Evaluate a patient's response to a treatment or a corrective procedure;
- Evaluate blood flow through the heart;
- Assess the heart condition prior to transplant;

  See if major blood vessels have been damaged by traumatic injury;
- Assess problems with the heart muscle (known as cardiomyopathy);
- Assess abnormal heart rhythms (arrhythmias);
- Assess bacterial endocarditis (BE—an infection of the valves and inner lining of the heart). This happens when bacteria from the skin, mouth, or intestines enter the bloodstream and infect the heart.
- Assess EF—ejection fraction levels (heart flow);
- Rule out any of the above mentioned abnormalities.

Why is heart ultrasound the most popular type of heart evaluation?

Heart ultrasound (echocardiography) has been the most widely used diagnostic test for heart disease for over 50 years.

- A sedative is not needed for the most common type of heart ultrasound

- Injection of a dye is not involved in the most common type of heart ultrasound. Injection of dye can be used to enhance the heart ultrasound in some circumstances, (contrast echocardiogram), but is not necessary for all heart ultrasound exams

- You aren't put in a claustrophobia-inducing machine to do the procedure. Heart ultrasounds are performed as you lie on a comfortable table

- Heart ultrasound scanning equipment is readily available in almost all hospitals and clinics. Other new technology may not be available in every healthcare setting

- Heart ultrasound is not a high priced procedure (typically cost $750–$1,500). Other technologies can be much more expensive than getting a heart ultrasound

- Heart ultrasound is helpful for the diagnosis of heart health, a variety of heart diseases and ailments. Heart ultrasounds can be used in all stages of life

- Ultrasound does not involve any radiation exposure

Why are you waiting?

Heart ultrasounds are not for everyone, but if you would like to protect your heart health because of a family history of heart disease, are in a high-risk group, or are experiencing any symptoms (shortness of breath, pain in your arm, etc., take the time to talk to your doctor today.

What types of heart ultrasounds are there?

The most common type of heart ultrasound performed is transthoracic, which is performed by placing a microphone-like device called the transducer on the outside of the chest wall with a gel-like substance to transmit sound waves into the body. There are also several other types:

- Doppler echocardiograms evaluate blood flow in the heart and blood vessels. This procedure measures the speed and direction of the blood flow within the heart. It screens the four valves for leaks. With Doppler echocardiograms, as the wand moves over your heart you will hear a "whooshing" sound much like that of a washing machine. This is the sound of blood moving within your heart.

- The stress echo or stress test combines the echo exam with a treadmill to walk on or a bike to pedal or medication that shows the effect of exercise on the heart. Stress tests are used to diagnose the narrowing of the coronary arteries.

- The contrast echocardiogram combines an echocardiogram with an IV that contains a solution which allows the sonographer or physician to see the inside of the heart more clearly. This is a harmless solution that has no known side effects. You will need to have an IV started to receive a contrast echocardiogram.

- Transesophageal echo is a form of echo where a miniature ultrasound camera is passed down the throat to coat the back of the heart. This allows the physician to obtain very high quality moving images. You can be sedated during the procedure if you wish. Transesophageal echocardiograms are typically performed to evaluate serious heart conditions.

What is it like?

A trained cardiac professional (a sonographer) will move a microphone-like object (a transducer—a hand-held device that sends and receives ultrasound signals) over the chest area. A small amount of gel used on the end of the transducer helps it glide over the skin. The transducer sends out high-frequency sound waves that are then shown (and captured) by equipment that includes a video screen and computer. Most people feel not much more than the presence of the gel on their skin during the procedure, but others may feel some pressure from the transducer being pressed down in order to obtain an enhanced image.

How safe is it?

Heart ultrasound is safer than some other heart imaging techniques because no radiation is involved. The sonographer taking your test will be right in the room next to you during the exam (without a protective vest or leaving the room). In fact, while she or he is taking a moving picture of your heart they will be talking to you. The final results will be reviewed by a specially trained physician to assure an accurate interpretation.

Who can have a heart ultrasound?

This exceptional view of your heart enables doctors to study your heart's functional and structural performance. Babies (even in the womb), children, adults, and the elderly all can safely experience cardiac ultrasound.

How do I find a qualified professional?

Looking for someone to perform or read a heart ultrasound? The designation Fellow of the American Society of Echocardiography (FASE) recognizes the experienced, dedicated ASE member with a diverse set of skills and comprehensive knowledge of all aspects of cardiac ultrasound (echocardiography). You can find a FASE in your area online at http://www.seemyheart.org/FindFASE.php.

How do I find an accredited echo lab?

Private offices, clinics, and departments within hospitals that are accredited by the Intersocietal Commission for the Accreditation of Echocardiography Laboratories (ICAEL) voluntarily submit to a review of their daily operations. This is a demonstration of a commitment to quality care.

How do I know if I'm at risk of heart failure?

Every year, 450,000 Americans die as the result of sudden cardiac death. But a safe, non-invasive procedure could save lives. Widely available heart ultrasounds are as easy on the patient as taking a blood pressure reading. The ejection fraction, or EF, measures the amount of blood pumped with each heartbeat. Recent medical research shows that people with hearts that pump poorly—that is, have a low EF—are at increased risk for sudden cardiac death.

What is EF?

Ejection fraction (EF) is a key indicator of heart health and is frequently used to determine the pumping function of the heart. Simply stated, EF is the amount of blood pumped out of the heart during each beat or contraction. In a healthy heart, 50–75% of the blood is pumped out during each beat. This indicates that the heart is pumping well and able to deliver an adequate supply of blood to the body and brain. Many people with heart failure and heart disease pump out less than 50%. Heart failure (also known as congestive heart failure) is a condition in which the heart is not able to pump enough blood to meet the oxygen demands of the body. For heart patients, knowing your EF is key first step to determining your risk for sudden cardiac arrest.

How is EF Measured?

A commonly used test to determine your EF is a heart ultrasound (echocardiogram). This is non-invasive and easy on the patient, and is often performed right in the doctor's office. By using ultrasound or sound waves, measurements are taken of the heart and with these measurements the pumping function the heart is calculated.

Should you know your EF number?

If you have heart disease, it is important to have your EF measured regularly, the same way that you have your blood pressure and cholesterol checked regularly. Keep in mind that your EF number can change, so it's important that you talk to your doctor about tracking it over time.

Where do I get a heart ultrasound?

A heart ultrasound can be performed in any setting, that is, wherever the patient is. While it is usually performed in a hospital or doctor's office, it can be performed bedside in the emergency room, an intensive care unit, or in an operating room. A cardiac sonographer, a health care professional specially trained and certified in cardiac ultrasound, usually performs the ultrasound, and the results are reviewed by a doctor.

What happens if the doctor finds a problem?

The heart ultrasound specialist physician will explain the findings of the heart ultrasound to your own doctor. You may need to undergo additional tests, or treatment may be recommended. Treatment for heart problems includes medication, surgery, and lifestyle modification.

What is the difference between heart ultrasound (echocardiogram) and an EKG?

Heart ultrasound shows a moving image of a beating heart on a television-like screen. An EKG, or electrocardiogram, measures the electrical currents in the heart. These are different diagnostic techniques

345

used to obtain different information. The EKG tells about the electrical health of the heart while the heart ultrasound health of the heart walls and valves.

How long has heart ultrasound (echocardiography) been around?

Ultrasounds began to be used on the heart in a clinical setting in the late 1960s. The technology is still going through improvements and developments. Live, moving pictures keep heart ultrasound as one of the most prescribed diagnostic tests.

Do health plans cover heart ultrasound?

Most health plans, HMO's, and Medicare cover echocardiography for established reasons.

The Most Common Heart Ultrasound: Transthoracic Echocardiogram

What is a heart ultrasound (transthoracic echocardiogram; TTE; echocardiogram; echo)?

A heart ultrasound is a useful tool to evaluate the structure and function of the heart and associated vessels. It is a fast, easy, and painless evaluation that uses ultrasound waves to produce images of the heart. In North America, the test is performed by a specially trained technologist, called a sonographer, and is interpreted by a specially trained physician, usually a cardiologist, trained in reading heart ultrasounds. Heart ultrasounds provide your doctor with moving pictures of your heart that allows your doctor to evaluate your heart's health. This ultrasound uses the same technology that allows doctors to see an unborn baby inside a pregnant mother.

Why has my doctor requested that I have a heart ultrasound (echocardiogram)?

There are many reasons that your physician may request that you have a heart ultrasound. Physicians use it evaluate your heart's performance as well as the structures of the heart, including the heart chambers and valves. An echo may sometimes also be used to look for the cause of a murmur, to check the size of the heart chambers, to check for fluid around the heart, or to inspect the pumping capability (the muscles) of the heart if a patient has short of breath or has complained of certain symptoms during exertion.

How do I prepare for an echo?

There is no special preparation required for a heart ultrasound. You should come as you are and eat or drink as you normally do. If you take medications, you should continue to take them as normal unless your doctor specifies otherwise. You should plan on being at the echocardiography lab for about forty-five minutes to one hour.

What should I expect?

Upon arrival at the lab the friendly staff will greet you. They may request you to provide additional insurance information, and will ask you to register. They may also ask that you provide a prescription or order for your exam.

You will then be escorted into an ultrasound room. The room will be dimly lit and will contain an examination table or bed and an ultrasound machine. You may be asked a few questions by the sonographer who will want to know why you are having the test, if you have had previous tests, and if you have ever had open heart surgery. Usually a brief explanation of the procedure will be given as well.

You will be asked to remove your clothing from the waist up and women will be given a gown to wear during the procedure. If you need help, the sonographer will assist you in getting onto the exam table, where you will be asked to lie on your left side. The sonographer will then attach ECG lead wires to electrodes adhered to your chest with simple medical tape.

The lights may be dimmed to allow the sonographer to see the monitor better.

The sonographer will apply ultrasound gel to a microphone-like device called a transducer. The transducer sends and receives the harmless ultrasound waves. The gel allows the ultrasound beams to penetrate your chest wall so that it is possible to "see" your heart.

Next, the sonographer will begin to acquire ultrasound images and audio recordings by methodically and precisely moving the transducer around on your chest, stomach, and neck. The sonographer will be viewing these images on a monitor and will take various recordings at several different locations or "views." During recording, you may be asked to change your position and to hold your breath. These variations in position and breathing allow the sonographer to obtain the best quality pictures. The sonographer will press the transducer

347

against your skin and this pressure may be moderate at times to facilitate the transmission of ultrasound waves. If it becomes uncomfortable, please let the sonographer know.

You should try to remain still and quiet during the exam. The imaging will take about 30 to 45 minutes. Often, the sonographer will review the study with a supervisor or physician while you are still in the room. You should not be alarmed; the technique to acquire images of the heart is technically demanding and sonographers frequently rely on the advice of others as they acquire these images.

The images and sounds of the exam will be recorded on a computer disk and/or videotape for later review.

What will I see and hear on the heart ultrasound machine during my exam?

Ultrasound waves used in performing the echocardiogram are not audible to the human ear, so you will not hear the sound waves.

Structures will be displayed in "real-time" and appear as white moving objects on the screen. For example, the valves of the heart will look like white flap-like moving structures. Areas of the heart where there is fluid or blood look black on the screen.

During the exam, you will notice the sonographer placing marks on the screen with small computer calipers. The sonographer uses the calipers to perform various measurements of the size, function, and blood flow of the heart.

An echocardiogram exam usually includes a Doppler recording of the blood movement or flow within the heart. When color flow Doppler is used in the exam it will appear as different colors moving within the white and black images on the monitor. The different colors represent the different speeds and directions of blood flow in the heart.

Doppler examinations often also include an audio signal of the blood flow. These audio signals can be heard and seen. During the audio Doppler recording, you will hear the sound of the blood moving through the heart and the sound of the heart valves opening and closing. The audio signals are also displayed as a graph on the monitor. These graphic recordings help the physician to determine valve function and heart pressures.

What happens after the exam?

Following the recording of the images, the sonographer will remove the ECG electrodes from your chest, will wipe off the ultrasound gel from your skin, will help you off the examination table, and escort you out of the lab.

The ultrasound images and Doppler recordings will be submitted to a cardiologist who is a specially trained physician in reading heart ultrasounds. He or she will interpret the images and will then provide your general physician with a written report. Often, you will not be given any results for one or two days. Generally, the sonographer will not provide you with any results at the time of the examination.

Pediatric and Fetal Ultrasound

A heart ultrasound provides your child's doctor with moving images of his or her heart and takes excellent pictures that will help your child's doctor evaluate his or her heart health. The most common type of heart ultrasound is non-invasive and very easy on your child.

Pediatric Heart Ultrasound (Also called Cardiovascular Ultrasound or Echocardiogram)

A specially trained technician (cardiac sonographer) uses a gel to slide a microphone-like device called a transducer over the chest area. This allows reflected sound waves to provide a live picture of your heart and valves. Heart ultrasound uses the same technology that allows doctors to see an unborn baby inside a pregnant mother. No radiation is involved in heart ultrasound, and the technology can be used on people of all ages. Cardiovascular ultrasound not only looks at the structure and function of the heart, but also all of the blood flow patterns through the valves, heart chambers, arteries, and veins. The heart ultrasound generally takes approximately 45–60 minutes, and is not painful.

Your child or adolescent may be referred for a cardiovascular ultrasound for a variety of reasons. These can include:

- A suspected heart murmur or other abnormal heart sound heard on examination;
- Abnormal oxygen saturation on examination;
- Concerns regarding heart function:
  - Following a heart infection such as myocarditis, rheumatic fever, or endocarditis,
  - Following treatment with specific chemotherapeutic agents (anthracyclines) for cancer,

- Cardiac symptoms such as chest pain, shortness of breath, decreasing exercise tolerance,

- Enlarged heart on chest x-ray,

- Receiving a medication which may affect heart function, or

- Persistent elevation in blood pressure;

- Family history of cardiomyopathy (dilated or thickened hearts);

- Concern regarding coronary arteries:

  - Kawasaki disease,

  - Chest pain with exercise, or

  - Syncope (fainting).

Fetal Heart Ultrasound (Fetal Echocardiogram)

An ultrasound of your fetus' heart provides your doctor with moving images of the heart and takes excellent pictures that will help your doctors evaluate your baby's heart health. A specially trained technician (sonographer) or cardiologist uses a gel to slide a microphone-like device called a transducer over your abdomen area. This allows reflected sound waves to provide a live picture of your baby's heart and valve structure and function. Heart ultrasound uses the same technology that allows doctors to see an unborn baby inside a pregnant mother. No radiation is involved in heart ultrasound, and the technology can be used on people of all ages. This test is safe and not painful. You may be referred for a fetal heart ultrasound during pregnancy by your obstetrician for a variety of reasons. These can include:

- Your obstetrician suspects a heart defect due to abnormal heart views on an obstetric scan;

- Abnormal fetal heart rate:

  - Tachycardia (too fast, over 200 beats per minute),

  - Bradycardia (too slow, less than 100 beats per minute), or

  - Persistently irregular (skipped or extra beats);

- Hydrops (heart failure);

- Family history (first degree relative) with a heart defect;

- Increased nuchal translucency (neck thickness) on a first trimester screening scan.

- You yourself have a disease that may increase the risk of a heart defect or abnormal rhythm in your fetus:

  - Diabetes mellitus, or

  - Sjögren syndrome or lupus (especially in the presence of SSA or SSB antibodies).

- Your fetus has an abnormality that can have an associated heart defect or by itself affect heart function such as:

  - Lung mass (can affect heart function and growth), diaphragmatic hernia, congenital cystic adenomatous malformation, sequestration, or

  - Intestinal abnormality, omphalocele, duodenal atresia, tracheoesophageal atresia;

- Twin-twin transfusion syndrome;

- Chromosomal abnormalities with associated heart problems.

Section 27.6

Vascular Ultrasound

"Vascular Testing and You," Copyright © Society for Vascular Ultrasound (www.svunet.org). Reprinted with permission.

Vascular ultrasound is an important diagnostic tool used in the diagnosis and detection of blood vessel problems. Ultrasound is also used to detect heart problems.

Your vascular lab visit will consist of a safe noninvasive ultrasound exam. Non-invasive means the ultrasound procedure does not require the use of needles, dyes, radiation, or anesthesia. Ultrasound uses sound wave frequencies too high to be heard by humans as a safe and harmless method to diagnose many medical conditions.

A qualified technologist will perform your procedure by applying a hypoallergenic water-gel to the area to be evaluated. Then a small phone-like device called a transducer is passed over the gel coated area to be examined, which produces an image on the screen of the ultrasound machine. Ultrasound is also used to blood flow in specific blood vessels. Noises might be heard while the technologist listens to the blood flow. Upon completion of the exam, a physician reviews and interprets all of the blood flow measurements.

Your Future Visit

To prepare for your vascular ultrasound examination, you should wear comfortable clothing. You may be given a hospital gown and asked to undress from the waist up or down. There is no special preparation for most exams except for abdominal vascular ultrasound exams.

Please arrive 15 minutes before your scheduled appointment for registration purposes. Most exams take 30–60 minutes to complete. After your exam is completed you will be free to go about your daily routine. The test results will generally be available within 24–48 hours for your referring physician's review.

Carotid Duplex

Ultrasound is used to evaluate the carotid arteries located in the neck that feeds the brain with blood. Gel will be applied to the skin of the neck. A transducer will be placed on the gel covered areas to obtain images and evaluate and listen to the blood flow in the arteries.

Transcranial Doppler (TCD)

The blood vessels that supply the brain within the skull are evaluated by transcranial Doppler. This exam is performed with a small transducer that is placed on the skin of the face and head. This exam takes approximately 60 minutes.

Venous Duplex

Ultrasound is used to evaluate the veins that carry blood to the heart from the legs or arms. Gel will be applied to the skin of the legs or arms. A transducer will be placed on the gel covered areas to obtain images and evaluate flow in the veins.

Arterial Duplex

Ultrasound is used to evaluate the arteries that feed the arms and legs with blood. Gel will be applied to the skin of the legs or arms. A transducer will be placed on the gel covered areas to obtain images and listen to the blood flow in the arms or legs.

Arterial Pressures and Waveforms

Ultrasound and blood pressure cuffs are used to evaluate the arteries that supply the arms and legs with blood. Several blood pressure cuffs will be placed at different segments of your legs or arms. When inflated, the cuffs will provide blood pressure readings as well as waveforms. This test will locate areas of block-age within the arteries.

Abdominal Vascular Duplex

Ultrasound is used to evaluate the blood vessels that bring blood to and away from your abdominal organs. Gel will be applied to the abdomen. A transducer will be placed on the gel covered areas to obtain images and listen to blood flow in the arteries and or veins.

Section 27.7

Carotid Ultrasound

From the *Diseases and Conditions Index,* National Heart Lung and Blood Institute (www.nhlbi.nih.gov), March 2007.

What Is Carotid Ultrasound?

Carotid ultrasound is a painless and harmless test that uses high-frequency sound waves to create images of the insides of the two large arteries in your neck. These arteries, called carotid arteries, supply your brain with blood. You have one carotid artery on each side of your neck.

Carotid ultrasound shows whether a material called plaque (plak) has narrowed your carotid arteries. Plaque is made up of fat, cholesterol, calcium, and other substances found in the blood. It builds up on the insides of your arteries as you age.

Too much plaque in a carotid artery can cause a stroke. The plaque can slow down or block the flow of blood through the artery, allowing a blood clot to form. A piece of the blood clot can break off and get stuck in the artery, blocking blood flow to the brain. This is what causes a stroke.

A standard carotid ultrasound shows the structure of your carotid artery. Your carotid ultrasound test may include a Doppler ultrasound. Doppler ultrasound is a special ultrasound that shows the movement of blood through your blood vessels. Your doctor often will need results from both types of ultrasound to fully assess if there is a problem with blood flow through your carotid arteries.

Other Names for Carotid Ultrasound

- Doppler ultrasound
- Carotid duplex ultrasound

Who Needs Carotid Ultrasound?

Carotid ultrasound checks for plaque buildup in the carotid arteries. This buildup can narrow or block your carotid arteries. You may need a carotid ultrasound if you:

- had a stroke or ministroke recently.
- have an abnormal sound in your carotid artery called a carotid bruit. Your doctor can hear a carotid bruit with the help of a stethoscope put on your neck over the carotid artery. A bruit can mean that there's a partial blockage in your carotid artery that could lead to a stroke.

Your doctor also may order a carotid ultrasound if he or she suspects you may have:

- blood clots that can slow blood flow in your carotid artery, or
- a split between the layers of your carotid artery wall that weakens the wall or reduces the blood flow to your brain.

A carotid ultrasound also may be done to see whether carotid artery surgery has restored normal blood flow. If you had a procedure called carotid stenting, your doctor may order a carotid ultrasound afterward to check the position of the stent put in your carotid artery. (The stent, a small mesh tube, helps prevent the artery from becoming narrowed or blocked again.)

Sometimes carotid ultrasound is used as a preventive screening test in people who have medical conditions that increase their risk of stroke, including high blood pressure and diabetes. People with these conditions may benefit from having their carotid arteries checked regularly even if they show no signs of plaque buildup.

What To Expect Before Carotid Ultrasound

Carotid ultrasound is a painless test, and typically there is little to do in advance. Your doctor will tell you how to prepare for your carotid ultrasound.

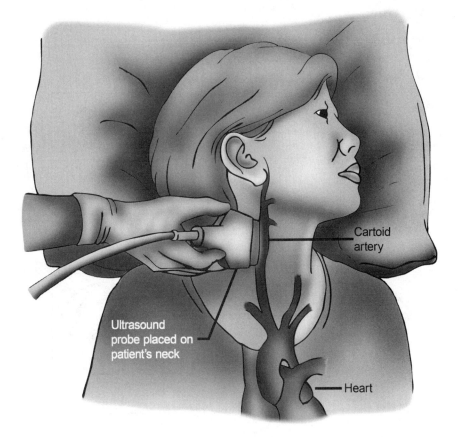

Figure 27.1. *Carotid Ultrasound: The ultrasound probe is placed over the carotid artery.*

What to Expect during Carotid Ultrasound

Carotid ultrasound is usually done in a doctor's office or hospital. The test is painless and usually doesn't take more than 30 minutes.

The ultrasound machine includes a computer, a video screen, and a transducer, which is a hand-held device that sends and receives ultrasound waves into and from the body.

You will lie down on your back on an exam table for the test. Your technician or doctor will put a gel on your neck where your carotid arteries are located. This gel helps the ultrasound waves reach the arteries better. Your technician or doctor will put the transducer against different spots on your neck and move it back and forth.

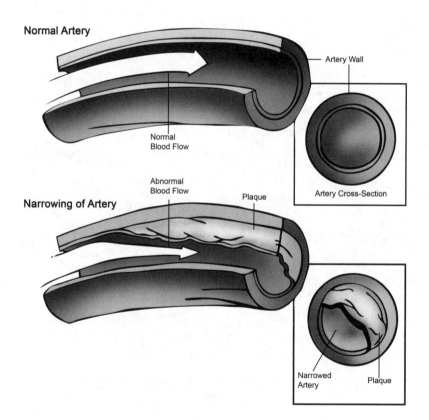

Figure 27.2. The illustration shows a normal artery with normal blood flow and an artery containing plaque buildup.

The transducer gives off ultrasound waves and detects their echoes after they bounce off the artery walls and blood cells. Ultrasound waves can't be heard by the human ear.

A computer uses the echoes of the ultrasound waves bouncing off the carotid arteries to create and record images of the insides of the arteries (usually in black and white) and your blood flowing through them (usually in color; this is the Doppler ultrasound). A video screen displays these live images for your doctor to review.

What to Expect after Carotid Ultrasound

Usually there is nothing special you have to do after a carotid ultrasound, and you should be able to return to normal activities immediately.

Often your doctor will be able to tell you the results of the carotid ultrasound when it occurs or soon afterward.

What Does a Carotid Ultrasound Show?

A carotid ultrasound can show whether buildup of a fatty material called plaque has narrowed one or both of your carotid arteries and reduced blood flow to your brain.

If your carotid arteries are narrowed by plaque, you may be at risk for having a stroke. That risk depends on how much of your artery is blocked and how much blood flow is restricted. To reduce your risk for stroke, your doctor may recommend medical or surgical treatments to reduce or remove the plaque buildup in your carotid arteries.

What Are the Risks of Carotid Ultrasound?

There are no risks linked to having a carotid ultrasound, because the test uses harmless sound waves. These are the same type of sound waves that doctors use to record pictures of fetuses in pregnant women.

Chapter 28

Computed Tomography

Chapter Contents

Section 28.1

What Is Computed Tomography (CT)?

U.S. Food and Drug Administration,
Center for Devices and Radiological Health, April 2002.

Conventional X-Ray Images

All x-ray imaging is based on the absorption of x-rays as they pass through the different parts of a patient's body. Depending on the amount absorbed in a particular tissue such as muscle or lung, a different amount of x-rays will pass through and exit the body. The amount of x-rays absorbed contributes to the radiation dose to the patient. During conventional x-ray imaging, the exiting x-rays interact with a detection device (x-ray film or other image receptor) and provide a 2-dimensional projection image of the tissues within the patient's body—an x-ray produced "photograph" called a "radiograph." The chest x-ray is the most common medical imaging examination. During this examination, an image of the heart, lungs, and other anatomy is recorded on the film.

Computed Tomography (CT)

Although also based on the variable absorption of x-rays by different tissues, computed tomography (CT) imaging, also known as "CAT scanning" (computerized axial tomography), provides a different form of imaging known as cross-sectional imaging. The origin of the word "tomography" is from the Greek word "tomos" meaning "slice" or "section" and "graphe" meaning "drawing." A CT imaging system produces cross-sectional images or "slices" of anatomy, like the slices in a loaf of bread. The cross-sectional images are used for a variety of diagnostic and therapeutic purposes.

How a CT System Works

1. A motorized table moves the patient through a circular opening in the CT imaging system.

2. As the patient passes through the CT imaging system, a source of x-rays rotates around the inside of the circular opening. A single rotation takes about one second. The x-ray source produces a narrow, fan-shaped beam of x-rays used to irradiate a section of the patient's body. The thickness of the fan beam may be as small as one millimeter or as large as ten millimeters. In typical examinations there are several phases; each made up of ten to 50 rotations of the x-ray tube around the patient in coordination with the table moving through the circular opening. The patient may receive an injection of a "contrast material" to facilitate visualization of vascular structure.

3. Detectors on the exit side of the patient record the x-rays exiting the section of the patient's body being irradiated as an x-ray "snapshot" at one position (angle) of the source of x-rays.

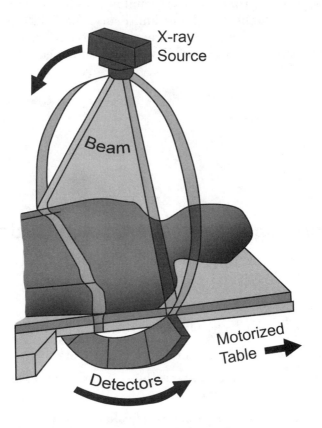

Figure 28.1. *Computed Tomography (CT) Fan Beam*

Many different "snapshots" (angles) are collected during one complete rotation.

4. The data are sent to a computer to reconstruct all of the individual "snapshots" into a cross-sectional image (slice) of the internal organs and tissues for each complete rotation of the source of x-rays.

Advances in Technology and Clinical Practice

Today most CT systems are capable of "spiral" (also called "helical") scanning as well as scanning in the formerly more conventional "axial" mode. In addition, many CT systems are capable of imaging multiple slices simultaneously. Such advances allow relatively larger volumes of anatomy to be imaged in relatively less time. Another advancement in the technology is electron beam CT, also known as EBCT. Although the principle of creating cross-sectional images is the same as for conventional CT, whether single- or multi-slice, the EBCT scanner does not require any moving parts to generate the individual "snapshots." As a result, the EBCT scanner allows a quicker image acquisition than conventional CT scanners.

Section 28.2

Questions and Answers about CT Scans

"Computed Tomography (CT): Questions and Answers,"
National Cancer Institute (www.cancer.gov), September 2003.

How is CT used in cancer?

Computed tomography is used in several ways:

- To detect or confirm the presence of a tumor;

- To provide information about the size and location of the tumor and whether it has spread;

- To guide a biopsy (the removal of cells or tissues for examination under a microscope);

- To help plan radiation therapy or surgery; and

- To determine whether the cancer is responding to treatment.

What can a person expect during the CT procedure?

During a CT scan, the person lies very still on a table. The table slowly passes through the center of a large x-ray machine. The person might hear whirring sounds during the procedure. People may be asked to hold their breath at times, to prevent blurring of the pictures.

Often, a contrast agent, or "dye," may be given by mouth, injected into a vein, given by enema, or given in all three ways before the CT scan is done. The contrast dye can highlight specific areas inside the body, resulting in a clearer picture.

Computed tomography scans do not cause any pain. However, lying in one position during the procedure may be slightly uncomfortable. The length of the procedure depends on the size of the area being x-rayed; CT scans take from 15 minutes to one hour to complete. For most people, the CT scan is performed on an outpatient basis at a hospital or a doctor's office, without an overnight hospital stay.

Are there risks associated with a CT scan?

Some people may be concerned about the amount of radiation they receive during a CT scan. It is true that the radiation exposure from a CT scan can be higher than from a regular x-ray. However, not having the procedure can be more risky than having it, especially if cancer is suspected. People considering CT must weigh the risks and benefits.

In very rare cases, contrast agents can cause allergic reactions. Some people experience mild itching or hives (small bumps on the skin). Symptoms of a more serious allergic reaction include shortness of breath and swelling of the throat or other parts of the body. People should tell the technologist immediately if they experience any of these symptoms, so they can be treated promptly.

What is spiral CT?

A spiral (or helical) CT scan is a new kind of CT. During a spiral CT, the x-ray machine rotates continuously around the body, following a spiral path to make cross-sectional pictures of the body. Benefits of spiral CT include:

- It can be used to make 3-dimensional pictures of areas inside the body;

- It may detect small abnormal areas better than conventional CT; and

- It is faster, so the test takes less time than a conventional CT.

What is total or whole body CT? Should a person have one?

A total or whole body CT scan creates images of nearly the entire body—from the chin to below the hips. This test has not been shown to have any value as a screening tool. ("Screening" means checking for signs of a disease when a person has no symptoms.)

The American College of Radiology (as well as most doctors) does not recommend scanning a person's body on the chance of finding signs of any sort of disease. In most cases abnormal findings do not indicate a serious health problem; however, a person must often undergo more tests to find this out. The additional tests can be expensive, inconvenient, and uncomfortable. The disadvantages of total body CT almost always outweigh the benefits.

For more information about whole body scanning, please visit the U.S. Food and Drug Administration's website at http://www.fda.gov/cdrh/ct/screening.html on the internet.

What is virtual endoscopy?

Virtual endoscopy is a new technique that uses spiral CT. It allows doctors to see inside organs and other structures without surgery or special instruments. One type of virtual endoscopy, known as CT colonography or virtual colonoscopy, is under study as a screening technique for colon cancer.

What is combined PET/CT scanning?

Combined PET/CT scanning joins two imaging tests, CT and positron emission tomography (PET), into one procedure. A PET scan creates colored pictures of chemical changes (metabolic activity) in tissues. Because cancerous tumors usually are more active than normal tissue, they appear different on a PET scan.

Combining CT with PET scanning may provide a more complete picture of a tumor's location and growth or spread than either test alone. Researchers hope that the combined procedure will improve health care professionals' ability to diagnose cancer, determine how far it has spread, and follow patients' responses to treatment. The combined PET/CT scan may also reduce the number of additional imaging tests and other procedures a patient needs. However, this new technology is currently available only at some facilities.

Where can people get more information about CT?

Additional information about CT is available from the CT Accreditation Department of the American College of Radiology, 1891 Preston White Drive, Reston, VA 20191-4397. The toll-free telephone number is 800-227-5463 (800-ACR-LINE). The CT Accreditation Department can be reached by e-mail at ctaccred@acr.org. The American College of Radiology website is located at http://www.acr.org on the internet.

Information about diagnostic radiology, including CT, is also available on the Radiology Info website at http://www.radiologyinfo.org on the internet. Radiology Info is the public information website of the Radiological Society of North America and the American College of Radiology.

Section 28.3

Cardiac CT

National Heart Lung and Blood Institute (www.nhlbi.nih.gov), July 2007.

What is cardiac CT?

Cardiac computed tomography, or cardiac CT, is a painless test that uses an x-ray machine to take clear, detailed pictures of your heart. It's a common test for showing problems of the heart. During a cardiac CT scan, the x-ray machine will move around your body in a circle and take a picture of each part of your heart.

Because an x-ray machine is used, cardiac CT scans involve radiation. However, the amount of radiation used is small. This test gives out a radiation dose similar to the amount of radiation you're naturally exposed to over three years. There is a very small chance that cardiac CT will cause cancer.

Each picture that the machine takes shows a small slice of the heart. A computer will put the pictures together to make a large picture of the whole heart. Sometimes an iodine-based dye is injected into one of your veins during the scan to help highlight blood vessels and arteries on the x-ray images.

Other Names for Cardiac CT

- CAT scan
- Coronary CT angiography
- Coronary artery scan
- CT angiography (CTA)

What should I expect before cardiac CT?

Your doctor will give you instructions before the cardiac computed tomography (CT) scan. Usually he or she will ask you to avoid drinks that contain caffeine before the test. Normally you'll be able to drink water, but you won't be able to eat for four hours before the scan.

If you take medicines for diabetes, ask your doctor whether you will need to change how you take them on the day of your cardiac CT scan.

Tell your doctor if you:

- Are pregnant or may be pregnant. Even though cardiac CT uses a low radiation dose, you shouldn't have the scan if you're pregnant. The x-rays may harm the developing fetus.

- Have asthma or kidney problems or are allergic to any medicines, iodine, and/or shellfish. These may increase your chance of having an allergic reaction to the contrast dye.

A technician will ask you to remove your clothes above the waist and wear a hospital gown. You also will be asked to remove any jewelry from around your neck or chest.

Taking pictures of the heart can be difficult because the heart is always beating (in motion). A slower heart rate will help produce better quality pictures. If you don't have asthma or heart failure, your doctor may give you a medicine called a beta blocker to help slow your heart rate. The medicine will be given by mouth or injected into a vein.

What should I expect during cardiac CT?

The cardiac computed tomography (CT) scan will take place in a hospital or outpatient office.

Because an x-ray machine is used, cardiac CT scans involve radiation. However, the amount of radiation used is small. This test gives out a radiation dose similar to the amount of radiation you're naturally exposed to over three years. There's a very small chance that cardiac CT will cause cancer. A doctor who has experience with CT scanning will supervise the test.

If your doctor wants to use contrast dye during the cardiac CT scan, a small needle connected to an intravenous (IV) line will be put in a vein in your hand or arm.

The contrast dye will be injected through the IV during the scan. You may have a warm feeling during the injection. The dye will highlight your blood vessels on the x-ray pictures from the cardiac CT scan.

The technician who operates the cardiac CT scanner will clean areas of your chest and place small sticky patches on those areas. The patches are attached to an EKG (electrocardiogram) machine to record the electrical activity of your heart during the exam.

The CT scanner is a large, square machine that has a hollow, circular tube in the middle. You will lie on your back on a sliding table that can move up and down and goes inside the tunnel-like machine.

Inside the scanner, an x-ray tube moves around your body to take pictures of different parts of your heart. These pictures can be shown on a computer as one large, three-dimensional picture. The technician controls the machine from the next room. The technician can see you through a glass window and talk to you through an intercom system.

Moving your body can cause the pictures to blur. You will be asked to lie still and hold your breath for short periods, while each picture is taken.

A cardiac CT scan usually takes about 15 minutes to complete. However, it can take over an hour to get ready for the test and for the medicine to slow your heart rate enough.

What should I expect after cardiac CT?

Once the cardiac computed tomography (CT) scan is done, you're able to return to your normal activities.

A doctor who has experience with CT will provide your doctor with the results of your test. Your doctor will discuss the findings with you.

What does cardiac CT show?

Many x-rays are taken while you're in the computed tomography (CT) scanner. Each picture that the machine takes shows a small slice of the heart. A computer can put the pictures together to make a large picture of the whole heart. This picture shows the inside of the heart and the structures that surround the heart.

Cardiac CT is a common test for finding and evaluating:

- **Problems in the heart:** Iodine-based dye used with a cardiac CT scan can show pictures of the coronary arteries. The coronary arteries are blood vessels on the surface of the heart. If these blood vessels are narrowed or blocked, you may have chest pain or a heart attack. The CT scan also can find problems with heart function and heart valves.

- **Problems with the aorta:** The aorta is the main artery that carries oxygen-rich blood from the heart to the body. Cardiac CT can detect two serious problems in the aorta:

  - *Aneurysms,* which are diseased areas of a weak blood vessel wall that bulge out. Aneurysms can be life threatening because they can burst.

  - *Dissections,* which can occur when the layers of the aortic artery wall peel away from each other. This condition can cause pain and also may be life threatening.

- **Blood clots in the lungs:** A cardiac CT scan also may be used to find a pulmonary embolism, a serious but treatable condition. A pulmonary embolism is a sudden blockage in a lung artery, usually due to a blood clot that traveled to the lung from the leg.

- **Pericardial disease:** This is a disease that occurs in the pericardium, a sac around your heart.

Because the heart is in motion, a fast type of CT scanner, called multidetector computed tomography (MDCT), is used to take high-quality pictures of the heart.

Another type of CT scanner, called electron-beam computed tomography (EBCT), is used to detect calcium in the coronary arteries. Calcium in the coronary arteries may be an early sign of coronary artery disease (CAD).

What are the risks of cardiac CT?

Cardiac computed tomography (CT) scans are safe, painless tests. Although cardiac CT uses radiation, the amount is small. This test gives out a radiation dose similar to the amount of radiation you're naturally exposed to over three years. There is a very small chance that cardiac CT will cause cancer.

Some people feel side effects from the contrast dye that's used during the cardiac CT scan, including the following:

- An itchy feeling or a rash may appear after the injection of the contrast dye. Neither one normally lasts for a long time, so medicine often isn't needed. If you do want medicine to relieve these symptoms, you can ask your doctor to prescribe you a medicine called an antihistamine, which is used to help stop allergic reactions.

- Although rare, it's possible to have a serious allergic reaction that may lead to breathing difficulties. Medicines are used to treat serious reactions.

People who have asthma or emphysema may have breathing problems during cardiac CT if they're given beta blockers to slow down their heart rates.

Section 28.4

Coronary Calcium Scan

National Heart Lung and Blood Institute (www.nhlbi.nih.gov), 2007.

What is a coronary calcium scan?

A coronary calcium scan is a test that can help show whether you have coronary artery disease (CAD). In CAD, a fatty material called plaque (plak) narrows your coronary (heart) arteries and limits blood flow to your heart. CAD is the most common type of heart disease in both men and women. It can lead to angina, heart attack, heart failure, and arrhythmia.

Coronary calcium scanning looks for specks of calcium (called calcifications) in the walls of the coronary arteries. Calcifications are an early sign of heart disease. The test can show, before other signs and symptoms occur, whether you're at increased risk for a heart attack or other heart problems.

A coronary calcium scan is most useful for people who are at moderate risk for a heart attack. You or your doctor can calculate your 10-year risk using the Risk Assessment Tool from the National Cholesterol Education Program. People at moderate risk have a ten to 20 percent chance of having a heart attack within the next ten years. The coronary calcium scan helps doctors decide who within this group needs treatment.

Two machines can show calcium in the coronary arteries—electron beam computed tomography (EBCT) and multidetector computed tomography (MDCT). Both use an x-ray machine to make detailed pictures of your heart. Doctors study the pictures to see whether you're at risk for heart problems in the next two to ten years.

A coronary calcium scan is simple and easy for the patient, who lies quietly in the scanner machine for about ten minutes. Pictures of the heart are taken that show whether the coronary arteries have calcifications.

Other Names for Coronary Calcium Scans

- Calcium scan test
- Cardiac CT for calcium scoring

Sometimes people refer to a coronary calcium scan by the name of the machine used to take pictures of the heart:

- Electron-beam computed tomography (EBCT) or electron-beam tomography (EBT)
- Multidetector computed tomography (MDCT)

What should I expect before a coronary calcium scan?

No special preparation is needed. You may be asked to avoid caffeine and smoking for four hours before the test. For the scan, you will remove your clothes above the waist and wear a hospital gown. You also will remove any jewelry from around your neck or chest.

What should I expect during a coronary calcium scan?

Coronary calcium scans are done in a hospital or outpatient office. The x-ray machine that's used is called a computed tomography (CT) scanner.

The technician who operates the scanner will clean areas of your chest and apply small sticky patches called electrodes. The electrodes are attached to an EKG (electrocardiogram) monitor. The EKG measures the electrical activity of your heart during the scan. This makes it possible to take pictures of your heart when it's relaxed, between beats.

The CT scanner is a large machine that has a hollow, circular tube in the center. You will lie on your back on a sliding table. The table can move up and down and goes inside the tunnel-like machine.

The table will slowly slide into the opening in the machine. Inside the scanner, an x-ray tube moves around your body to take pictures of your heart. You may be asked to hold your breath for ten to 20 seconds while the pictures are taken. This prevents movement in the image.

During the test, the technician will be in a nearby room with the computer that controls the CT scanner. The technician can see you through a window and talk to you through an intercom system.

You may be given medicine to slow down a fast heart rate. This helps the machine take better pictures of your heart. The medicine will be given by mouth or injected into a vein.

A coronary calcium scan takes about five to ten minutes. During the test, the machine makes clicking and whirring sounds as it takes pictures. It causes no discomfort, but the exam room may be chilly to keep the machine working properly.

If you become nervous in enclosed spaces, you may need to take medicine to stay calm. This isn't a problem for most people, because your head will remain outside the opening in the machine.

What should I expect after a coronary calcium scan?

You're able to return to your normal activities after the coronary calcium scan is done. A doctor who is trained in reading these scans will discuss the results with you.

What does the coronary calcium scan show?

After the coronary calcium scan, you will get a calcium score called an Agatston score. The score is based on the amount of calcium found in your coronary arteries. You may get an Agatston score for each major artery and a total score.

The test is negative if no sign of calcium deposits (calcifications) is found in your arteries. This means your chance of having a heart attack in the next two to five years is low.

The test is positive if calcifications are found in your arteries. Calcifications are a sign of atherosclerosis and coronary artery disease. (Atherosclerosis is when the arteries harden and narrow due to plaque buildup.) The higher your Agatston score, the greater the amount of atherosclerosis.

What are the risks of a coronary calcium scan?

Coronary calcium scanning has very few risks. The test isn't invasive, which means that no surgery is done and no instruments are inserted into your body. Coronary calcium scanning doesn't require an injection of contrast dye to make your heart or arteries visible on the x-ray images.

Because an x-ray machine is involved, you will be exposed to a small amount of radiation. Electron-beam computed tomography (EBCT) uses less radiation than multidetector computed tomography (MDCT). In either case, the amount of radiation is less than or equal to the amount of radiation you're naturally exposed to in a single year.

Section 28.5

Full-Body CT Scans: What You Need to Know

U.S. Food and Drug Administration,
DHHS Pub. No. (FDA) 03-0001, March 2003.

Using a technology that "takes a look" at people's insides and promises early warnings of cancer, cardiac disease, and other abnormalities, clinics and medical imaging facilities nationwide are touting a new service for health-conscious people: whole-body CT screening. This typically involves scanning the body from the chin to below the hips with a form of x-ray imaging that produces cross-sectional images.

The technology used is called x-ray computed tomography (CT), sometimes referred to as computerized axial tomography (CAT). A number of different types of x-ray CT systems are being promoted for various types of screening. For example, multi-slice CT (MSCT) and electron beam CT (EBCT)—also called electron beam tomography

(EBT)—are x-ray CT systems that produce images rapidly and are often promoted for screening the buildup of calcium in arteries of the heart.

CT, MSCT, and EBCT all use x-rays to produce images representing "slices" of the body—like the slices of a loaf of bread. Each image slice corresponds to a wafer-thin section which can be viewed to reveal body structures in great detail.

CT is recognized as an invaluable medical tool for the diagnosis of disease, trauma, or abnormality in patients with signs or symptoms of disease. It's also used for planning, guiding, and monitoring therapy. What's new is that CT is being marketed as a preventive or proactive health care measure to healthy individuals who have no symptoms of disease.

No Proven Benefits for Healthy People

Taking preventive action, finding unsuspected disease, uncovering problems while they are treatable—these all sound great, almost too good to be true. In fact, at this time the Food and Drug Administration (FDA) knows of no scientific evidence demonstrating that whole-body scanning of individuals without symptoms provides more benefit than harm to people being screened. The FDA is responsible for assuring the safety and effectiveness of such medical devices, and it prohibits manufacturers of CT systems to promote their use for whole-body screening of asymptomatic people. The FDA, however, does not regulate practitioners and they may choose to use a device for any use they deem appropriate.

Compared to most other diagnostic x-ray procedures, CT scans result in relatively high radiation exposure. The risks associated with such exposure are greatly outweighed by the benefits of diagnostic and therapeutic CT. However, for whole-body CT screening of asymptomatic people, the benefits are questionable:

- Can it effectively differentiate between healthy people and those who have a hidden disease?

- Do suspicious findings lead to additional invasive testing or treatments that produce additional risk with little benefit?

- Does a "normal" finding guarantee good health?

Many people don't realize that getting a whole body CT screening exam won't necessarily give them the "peace of mind" they are hoping for or the information that would allow them to prevent a health problem. An abnormal finding, for example, may not be a serious one, and a normal finding may be inaccurate. CT scans, like other medical procedures, will miss some conditions, and "false" leads can prompt further, unnecessary testing.

Points to Consider

If you are thinking of having a whole-body screening, consider these points:

- CT screening has not been demonstrated to meet generally accepted criteria for an effective screening procedure.

- Medical professional societies have not endorsed CT scanning for individuals without symptoms.

- CT screening of high-risk individuals for specific diseases, such as lung cancer or colon cancer, is currently being studied, but results are not yet available.

- The radiation from a CT scan may be associated with a very small increase in the possibility of developing cancer later in a person's life.

- The FDA provides additional information regarding whole-body CT screening on its website at: www.fda.gov/cdrh/ct/

FDA's Recommendation

Before having a CT screening procedure, carefully investigate and consider the potential risks and benefits and discuss them with your physician.

Chapter 29

Magnetic Resonance Imaging (MRI)

Chapter Contents

Section 29.1

MRI: An Introduction

This section includes "Magnetic Resonance Imaging" and "Magnetic Resonance Safety," © 2008, the American Society of Radiologic Technologists. All rights reserved. Reprinted with permission of the ASRT.

Magnetic Resonance Imaging

Magnetic resonance imaging (MRI) is a sophisticated diagnostic technique that uses a magnetic field, radiowaves, and a computer to generate detailed, cross-sectional images of human anatomy. Because it produces better soft-tissue images than x-rays can, MRI is most commonly used to image the brain, spine, thorax, vascular system, and musculoskeletal system (including the knee and shoulder).

During an MRI exam, the patient is placed inside a scanner that produces a static magnetic field up to 8,000 times stronger than the earth's own magnetic field. Exposure to this force causes the hydrogen protons within the patient's body to align with the magnetic field. When a radiofrequency pulse is applied, the protons spin perpendicular to the magnetic field. As the protons relax back into alignment with the magnetic field, a signal is sent to a radiofrequency coil that acts as an antenna. This signal then is processed by a computer. Different tissues produce different signals. For example, protons in water relax more slowly than those in fat. This differentiation can be detected, measured and converted into a cross-sectional image of the patient's anatomy.

Patient Preparation

MRI is a safe procedure for most patients, although it generally is not recommended for pregnant women. If you are pregnant, let your physician know. Also, because the body is exposed to a strong magnetic field, patients who have a pacemaker, cochlear implants, or aneurysm clips should check with a physician before undergoing an MRI examination. Patients who have other types of metal implants and patients who have been exposed to shrapnel or whose eyes have been exposed to metal shavings also might not be candidates for MRI; it's important to let your physician know if these conditions apply to you. For similar reasons, women undergoing an MRI exam should not wear eyeshadow, because it sometimes contains metallic substances.

If you are claustrophobic or experience pain when lying on your back for more than 30 minutes, let your doctor know. He or she may be able to prescribe a relaxant or pain medication. If you are sedated for the examination, a friend will have to drive you home afterward. In some facilities, you can arrange for your scan to be performed in an "open" magnet. Open MR units are less confining than traditional MRI machines. Instead of sliding the patient into a long metal tube, the magnet is suspended above the patient. Keep in mind, however, that open magnets are a new technology and not all facilities have them.

Before your examination, an MR technologist will explain the procedure to you and answer any questions you might have. An MR technologist, also known as a radiologic technologist, is a skilled medical professional who has received specialized education in the areas of anatomy, patient positioning, patient care, imaging techniques, and MR procedures.

During the Examination

Examination time depends upon the part of the body being examined, but typically ranges from 30 minutes to an hour. You will be asked to undress, remove all jewelry, and put on a hospital gown. Remember, the magnet will damage wristwatches and erase credit cards and bank cards, so don't take them into the exam room with you. You will be provided a secure place to store these items during your examination.

For most types of exams, the MR technologist will wrap a special coil around the body part that is being examined. This coil helps concentrate the radiofrequency pulses. The MR technologist then will position you on a padded, movable table that will slide into the opening of the scanner.

You may be given a contrast agent to highlight internal organs and structures. The contrast changes the relaxation rate of protons in the body, illuminating organs and tissues, and making tumors, vessels, and scar tissue appear brighter.

You won't feel anything during the scan, but you may hear intermittent humming, thumping, clicking, and knocking sounds. These are the sounds of the magnetic gradients turning on and off. Some MR centers provide patients with headphones or earplugs to help mask the noise.

The MR technologist will not be in the room during the scan, but will be able to observe you through a window from a room next door and will be able to hear you and talk to you through a two-way microphone system. The technologist will tell you when each scan sequence is beginning and how long it will last. You will be asked to remain as still as possible throughout the sequence.

When the exam is complete, your MR scans obtained will be given to a radiologist—a physician who specializes in the diagnostic interpretation of medical images.

Post-Examination Information

After your films have been reviewed by a radiologist, your personal physician will receive a report of the findings. Your physician then will advise you of the results and discuss what further procedures, if any, are needed.

Magnetic resonance imaging is a noninvasive procedure, and there are no known side effects or after effects. If a contrast agent was administered, you may experience nausea, headache, or dizziness following your examination. It's important to increase your water consumption in the days following the examination. If these symptoms persist, contact your physician.

Please remember that the material presented here is for informational purposes only. If you have specific questions about a medical imaging procedure, contact your physician or the radiology department of the institution where your test will be performed.

About Magnetic Resonance Angiography and Other MR Procedures

In addition to MRI, magnetic resonance has other diagnostic applications. One rapidly advancing technique is magnetic resonance angiography, or MRA. Angiography is the imaging of blood vessels. Usually, it is performed to evaluate aneurysms or to determine whether vessels in the brain, neck, legs, or other areas have become narrowed due to atherosclerosis ("hardening of the arteries"). During conventional x-ray angiography, a catheter is inserted into the body through the groin and an iodine-based contrast agent is injected into the blood vessel while a series of x-rays are taken. MRA allows physicians to view blood vessels and the flow of blood through arteries without the need to introduce a catheter or a contrast agent into the patient's artery.

Neurological and intracranial applications for magnetic resonance technology include functional MR and MR spectroscopy. Functional

MR uses magnetic resonance to map the brain, matching motor and sensory activities with corresponding areas of brain activation. Functional MR detects changes in the blood supply to specific areas of the brain. Using it, researchers can "watch" changes that occur in the brain when a patient speaks, recalls a past event, or moves a body part. Functional MR is still in its early stages of development, but it shows promise as a method to study stroke, multiple sclerosis, epilepsy, Alzheimer disease, and Parkinson disease.

MR spectroscopy uses magnetic resonance to measure metabolites, creating a chemical spectrum (map) of the brain. Metabolites are byproducts of metabolism that are present in the brain matter. By measuring their concentrations in different areas of the brain, researchers can determine how the brain works at an unprecedented level of detail. Applications include measurement of the volume and flow of blood to brain tumors, assessment of brain tissue, and study of sleep disorders and Alzheimer disease.

Magnetic Resonance Safety

Unlike x-ray exams, which use radiation, magnetic resonance (MR) images are created with magnetic fields and radio waves. MR scanning is a very safe and effective technique for examining the body's soft tissues, such as organs, muscles, ligaments, and tendons. However, because MR scanning uses a powerful magnet, patients need to know about some special precautions and check-in procedures.

No metal is allowed in the room where MR scans are performed because metal objects are attracted to the magnet. The magnet is always on, whether or not scanning is going on. On rare occasions, patients and health care professionals have been injured when an object suddenly was drawn to the magnet. Also, metal objects can create artifacts on MR scans, making it difficult or impossible to see the patient's anatomy. For your own safety and comfort, for the safety of the staff who will care for you, and to ensure a high-quality diagnostic exam, please follow these guidelines.

You will not be allowed to wear a watch or any jewelry, including body piercing, during the exam. It may be best to leave these items at home, although some facilities provide a safe place to store your valuables during your exam. Barrettes, hairpins, eyeglasses, dentures, and hearing aids also must be removed. Some types of cosmetics contain small amounts of metal, so avoid wearing any makeup the day of your exam. Also avoid clothing with metal zippers, rivets, buttons, or metallic fabric. Empty your pockets of all metal items, including coins, money clips, credit cards, pens, pocket knives, keys, safety pins, and paper clips. Permanent metal dental work, such as crowns, fillings, and non-removable braces, do not normally cause a problem during MR scans.

Metal wheelchairs and oxygen tanks are not permitted near the MR magnet. However, special MR-safe versions may be available at the facility where your exam will be performed. If you have questions about any medical equipment you use, ask the MR technologist who will perform your exam. He or she is a skilled professional educated in anatomy, positioning and the safe use of magnetic resonance technology.

The technologist will screen you before your exam. He or she will check you for metal objects and ask you a series of questions about metal that might be in or on your body. Think carefully about these questions, answer them truthfully, and ask the technologist if there is anything you don't understand.

Be sure to tell the technologist if you have any of the following:

- A pacemaker or artificial valve in your heart
- Metal pins, plates, rods, screws, or nails anywhere in your body
- Wire sutures or surgical staples
- An intrauterine device (IUD) or diaphragm
- An insulin pump
- An aneurysm clip
- A joint replacement
- An ear implant
- A stent, filter, or coil in any blood vessel
- Any type of prosthesis, including a penile implant or artificial eye
- Permanent (tattooed) makeup, such as eyeliner or lip coloring

It also is important to tell the technologist if you ever have suffered a gunshot wound or any type of accident that may have left metallic particles in your body. Depending on the type of metal and where it is located, you may not be able to have an MR exam. A radiologist, a physician trained in interpreting medical images, will decide if you should have the exam.

By knowing these important precautions and cooperating fully with the MR technologist, patients can help ensure that they have a safe and useful exam.

Section 29.2

Cardiac MRI

Diseases and Conditions Index,
National Heart Lung and Blood Institute, August 2007.

What Is Cardiac MRI?

Magnetic resonance imaging (MRI) is a safe, noninvasive test that creates detailed images of your organs and tissues. "Noninvasive" means that no surgery is done and no instruments are inserted into your body.

MRI uses radio waves and magnets to create images of your organs and tissues. Unlike computed tomography scans (also called CT scans) or conventional x-rays, MRI imaging doesn't use ionizing radiation or carry any risk of causing cancer.

Cardiac MRI uses a computer to create images of your heart as it's beating, producing both still and moving pictures of your heart and major blood vessels. Doctors use cardiac MRI to get images of the beating heart and to look at the structure and function of the heart. These images can help them decide how best to treat patients with heart problems.

Cardiac MRI is a common test for diagnosing and evaluating a number of diseases and conditions, including the following:

- Coronary artery disease
- Damage caused by a heart attack
- Heart failure
- Heart valve problems
- Congenital heart defects
- Pericardial disease (a disease that affects the tissues around the heart)
- Cardiac tumors

Cardiac MRI images can help explain results from other tests, such as x-ray and CT scans. Cardiac MRI is sometimes used to avoid the need for other tests that use radiation (such as x-rays), invasive procedures, and dyes containing iodine (these dyes may be harmful to people who have kidney problems).

Sometimes during cardiac MRI, a special dye is injected into a vein to help highlight the heart or blood vessels on the images. Unlike the case with x-rays, the special dyes used for MRI don't contain iodine, so they don't present a risk to people who are allergic to iodine or have kidney problems.

Other Names for Cardiac MRI

- Heart MRI

- Cardiovascular MRI

- Cardiac nuclear magnetic resonance (NMR)

What to Expect before Cardiac MRI

You'll be asked to fill out a screening form before the test takes place. The form may ask whether you've had previous surgeries, whether you have any metal objects in your body, and whether you have any medical devices (like a cardiac pacemaker) surgically implanted in your body.

Most, but not all, implanted medical devices are allowed near the magnetic resonance imaging (MRI) machine. Ask your doctor or the technician operating the machine if you have concerns about any implanted devices or conditions that may interfere with the MRI.

MRI can interfere seriously with some types of implanted medical devices.

- Implanted cardiac pacemakers and defibrillators can malfunction.

- Cochlear (inner-ear) implants can be damaged. Cochlear implants are small electronic devices that are used to help people who are deaf or who can't hear well to get an idea of the sounds around them.

- Brain aneurysm clips can move due to MRI's strong magnetic field. This can cause severe injury.

Your doctor will let you know if you shouldn't have a cardiac MRI because of a medical device.

Your doctor or technician will tell you whether you need to change into a hospital gown for the test. Don't bring hearing aids, credit cards, jewelry and watches, eyeglasses, pens, removable dental work, and anything that's magnetic near the MRI machine.

Tell your doctor if you have a history of becoming anxious or fearful when in a fairly tight or confined space. This fear is called claustrophobia. In this case, your doctor might give you medicine to help you relax. Your doctor may ask you to stop eating six hours before you take this medicine on the day of the test.

Some of the newer cardiac MRI machines are open on all sides. Ask your doctor to help you find a facility that has an open MRI machine if you're fearful in tight or confined spaces.

Your doctor will let you know if you need to arrange for a ride home after the test.

What to Expect during Cardiac MRI

Magnetic resonance imaging (MRI) machines are usually located at a hospital or at a special medical imaging facility. A radiologist or other physician with special training in medical imaging oversees MRI testing.

Cardiac MRI usually takes 45 to 90 minutes, depending on how many images are needed. The test may take less time with some newer MRI machines.

The MRI machine will be located in a specially constructed room. This will prevent radio waves from disrupting the machine and will prevent the strong magnetic fields generated by the MRI machine from interfering with other equipment.

Traditional MRI machines look like a long, narrow tunnel. Newer MRI machines called short-bore systems are shorter, wider, and don't completely surround you. Some of the newer machines are open on all sides. Your doctor will help decide which machine type is best for you.

Cardiac MRI is painless and harmless. You will lie on your back on a sliding table that goes inside the tunnel-like machine. The technician will control the machine from the next room. He or she will be able to see you through a glass window and will be able to talk to you through an intercom system. Tell the technician if you have a hearing problem.

The MRI machine makes loud humming, tapping, and buzzing noises. Earplugs may help lessen the noises made by the MRI machine. Some facilities let you listen to music during the test.

Remaining very still during the test is important. Any movement may blur the images. If you're unable to lie still, you may be given medicine to help you relax. You may be asked to hold your breath for 10 to 15 seconds at a time while the technician takes pictures of your heart. Researchers are studying ways that will allow someone having a cardiac MRI to breathe freely during the exam, while achieving the same image quality.

A contrast dye, such as gadolinium, may be used to highlight your blood vessels or heart in the images. Contrast dye is usually injected into a vein in your arm with a needle. You may feel a cool sensation during the injection, and you may feel discomfort where the needle was inserted. Gadolinium doesn't contain iodine so it won't create problems for people who are allergic to iodine.

If your cardiac MRI includes a stress test to detect blockages in your coronary arteries, you will receive other medicines to increase the blood flow in your heart or to increase how fast your heart beats.

What to Expect after Cardiac MRI

Once the cardiac magnetic resonance imaging (MRI) is done, if you haven't received medicine to help you relax, you will be able to return to normal activities immediately.

If you did receive medicine to help you relax during the test, your doctor will tell you when you can return to normal activities. You will need someone to drive you home.

What Does Cardiac MRI Show?

The doctor supervising your scan will provide your doctor with the results of your cardiac MRI. Your doctor will discuss the findings with you.

Cardiac MRI can reveal various heart conditions and disorders, such as the following:

- Coronary artery disease
- Damage caused by a heart attack
- Heart failure
- Heart valve problems
- Congenital heart defects
- Pericardial disease (a disease that affects the tissues around the heart)
- Cardiac tumors

Cardiac MRI is a fast, accurate tool that can help diagnose a heart attack by detecting areas of the heart that don't move normally, have poor blood supply, or are scarred. Cardiac MRI can show whether any of the coronary arteries are blocked, causing reduced blood flow to your heart muscle.

Currently, coronary angiography is the procedure most commonly used to look at blockages in the coronary arteries. Coronary angiography is an invasive procedure that uses x-rays and iodine-based contrast dye. Researchers have found that cardiac MRI can replace coronary angiography in some cases, avoiding the need to use x-ray radiation and iodine-based dyes.

Researchers are discovering new ways to use cardiac MRI. In the future, cardiac MRI may be able to replace x-rays as the main way to guide invasive procedures such as cardiac catheterization. Also, improvements in cardiac MRI are likely to lead to better methods for detecting heart disease in the future.

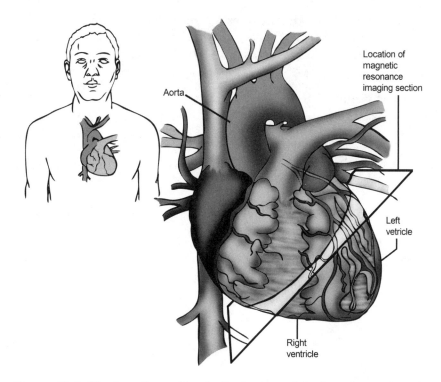

Figure 29.1. *The heart's position in the body and the location and angle of a example cross-sectional image of the heart.*

What Are the Risks of Cardiac MRI?

Cardiac magnetic resonance imaging (MRI) produces no side effects from the magnetic fields and radio waves. This method of obtaining images of organs and tissues doesn't carry a risk of causing cancer or birth defects.

Serious reactions to the special contrast dyes used for MRI are very rare. However, side effects are possible and include the following:

- Headache
- Nausea
- Dizziness
- Changes in taste
- Allergic reactions

Rarely, the contrast dyes can be harmful in patients with severe kidney disease.

If your cardiac MRI includes a stress test, more medicines will be used during the test. These medicines may have additional side effects such as the following that aren't expected during a regular MRI scan:

- Arrhythmias (irregular heartbeats)
- Chest pain
- Shortness of breath
- Palpitations (a sensation of the heart beating hard or fast)

Section 29.3

MR Angiography

Magnetic resonance imaging (MRI) is a method of producing extremely detailed pictures of body tissues and organs without the need for x-rays. The electromagnetic energy that is released when exposing a patient to radio waves in a strong magnetic field is measured and analyzed by a computer, which forms two- or three-dimensional images that may be viewed on a TV monitor. MR angiography (MRA) is an MRI study of the blood vessels. The procedure is performed in the MRI machine so it uses MRI technology to detect, diagnose, and aid the treatment of heart disorders, stroke, and blood vessel diseases. MRA provides detailed images of blood vessels without using any contrast material, although today a special form of contrast usually is given to make the MRI images even clearer. The procedure is painless, and the magnetic field is not known to cause tissue damage of any kind.

What are some common uses of the procedure?

- Many patients with arterial disease now have it treated in the radiology department rather than undergoing surgery in an operating room. MRA is a very useful way of finding problems with blood vessels and determining how to best to treat those problems.

- The carotid arteries in the neck that conduct blood to the brain are a common site of atherosclerosis, which may severely narrow or block off an artery, reducing blood flow to the brain and even causing a stroke. If an ultrasound study shows that such disease is present, many surgeons now will do the necessary operation after confirmation by MRA, doing away with the need for catheter angiography.

- MRA has found wide use in checking patients for diseased intracranial (in the head) arteries, so that only those with positive findings will need to have a more invasive catheter study.

- MRA also is used to detect disease in the aorta and in blood vessels supplying the kidneys, lungs, and legs.

- Patients with a family history of arterial aneurysm, a ballooning out of a segment of the vessel wall, can be screened by MRA to see if they have a similar disorder that has not produced symptoms. If an aneurysm is found, it may be eliminated surgically, possibly avoiding serious or fatal bleeding.

How should I prepare for the procedure?

The magnetic field used for MRA will pull on any ferromagnetic metal object in the body, such as a heart pacemaker, intrauterine device, vascular access port, metal plate, or pins, screws, or staples. You will be given a questionnaire to answer regarding these issues. The radiologist or technologist should know about any such item and also whether you have ever had a bullet in your body, whether you ever worked with metals, or if you have had a joint replacement. If there is any question, an x-ray can be taken to detect metal objects. The radiologist also should know if you have fillings in your teeth, which could distort images of the facial region or brain. Braces make it harder to properly adjust the MRI unit. You will be asked to remove hairpins, jewelry, eyeglasses, hearing aids, and any dental work that can be taken out. Some wigs contain metal and must be removed. Red dyes used in tattoos and permanent eyeliner may contain metallic iron, but this is rarely a problem. You should report any drug allergies to the radiologist or technologist, and should mention if there's any possibility that you might be pregnant.

You can eat normally before the exam unless you are instructed otherwise. Medications may be taken as usual. Some patients will feel uncomfortably confined (claustrophobic) when enclosed in an MRI unit. You should discuss this with your physician prior to your exam. If necessary, a mild sedative may be prescribed to help easy your anxiety.

What does the equipment look like?

The traditional MRI unit is a large tube surrounded by a circular magnet, in which the patient lies without moving for the duration of the scan. In recent years patient-friendly units have been designed, and examination in such units is becoming increasingly available.

An MRI uses high field-strength magnets and special coils to produce detailed images of body tissues without the use of x-rays. A moving table will position you inside a hollow tube that is open at both ends at all times. You will hear a series of loud, "knocking" sounds. This is the instrument positioning its internal components to get the very best view. You can listen to music or use the earplugs provided, and the technologist will communicate with you throughout the 30–45 minute procedure.

How does the procedure work?

Exposing the patient to radio waves in a strong magnetic field generates data that are used by a computer to create images of tissue slices that may be viewed in any plane or from any direction. The magnetic field lines up atomic particles called protons in the tissues, which are then spun by a beam of radio waves and produce signals that are picked up by a receiver in the scanner. It is these signals that are processed by the computer to produce images. The resulting images are very sharp and detailed, and so are able to detect tiny changes from the normal pattern that are caused by disease or injury. Special settings are used to image various structures, such as arteries in the case of MRA.

How is the procedure performed?

The patient is placed on a special table and positioned inside the opening of the MRI unit. A typical exam consists of two to six imaging sequences, each taking two to 15 minutes. Each sequence provides a specific image orientation and a specified degree of image clarity or contrast. Depending on the type of exam being done, the total time needed can range from 10 to 60 minutes, not counting the time needed to change clothing, have an IV put in, and answer questions. When contrast material is needed, a substance called gadolinium is given by IV injection during one of the imaging sequences. It highlights blood vessels, making them stand out from surrounding tissues.

What will I experience during the procedure?

The technologist will make you as comfortable as possible. For those who become very uncomfortable when enclosed in a small space, a mild sedative is nearly always effective. Speak to your physician about your discomfort in small spaces before you go into the exam. You may notice a warm feeling in the area being studied. This is normal, but do not hesitate to report it if it bothers you. The loud tapping or knocking noises that are heard during certain parts of the exam disturb some patients; earplugs are provided to reduce this noise.

Who interprets the results and how do I get them?

A radiologist experienced in MRI will analyze the results and send a report to your physician, along with an interpretation of the findings. Your physician in turn will discuss the MRA findings with you. Some centers now send diagnostic reports and images over the internet, speeding up the process.

Section 29.4

Abdominal MRI

© 2008 A.D.A.M., Inc. Reprinted with permission.

Abdominal magnetic resonance imaging (MRI) is a noninvasive test that uses powerful magnets and radio waves to create pictures of the inside of the belly area. It does not use radiation (x-rays).

How the Test Is Performed

You will be asked to lie on a narrow table, which slides into a large tunnel-like tube. The health care provider may inject a dye through one of your veins. This helps certain diseases and organs show up better on the images. Small devices, called coils, may be placed around certain body areas to be studied. They also help produce better images.

Unlike and computed tomographic (CT) scans, MRI does not use radiation. Instead, it uses powerful magnets and radio waves. The magnetic field produced by an MRI forces certain atoms in your body to line up in a certain way. It's similar to how the needle on a compass moves when you hold it near a magnet.

The radio waves are sent toward these atoms and bounce back, and a computer records the signal. Different types of tissues send back different signals. For example, healthy tissue sends back a slightly different signal than cancerous tissue.

A technologist will operate the machine from a room next door and watch you during the entire study.

Several sets of images are usually needed. Each one takes about two to 15 minutes. A complete scan may take up to one hour. Newer scanners may complete the process in less time.

How to Prepare for the Test

There is usually no preparation needed, unless your doctor says you must clean out your bowels. This is often done using a laxative or enema.

You may be asked to wear a hospital gown.

The strong magnetic fields created during an MRI can interfere with certain implants, particularly cardiac pacemakers. People with cardiac pacemakers can not have an MRI and should not enter the MRI area.

If you have any of the following metallic objects in your body, you should not get an MRI:

- Brain aneurysm clips

- Certain artificial heart valves

- Inner ear (cochlear) implants

- Older vascular stents

- Recently placed artificial joints

You will be asked to sign a consent form that says you do not have any of these items in your body.

Before an MRI, sheet metal workers or any person that may have been exposed to small metal fragments should receive a skull x-ray to check for metal in the eyes.

MRI can easily be performed through clothing. However, because the magnet is very, very strong, certain types of metal can cause significant errors, called artifacts, in the images. Also, certain metallic objects are not allowed into the room.

- Items such as jewelry, watches, credit cards, and hearing aids can be damaged.

- Pins, hairpins, metal zippers, and similar metallic items can distort the images.

- Removable dental work should be taken out just prior to the scan.

The MRI magnet is always turned on. Pens, pocketknives, and eyeglasses may fly across the room if they are too close to the magnet.

391

This can be dangerous, so such items are not allowed into the scanner area.

How the Test Will Feel

An MRI exam causes no pain. Some people may become anxious when inside the scanner. If you have difficulty lying still or are very anxious, you may be given a mild sedative. Excessive movement can blur MRI images and cause errors.

The table may be hard or cold, but you can request a blanket or pillow. The machine produces loud thumping and humming noises when turned on. Ear plugs are usually given to help reduce the noise.

An intercom in the scanner allows you to speak to the person operating the exam at any time. Some MRIs have televisions and special headphones that you can use to help the time pass.

There is no recovery time, unless sedation was necessary. After an MRI scan, you can resume your normal diet, activity, and medications.

Why the Test Is Performed

An abdominal MRI provides detailed pictures of the belly area from many different views. It is often used to clarify findings from previous x-rays or CT scans.

This test may be used to diagnose or evaluate:

- Abnormal growths and tumors
- Blood flow
- Blood vessels
- Lymph nodes
- How certain organs work

MRI can distinguish tumors from normal tissues and can help the doctor determine the tumor's size, severity, and spread. This is called staging.

MRI is sometimes used to avoid the dangers of angiography, repeated radiation exposure, iodine-related allergic reactions.

What Abnormal Results Mean

The sensitivity of MRI depends, in part, on the experience of the radiologist.

Abdominal MRI may reveal many medical conditions, including the following:

- Abscess
- Acute tubular necrosis
- Adrenal masses
- Cancer
- Enlarged spleen or liver
- Gallbladder or bile duct problems
- Gallstones, bile duct stones
- Glomerulonephritis (inflammation of the kidney glomeruli)
- Hemangiomas, or others
- Hydronephrosis (kidney enlargement from reflux of urine)
- Kidney damage
- Lymphadenopathy (abnormalities of the lymph nodes)
- Obstructed vena cava
- Pancreatic cancer
- Portal vein obstruction (liver)
- Renal arterial obstruction
- Renal vein thrombosis
- Transplant rejection
- Tumor of the gallbladder

Additional conditions under which the test may be performed:

- Abdominal aortic aneurysm
- Acute renal failure
- Adenomyosis
- Atheroembolic renal disease
- Carcinoma of the renal pelvis or ureter
- Chronic renal failure
- Cystinuria
- Hydatidiform mole
- Injury of the kidney and ureter

- Insulinoma
- Islet of Langerhans tumor
- Medullary cystic disease
- Multiple endocrine neoplasia (MEN) II
- Multiple endocrine neoplasia (MEN) I
- Nephrolithiasis
- Ovarian cancer
- Pheochromocytoma
- Skin lesion of histoplasmosis

Risks

There is no ionizing radiation involved in MRI, and there have been no documented significant side effects of the magnetic fields and radio waves used on the human body to date.

The most common type of contrast (dye) used is gadolinium. It is very safe. Allergic reactions to the substance rarely occur. The person operating the machine will monitor your heart rate and breathing as needed.

People have been harmed in MRI machines when they did not remove metal objects from their clothes or when metal objects were left in the room by others.

MRI is usually not recommended for acute trauma situations, because traction and life-support equipment cannot safely enter the scanner area and scan times are relatively lengthy.

Section 29.5

MRI of the Skeletal System

What is MR imaging (MRI) of the musculoskeletal system?

MRI (magnetic resonance imaging) uses radio waves and a strong magnetic field rather than x-rays to provide clear and detailed pictures of internal organs and tissues. The parts of the musculoskeletal system that are most frequently imaged with MRI are the knee and shoulder. However, MRI has also been used to study almost every joint in the body, including the spine, hips, wrists, and hands. MRI requires specialized equipment and expertise and allows evaluation of some body structures that may not be as visible with other imaging methods.

What are some common uses of the procedure?

Because MRI can give such clear pictures of soft tissue structures near and around bones, it is usually the best choice for examination of the body's major joints, the spine for disk disease, and soft tissues of the extremities. MRI is widely used to diagnose sports-related injuries, as well as work-related disorders caused by repeated strain, vibration, or forceful impact.

Using MRI images, physicians can locate and identify the cause of pain, swelling, or bleeding in the tissues in and around the joints and bones. The images allow the physician to clearly see even very small tears and injuries to tendons, ligaments and muscles, and even some fractures that cannot be seen on x-rays.

In addition, MRI images can give physicians a clear picture of degenerative disorders such as arthritis, deterioration of joint surfaces, or a herniated disc. Neurosurgeons often use MRI to evaluate the integrity of the spinal cord after trauma.

Finally, MRI is also useful for the diagnosis and characterization of infections (for example osteomyelitis) and tumors (for example metastases) involving bones and joints.

How should I prepare for the procedure?

Because the strong magnetic field used for MRI will pull on any ferromagnetic metal object implanted in the body, MRI staff will ask whether you have a prosthetic hip, an aneurysm clip in the brain, heart pacemaker (or artificial heart valve), implanted port (brand names Port-o-cath, Infusaport, Lifeport), intrauterine device (IUD), or any metal plates, pins, screws, or surgical staples in your body. In most cases, surgical staples, plates, pins, and screws pose no risk during MRI if they have been in place for more than four to six weeks. Dyes used in tattoos and permanent eyeliner may contain metallic iron oxide and could heat up during MRI; however, this is rare. You will be asked if you have ever had a bullet or shrapnel in your body, or ever worked with metal. If there is any question of metal fragments, especially in the orbit, you may be asked to have an x-ray that will detect any such metal objects. Tooth fillings usually are not affected by the magnetic field, but they may distort images of the facial area or brain, so the radiologist should be aware of them. The same is true of braces, which may make it hard to "tune" the MRI unit to your body. You will be asked to remove anything that might degrade MRI images of the head, including hairpins, jewelry, eyeglasses, hearing aids, and any removable dental work.

The technologist may ask if you have any drug allergies and whether you have undergone any surgery in the past. If you are or might be pregnant, mention it to the MRI staff.

Some patients who undergo MRI in an enclosed unit may feel confined or claustrophobic. You should discuss this with your physician prior to your MRI exam. A mild sedative may be prescribed to help ease your anxiety.

What does the equipment look like?

The conventional MRI unit is a closed cylindrical magnet in which the patient must lie totally still for several seconds at a time, and consequently may feel "closed-in" or truly claustrophobic. However new "patient-friendly" designs are rapidly coming into routine use. The "short-bore" systems are wider and shorter and do not fully enclose the patient.

An MRI uses high field-strength magnets and special coils to produce detailed images of body tissues without the use of x-rays. A moving table will position you inside a hollow tube that is open at both ends at all times. You will hear a series of loud, "knocking" sounds. This is the instrument positioning its internal components to get the very best view. You can listen to music or use the earplugs provided, and the technologist will communicate with you throughout the 30–45 minute procedure.

How does the procedure work?

MRI is a unique imaging method because, unlike the usual radiographs (x-rays), radioisotope studies, and even CT, it does not rely on ionizing radiation. Instead, radio waves are directed at protons, the nuclei of hydrogen atoms, in a strong magnetic field. The protons are first "excited" and then "relaxed," emitting radio signals, which can be computer-processed to form an image. In the body, protons are most abundant in the hydrogen atoms of water—the "H" of H_2O—so that an MRI image shows differences in the water content and distribution in various body tissues. Even different types of tissue within the same organ, such as the gray and white matter of the brain, can easily be distinguished. Typically an MRI exam consists of two to six imaging sequences, each lasting two to 15 minutes. Each sequence has its own degree of contrast and shows a cross section of the body in one of several planes (right to left, front to back, upper to lower).

How is the procedure performed?

The patient is comfortably positioned on a special table which slides into the MRI system opening where the magnetic field is created. Then the technologist leaves the room and the individual MRI sequences are performed. The patient will hear tapping noises during the exam. The tapping is created when magnetic field gradient coils are switched on and off to measure the MRI signal reflecting back out of the patient's body. The patient is able to communicate with the technologist at any time using an intercom.

Depending on how many images are needed, the exam will generally take from 15 to 45 minutes, although a very detailed study may take longer. You will be asked not to move during the actual imaging process, but between sequences some movement is allowed. Patients are generally required to remain still for only a few seconds to a few minutes at a time.

Depending on the part of the body being examined, a contrast material may be used to enhance the visibility of certain tissues or blood vessels.

What will I experience during the procedure?

MRI causes no pain, but some patients can find it uncomfortable to remain still during the examination. Others experience a sense of being "closed in," though the more open construction of newer MRI systems has done much to reduce that reaction. You may notice a warm feeling in the area under examination; this is normal, but if it bothers you, the radiologist or technologist should be told. If an injection of contrast material is needed, there may be discomfort at the injection site, and you may have a cool sensation at the site during the injection. Most bothersome to many patients are the loud tapping or knocking noises heard at certain phases of imaging. Ear plugs are provided to reduce the noise.

Who interprets the results and how do I get them?

A radiologist, who is a physician experienced in MRI and other radiology examinations, will analyze the images and send a signed report with his or her interpretation to the patient's personal physician. The personal physician's office will inform the patient on how to obtain their results. New technology also allows for distribution of diagnostic reports and referral images over the internet at some facilities.

Section 29.6

MRI of the Head

What is MR imaging (MRI) of the head?

MRI (magnetic resonance imaging) uses radio waves and a strong magnetic field rather than x-rays to provide remarkably clear and detailed pictures of internal organs and tissues. This technique has proved very helpful to radiologists in diagnosing tumors of the brain as well as disorders of the eyes and the inner ear. It requires specialized equipment and expertise and allows evaluation of some body structures that may not be as visible with other imaging methods.

What are some common uses of the procedure?

MRI is the most sensitive exam for brain tumors, strokes, and certain chronic disorders of the nervous system such as multiple sclerosis. In addition, it is a useful means of documenting brain abnormalities in patients with dementia, and it is commonly used for patients with disease of the pituitary gland. MRI can detect tiny areas of tissue abnormality in patients with disease of the eyes or the inner ear.

How should I prepare for the procedure?

Because the strong magnetic field used for MRI will pull on any ferromagnetic metal object implanted in the body, MRI staff will ask whether you have a prosthetic hip, heart pacemaker (or artificial heart valve), implanted port (brand names Port-o-cath, Infusaport, Lifeport), intrauterine device (IUD), or any metal plates, pins, screws, or surgical staples in your body. Tattoos and permanent eyeliner may also create a problem. You will be asked if you have ever had a bullet or shrapnel in your body, or ever worked with metal. If there is any question of metal fragments, you may be asked to have an x-ray that will

399

detect any such metal objects. Tooth fillings usually are not affected by the magnetic field, but they may distort images of the facial area or brain, so the radiologist should be aware of them. The same is true of braces, which may make it hard to "tune" the MRI unit to your body. You will be asked to remove anything that might degrade MRI images of the head, including hairpins, jewelry, eyeglasses, hearing aids, and any removable dental work.

What does the equipment look like?

The conventional MRI unit is a closed cylindrical magnet in which the patient must lie still, and consequently may feel "closed-in" or truly claustrophobic. However new "patient-friendly" designs are rapidly coming into routine use. Frederick Memorial Healthcare (FMH) offers the "short-bore" systems which are wider and shorter and do not fully enclose the patient.

An MRI uses high field-strength magnets and special coils to produce detailed images of body tissues without the use of x-rays. A moving table will position you inside a hollow tube that is open at both ends at all times. You will hear a series of loud, "knocking" sounds. This is the instrument positioning its internal components to get the very best view. You can listen to music or use the earplugs provided, and the technologist will communicate with you throughout the 30–45 minute procedure.

How does the procedure work?

MRI is a unique imaging method because, unlike the usual radiographs (x-rays), radioisotope studies, and even CT scanning, it does not rely on radiation. Instead, radio waves are directed at protons, the nuclei of hydrogen atoms, in a strong magnetic field. The protons are first "excited" and then "relaxed," emitting radio signals, which can be computer-processed to form an image.

In the body, protons are most abundant in the hydrogen atoms of water—the "H" of H_2O—so that an MRI image shows differences in the water content and distribution in various body tissues. Even different types of tissue within the same organ, such as the gray and white matter of the brain, can easily be distinguished. Typically an MRI exam consists of two to six imaging sequences, each lasting two to 15 minutes. Each sequence has its own degree of contrast and shows a cross section of the head in one of several planes (right to left, front to back, upper to lower).

400

How is the procedure performed?

The patient is placed on a sliding table and a radio antenna device called a surface coil is positioned around the upper part of the head. After positioning the patient with the head inside the MRI gantry, the technologist leaves the room and the individual MRI sequences are performed. The patient is able to communicate with the technologist at any time using an intercom.

Depending on how many images are needed, the exam will generally take from 15 to 45 minutes, although a very detailed study may take longer. You will be asked not to move during the actual imaging process, but between sequences some movement is allowed. Some patients will require an injection of a contrast material to enhance the visibility of certain tissues or blood vessels. A small needle connected to an intravenous line is placed in an arm or hand vein.

What will I experience during the procedure?

MRI causes no pain, but there may be discomfort from being closed in or from the need to remain still. You may notice a warm feeling in the area under examination. This is normal, but if it bothers you the radiologist or technologist should be told. If a contrast injection is needed, there may be discomfort at the injection site, and you may have a cool sensation at the site during the injection. Most bothersome to many patients are the loud tapping or knocking noises heard at certain phases of imaging. Ear plugs will be provided.

Who interprets the results and how do I get them?

A radiologist, who is a physician experienced in MRI and other radiology examinations, will analyze the images and send a signed report with his or her interpretation to the patient's personal physician. The personal physician's office will inform the patient on how to obtain their results.

Chapter 30

Nuclear Imaging Tests

Chapter Contents

Section 30.1

Nuclear Medicine: An Overview

From "Common Imaging Tests," © 2008 Sue Stiles Program in Integrative Oncology at the University of California Los Angeles Jonsson Comprehensive Cancer Center (www.canceralternatives.com). Reprinted with permission.

Radiological studies—x-rays and CT scans—send radiation from an exterior source through the body to be detected and recorded on film or by computer. Nuclear medicine studies are based on a reverse principle, a radioactive substance is introduced into the body (orally or intravenously by injection or by inhalation for some lung studies). The radioactive substance emits gamma rays (similar to x-rays, although with a shorter wavelength) as it travels through the body. A device known as a gamma camera detects the gamma rays, which are converted into a computer signal and reconstructed as an image.

The radioactive substances (called radionuclides) are formulated to be temporarily collected by the specific part of the body being studied. As the radionuclide is taken up by organs in the body, faint radiation signals are emitted and detected by the gamma camera's scintillation crystal. The scintillation crystal converts the radiation signal into faint light, which is in turn converted to an electric signal. The electric signal is then digitized (converted to a computer signal) and reconstructed as an image. The image can be viewed on a monitor and imaged on film or saved on a disk.

The images produced by nuclear medicine studies show not only the anatomy or structure of an organ or other body part, but also the functioning of the organ. The radionuclides introduced into the body for nuclear medicine studies are absorbed at varying rates or in different concentrations by different tissue types. (For example, the thyroid gland absorbs more radioactive iodine than other tissues.) The amount of radionuclide absorbed and then emitted by tissues is linked to the cellular function (metabolic activity) of that tissue. Where cancer is present or suspected, cells which are dividing rapidly, like cancer tissue cells, will been seen as "hot spots" of metabolic activity since such cells will absorb more of the radionuclide. Also, diseased or poorly functioning tissue emits a signal different from that emitted by healthy tissue, thus giving an indication of pathology sooner than other forms of imaging. This early indication of pathology is the result of the propensity of disease to affect the function of the tissue before it affects the anatomy of that tissue.

Nuclear Medicine Imaging

Nuclear medicine imaging allows visualization of organs and portions within organs that cannot be visualized on conventional x-ray images. Space occupying lesions (an injury or abnormality) stand out on nuclear medicine images, being seen as "cold spots" or areas of reduced radioactivity and indicative of abnormal tissue function. By contrast, rapidly dividing cells, often indicative of cancerous tissue, appear as "hot spots" because of increased radioactivity.

Nuclear medicine imaging can show the function of a variety of organs and parts of the body:

- **Abdomen:** To test for gastrointestinal bleeding or bowel obstruction.

- **Blood:** To test for blood cell disorders.

- **Bone:** To test for bony metastases or degenerative arthritis.

- **Brain:** To image tumors or aneurysms and evaluate stroke.

- **Breast:** To image breast tumors.

- **Heart:** To check for coronary artery disease, myocardial infarction, or valve disease.

- **Hepatobiliary system:** To test gallbladder and bile duct function.

- **Kidneys:** To test renal function, detect renal tumors.

- **Liver and spleen:** To test for cirrhosis or metastatic disease.

- **Lung:** To test for pulmonary embolism, lung tumors, or metastatic disease.

- **Lymph system:** To test for the spread of cancer to the lymph nodes (lymphadenopathy).

- **Stomach:** To test stomach function or to confirm peptic ulcer or gastric cancer.

- **Thyroid and parathyroid:** To test for abnormal function or tumor.

Procedures for nuclear medicine imaging studies are broadly similar regardless of the type of study.

- Some studies require preparation in advance of the study, such as fasting or ingesting pharmaceuticals prior to the study.

- On arrival the patient will be asked to remove clothing or jewelry that might interfere with the imaging process. In some instances, the patient is asked to wear a gown.

- Patients should tell the physician or technologist if any prosthetic implants are present in the body, of all current medications, of any allergies, of any chronic conditions such as diabetes.

- Pregnant or nursing women should consult their physician prior to any imaging study.

- A pharmaceutical radionuclide is administered either orally, by intravenous injection, or inhalation (for lung imaging). The type and dose of radionuclide administered is based upon the organ to be imaged and the patient's body weight.

- In many studies, the patient is imaged shortly after the administration of the radionuclide. In some studies, such as a bone scan, there is a waiting period between administration of the radionuclide and the actual study. A few studies, such as a gallium scan, require that the radionuclide be administered the day before the study. Since different organs and systems absorb the pharmaceutical radionuclides differently, waiting times vary.

- Immediately before imaging begins the patient is placed on an examination table or, for some studies seated in a chair, and the gamma camera is placed in position over the area to be imaged. In some studies such as PET, the examining table passes through a doughnut hole-like aperture similar to a CT scanner. The patient is asked to relax and remain still through the course of the study. The duration of nuclear medicine studies varies from 15 to 60 minutes.

- At the conclusion of the study, the images are reviewed, and if no further images are needed, the patient is free to leave.

- The low level radioactivity is retained for a relatively short period. The radioactive energy will dissipate on its own, and is eliminated from the body through excretion. There are no reported side effects to nuclear medicine imaging.

Bone Scan

This study creates a "picture" of the complete skeletal system. The patient receives an injection of the radioactive tracer. Approximately two hours later, the scan is performed. When completed, abnormalities of the bony structure appear as "uptakes" or "hot spots," which may indicate the presence of tumor, or may be the result of other causes, such as arthritis. The bone scan is also useful for analysis of bony healing. No preparation is required. During the two hour interval between the injection and the scan the patient is free to do as desired. The scan itself lasts about 45 minutes.

Gallium Scan

A study of the mediastinum (the cavity around the lungs) using radioactive Gallium 67, used for patients with an history of lung disease or lymphoma to rule out the presence of residual disease in the thoracic cavity. No preparation is required. The patient is injected on day one, and returns after 48 or 72 hours for imaging. The imaging time is less than 30 minutes.

MUGA Scan (Multiple Gated Radionuclide Cardiac Scan)

A study to assess cardiac function, particularly left ventricle ejection fraction. Requested prior to and following certain chemotherapy regimens with possible cardiac effects in some patients. No preparation is required. Imaging time is about 30 minutes.

PET Scan (Positron Emission Tomography)

Creates "pictures" showing the body's metabolism and other biological functions. The patient is injected with a small amount of glucose tagged with a radioactive tracer. About one hour after injection, the patient is scanned. As the glucose compound is distributed and processed throughout the body, the scanner detects the radioactive tag and shows its metabolic activity within all organ systems. PET provides information for evidence of the location of malignancy, the effect of treatment, and recurrence of disease. Patients may drink small amounts of black coffee, clear tea, or water before the scan but may not eat solid food within six hours prior to the scan. Imaging time is less than one hour.

Section 30.2

Positron Emission Tomography (PET Scan)

What is positron emission tomography?

Positron emission tomography, also called PET imaging or a PET scan, is a diagnostic examination that involves the acquisition of physiologic images based on the detection of subatomic particles. These particles are emitted from a radioactive substance given to the patient. The subsequent views of the human body are used to evaluate function.

PET Scans use a technology that is completely different from either the CT Scan (x-ray), or the MRI. P.E.T. stands for positron emission tomography—and once again, as it images your body's soft tissues—it sends back images that tell the physician how certain clusters of cells may—or may not—be behaving. The procedure does require the injection of a radio isotope in a sugar solution, and while the injection may be only momentarily uncomfortable—the scan itself is quite unremarkable.

What are some common uses of the procedure?

PET scans are used most often to detect cancer and to examine the effects of cancer therapy by characterizing biochemical changes in the cancer. These scans are performed on the whole body. PET scans of the heart can be used to determine blood flow to the heart muscle and help evaluate signs of coronary artery disease. Combined with a myocardial metabolism study, PET scans differentiate non-functioning heart muscle from heart muscle that would benefit from a procedure, such as angioplasty or coronary artery bypass surgery, which would re-establish adequate blood flow. PET scans of the brain are used to evaluate patients who have memory disorders of an undetermined cause; who have suspected or proven brain tumors; or who have seizure disorders that are not responsive to medical therapy, and therefore, are candidates for surgery.

How should I prepare for the procedure?

PET is usually done on an outpatient basis. Your doctor will give you detailed instructions on how to prepare for your examination. You should wear comfortable, loose-fitting clothes. You should not eat for four hours before the scan. You will be encouraged to drink water. Your doctor will instruct you regarding the use of medications before the test.

Note: Diabetic patients should discuss specific diet guidelines to control glucose levels during the day of the test.

What does the equipment look like?

You will be taken to an examination room that houses the PET scanner, which has a hole in the middle and looks like a large, doughnut. Within this machine are multiple rings of detectors that record the emission of energy from the radioactive substance in your body. While lying on a cushioned examination table, you will be moved into the hole of the machine. The images are displayed on the monitor of a nearby computer, which is similar in appearance to the personal computer you may have in your home.

How does the procedure work?

Before the examination begins, a radioactive substance is produced in a machine called a cyclotron and attached, or tagged, to a natural body compound, most commonly glucose, but sometimes water or ammonia. This process is called radiolabeling. Once this attached substance is administered to the patient, the radioactivity localizes in the appropriate areas of the body and is detected by the PET scanner.

Different colors or degrees of brightness on a PET image represent different levels of tissue or organ function. For example, because healthy tissue uses glucose for energy, it accumulates some of the radiolabeled glucose, which will show up on the PET images. However, cancerous tissue, which uses more glucose than normal tissue, will absorb more of the substance and appear brighter than normal tissue on the PET images.

Scientifically speaking, the radioactive substance decay leads to the ejection of positive particles called positrons. A positron travels about one to two millimeters before colliding with an electron. The collision results in a conversion from mass to energy, resulting in the emission of two gamma rays heading off in exact opposite directions.

Special crystals, called photomultiplier-scintillator detectors, within the PET scanner detect the gamma rays. The scanner's special camera records the millions of gamma rays being emitted, and a connected computer uses the information and complicated mathematical formulas, called algorithms, to map an image of the area where the radioactive substance has accumulated.

How is the procedure performed?

A technologist will take you into a special PET examination room. You will lie down on an examination table and be given the radioactive substance as an intravenous injection (although, in some cases, it will be given through an existing intravenous line). It will then take approximately 30 to 60 minutes for the substance to travel through your body and be absorbed by the tissue under study. During this time, you will be asked to rest quietly in a partially darkened room and to avoid significant movement or talking, which may alter the localization of the administered substance. After that time, scanning begins. This takes an additional 30 to 45 minutes.

Some patients, specifically those with heart disease, may undergo a stress test in which PET scans are obtained while they are at rest, then after undergoing the administration of a pharmaceutical to alter the blood flow to the heart.

Usually, there are no restrictions on daily routine after the test, although you should drink plenty of fluids to flush the radioactive substance from your body.

What will I experience during the procedure?

The administration of the radioactive substance will feel like a slight pinprick if given by intravenous injection. You will then be made as comfortable as possible on the examination table before you are positioned in the PET scanner for the test. You will be asked to remain still for the duration of the examination. You will not feel anything related to the radioactivity of the substance in your body.

Who interprets the results and how do I get them?

Patients undergo PET because their referring physician has recommended it. A radiologist who has specialized training in PET will interpret the images and forward a report to your referring physician. It usually takes one to three days to interpret, report, and deliver the results.

Section 30.3

Nuclear Heart Scan

National Heart Lung and Blood Institute, July 2007.

What is a nuclear heart scan?

A nuclear heart scan is a type of medical test that allows your doctor to get important information about the health of your heart. During a nuclear heart scan, a safe, radioactive material called a tracer is injected through a vein into your bloodstream. The tracer then travels to your heart. The tracer releases energy, which special cameras outside of your body detect. The cameras use the energy to create pictures of different parts of your heart.

Nuclear heart scans are used for three main purposes:

- To provide information about the flow of blood throughout the heart muscle. If the scan shows that one part of the heart muscle isn't receiving blood, it's a sign of a possible narrowing or blockage in the coronary arteries (the arteries that supply blood and oxygen to your heart). Decreased blood flow through the coronary arteries may mean you have coronary artery disease (CAD). CAD can lead to angina, heart attack, and other heart problems. When a nuclear heart scan is performed for this purpose, it's called myocardial perfusion scanning.

- To look for damaged heart muscle. Damage may be due to a previous heart attack, injury, infection, or medicine. When a nuclear heart scan is performed for this purpose, it's called myocardial viability testing.

- To see how well your heart pumps blood out to your body. When a nuclear heart scan is performed for this purpose, it's called ventricular function scanning.

Usually, two sets of pictures are taken during a nuclear heart scan. The first set is taken when the heart is beating fast due to you exercising. This is called a cardiac stress test. If you can't exercise, your heart rate can be increased using medicines such as adenosine, dipyridamole, or dobutamine.

The second set of pictures is taken later, when the heart is at rest and beating at a normal rate.

What are the types of nuclear heart scanning?

There are two main types of nuclear heart scanning:

- Single positron emission computed tomography (SPECT)
- Cardiac positron emission tomography (PET)

SPECT is the most well-established and widely used type, while PET is newer. There are specific reasons for using each, which are discussed in the following paragraphs.

Single positron emission computed tomography: Cardiac SPECT is the most commonly used nuclear scanning test for diagnosing coronary artery disease (CAD). Combining SPECT with a cardiac stress test can show problems with blood flow to the heart that can be detected only when the heart is working hard and beating fast.

SPECT also is used to look for areas of damaged or dead heart muscle tissue, which may be due to a previous heart attack or other cause of injury.

SPECT also can show how well the heart's left ventricle pumps blood to the body. Weak pumping ability may be the result of heart attack, heart failure, and other causes.

The most commonly used tracers in SPECT are called thallium-201, technetium-99m sestamibi (Cardiolite®), and technetium-99m tetrofosmin (Myoview™).

Positron emission tomography: PET uses different kinds of tracers than SPECT. PET can provide more detailed pictures of the heart. However, PET is newer and has some technical limits that make it less available than SPECT. Research into advances in both SPECT and PET is ongoing. Right now, there is no clear cut advantage of using one over the other in all situations.

PET can be used for the same purposes as SPECT—to diagnose CAD, check for damaged or dead heart muscle, and evaluate the heart's pumping strength.

PET takes a clearer picture through thick layers of tissue (such as abdominal or breast tissue). PET also is better than SPECT at showing whether CAD is affecting more than one of your heart's blood vessels. A PET scan also may be used if a SPECT scan wasn't able to produce good enough pictures.

What are other names for nuclear heart scans?

- Nuclear stress test
- SPECT scan
- PET scan

What should I expect before a nuclear heart scan?

Talk to your doctor about how the nuclear heart scan is done. Discussing your overall health, including health problems such as asthma, chronic obstructive pulmonary disease (COPD), diabetes, and kidney disease, is important. If you have lung disease or diabetes, your doctor will give you special instructions before the nuclear heart scan.

Also, let your doctor know about any medicines you take, including prescription and over-the-counter medicines, vitamins, minerals, and other supplements. Some medicines and supplements can cause problems when used with adenosine, dipyridamole, or dobutamine (medicines used to increase your heart rate during a stress test).

If you are having a stress test as part of your nuclear heart scan, wear comfortable walking shoes and loose-fitting clothes for the test. You may be asked to wear a hospital gown during the test.

A nuclear heart scan can take a lot of time. Most take between two to five hours, especially if two sets of pictures are needed.

What should I expect during a nuclear heart scan?

Many, but not all, nuclear medicine centers are located in hospitals. A doctor who has special training in nuclear heart scans—a cardiologist or radiologist—will oversee the test. (Cardiologists are doctors who specialize in diagnosing and treating heart problems. Radiologists are doctors who specialize in diagnostic techniques such as nuclear scans.)

Before the test begins, the doctor or a technician will use a needle to insert an intravenous (IV) line into a vein in your arm. Through this IV line, he or she will put the radioactive tracers into your bloodstream at the right time. You also will have EKG (electrocardiogram) patches attached to your body to check your heart rate during the test.

If you're having an exercise stress test as part of your nuclear scan, you will walk on a treadmill or pedal a stationary bicycle, while attached to EKG and blood pressure monitors.

You will be asked to exercise until you're too tired to continue, short of breath, or having chest or leg pain. You can expect that your heart will beat faster, you will breathe faster, your blood pressure will increase, and you will sweat. Report any chest, arm, or jaw pain or discomfort; dizziness; lightheadedness; or any other unusual symptoms.

If you're unable to exercise, your doctor can give you medicine to make your heart beat faster. This is called a chemical stress test. The medicine used may make you feel anxious, sick, dizzy, or shaky for a short time. If the side effects are severe, other medicine can be given for relief.

Before the exercise or the chemical stress test stops, the tracer is injected through the IV line.

The nuclear heart scan will start shortly after the exercise or chemical stress test. You will be asked to lie very still on a padded table.

The nuclear heart scan camera, called a gamma camera, is enclosed in a metal housing. The part of the camera that detects the radioactivity from the tracer can be put in several positions around your body as you lie on the padded table. For some nuclear heart scans, the metal housing is shaped like a doughnut and you lie on a table that goes slowly through the doughnut hole. The computer used to collect the pictures of your heart is nearby or in another room.

Two sets of pictures will be taken. One will be taken right after your exercise or chemical stress test and the other will be taken after a period of rest. The pictures may be taken all in one day or over two days. Each set of pictures takes about 15 to 30 minutes to do.

Some people find it hard to stay in one position for some time. Others may feel anxious while lying in the doughnut-shaped scanner. The table may feel hard. Sometimes, the room feels chilly because of the air conditioning needed to maintain the machines.

Let the person performing the test know how you're feeling during the test so he or she can respond as needed.

What should I expect after a nuclear heart scan?

You may be asked to return to the nuclear medicine center the next day for more pictures. Outpatients will be allowed to go home after the scan or leave the nuclear medicine center between the two scans.

Most people can go back to daily activities after a nuclear heart scan. The radioactivity will naturally leave the body in the urine or stool. It's helpful to drink plenty of fluids after the test.

The cardiologist or radiologist will read and interpret the results of the test within one to three days. Results will be reported to your doctor, who will contact you to discuss the results. Or, the cardiologist may discuss the results directly with you.

What are the risks of a nuclear heart scan?

The radioactive tracers used during a nuclear heart scan expose the body to a very small amount of radiation. No long-term effects have been reported from these doses.

If you have coronary artery disease, you may have chest pain during exercise or when you take medicine to increase your heart rate. Medicine can be given to relieve this symptom.

Some people may be allergic to the radioactive tracers, but this is very rare.

Women who are pregnant should tell their doctor and technician before the scan is done. It may be postponed until after the pregnancy.

Part Five

Electrical, Endoscopic, and Functionality Exams

Chapter 31

Electrocardiograms (EKGs)

What is an electrocardiogram?

An electrocardiogram, also called an EKG or ECG, is a simple test that detects and records the electrical activity of the heart. It is used to detect and locate the source of heart problems.

Electrical signals in the heart trigger heartbeats. These signals start at the top of the heart in an area called the right atrium. The electrical signals travel from the top of the heart to the bottom. They cause the heart muscle to contract as they travel through the heart. As the heart contracts, it pumps blood out to the rest of the body.

An EKG shows how fast the heart is beating. It shows the heart's rhythm (steady or irregular) and where in the body the heartbeat is being recorded. It also records the strength and timing of the electrical signals as they pass through each part of the heart.

An EKG is sometimes called a 12-lead EKG (or 12-lead ECG) because the electrical activity of the heart is most often recorded from 12 different places on the body at the same time.

What does an EKG reveal?

Many heart problems change the electrical signature of the heart in distinct ways. EKG recordings of this electrical activity can help reveal a number of heart problems; these include the following:

"Electrocardiogram," National Heart Lung and Blood Institute, March 2007.

- Heart attack
- Lack of blood flow to the heart muscle
- A heart that is beating irregularly, or too fast or too slow
- A heart that does not pump forcefully enough

EKG recordings can help doctors diagnose a heart attack that is happening now or has happened in the past. This is especially true if doctors can compare a current EKG recording to an older one. EKG recordings can also reveal problems such as these:

- Heart muscle that is too thick or parts of the heart that are too big
- Birth defects in the heart
- Disease in the heart valves between the different heart chambers

An EKG also reveals whether the heartbeat starts at the top right part of the heart like it should. It shows how long it takes for the electrical signals to travel through the heart.

How does the heart works?

The heart is a muscle about the size of your fist. It works like a pump and beats 100,000 times a day.

The heart has two sides, separated by an inner wall called the septum. The right side of the heart pumps blood to the lungs to pick up oxygen. Then, oxygen-rich blood returns from the lungs to the left side of the heart, and the left side pumps it to the body.

The heart has four chambers and four valves and is connected to various blood vessels. Veins are the blood vessels that carry blood from the body to the heart. Arteries are the blood vessels that carry blood away from the heart to the body.

Heart chambers: The heart has four chambers or "rooms."

- The atria are the two upper chambers that collect blood as it comes into the heart.
- The ventricles are the two lower chambers that pump blood out of the heart to the lungs or other parts of the body.

Heart valves: Four valves control the flow of blood from the atria to the ventricles and from the ventricles into the two large arteries connected to the heart.

- The tricuspid valve is in the right side of the heart, between the right atrium and the right ventricle.

- The pulmonary valve is in the right side of the heart, between the right ventricle and the entrance to the pulmonary artery, which carries blood to the lungs.

- The mitral valve is in the left side of the heart, between the left atrium and the left ventricle.

- The aortic valve is in the left side of the heart, between the left ventricle and the entrance to the aorta, the artery that carries blood to the body.

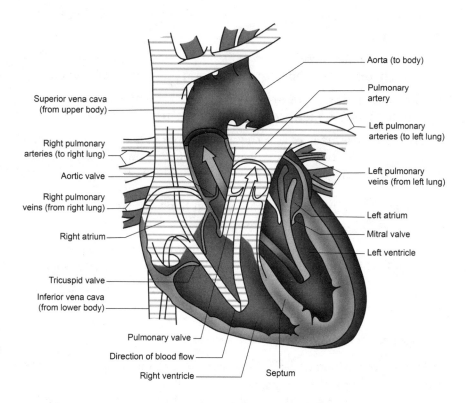

Figure 31.1. *A cross-section of a healthy heart and its inside structures. The striped arrow shows the direction in which oxygen-poor blood flows from the body to the lungs. The shaded arrow shows the direction in which oxygen-rich blood flows from the lungs to the rest of the heart.*

Valves are like doors that open and close. They open to allow blood to flow through to the next chamber or to one of the arteries, and then they shut to keep blood from flowing backward.

When the heart's valves open and close, they make a "lub-DUB" sound that a doctor can hear using a stethoscope.

- The first sound—the "lub"—is made by the mitral and tricuspid valves closing at the beginning of systole. Systole is when the ventricles contract, or squeeze, and pump blood out of the heart.

- The second sound—the "DUB"—is made by the aortic and pulmonary valves closing at beginning of diastole. Diastole is when the ventricles relax and fill with blood pumped into them by the atria.

Arteries: The arteries are major blood vessels connected to your heart.

- The pulmonary artery carries blood pumped from the right side of the heart to the lungs to pick up a fresh supply of oxygen.

- The aorta is the main artery that carries oxygen-rich blood pumped from the left side of the heart out to the body.

- The coronary arteries are the other important arteries attached to the heart. They carry oxygen-rich blood from the aorta to the heart muscle, which must have its own blood supply to function.

Veins: The veins are also major blood vessels connected to your heart.

- The pulmonary veins carry oxygen-rich blood from the lungs to the left side of the heart so it can be pumped out to the body.

- The vena cava is a large vein that carries oxygen-poor blood from the body back to the heart.

Why is an electrocardiogram done?

An electrocardiogram (EKG) is done to evaluate signs and symptoms that could indicate heart problems. Some of the signs and symptoms that might be evaluated with an EKG include the following:

- Chest pain

- Heart pounding, racing, or fluttering, or the sense that your heart is beating unevenly

- Difficulty breathing
- Feeling tired and weak (fatigue)
- Unusual heart sounds when the doctor listens to your heartbeat

When an adult—usually someone who is older than 40 or 50 years of age—has a routine health exam, the doctor may order an EKG to screen for early heart disease that has no symptoms. The doctor is more likely to look for early heart disease if the person has a family history of heart disease in a mother, father, brother, or sister—especially if the heart disease developed early in those family members' lives.

Doctors also use EKGs to check how well heart treatments, such as drugs or medical devices, are working.

What happens during an electrocardiogram?

An electrocardiogram (EKG) is painless and harmless. A technician first attaches 12 soft patches called electrodes to the skin of the chest, arms, and legs. These electrodes are about the size of a quarter. To help an electrode stick to the skin, the technician may have to shave a patch of hair where the electrode will be attached.

After the electrodes are placed on the skin, the patient lies still on a table for a few minutes while the electrodes detect the electrical signals of the heart. A machine then records these signals on graph paper or displays them on a screen.

The entire test takes about 10 minutes. After the test, the electrodes are removed from the skin and discarded.

What are other types of EKGs?

The common EKG described above, called a resting 12-lead EKG, records only a few minutes of heart signals at a time. It will show a heart problem only if the problem is present during the few minutes that the test is being run. Many heart problems are present all the time and will be found by a resting 12-lead EKG. But some heart problems, like those related to irregular heartbeat, can come and go. They may be present for only a few minutes out of the day or only while exercising.

Special types of EKGs are used to help diagnose those kinds of problems. Three of these special EKGs are stress test, Holter monitor, and event monitor. Holter and event monitors are discussed in Chapter 36.

Stress test: Some heart problems are easier to diagnose when your heart is working harder and beating faster than when it's at rest. During stress testing, you exercise (or are given medicine if you are unable to exercise) to make your heart work harder and beat faster while heart tests are performed.

During exercise stress testing, your blood pressure and EKG readings are monitored while you walk or run on a treadmill or pedal a bicycle. Other heart tests, such as nuclear heart scanning or echocardiography, also can be done at the same time. These would be ordered if your doctor needs more information than the exercise stress test can provide about how well your heart is working.

If you are unable to exercise, a medicine can be injected through an intravenous line (IV) into your bloodstream to make your heart work harder and beat faster, as if you are exercising on a treadmill or bicycle. Nuclear heart scanning or echocardiography is then usually done.

During nuclear heart scanning, radioactive tracer is injected into your bloodstream, and a special camera shows the flow of blood through your heart and arteries. Echocardiography uses sound waves to show blood flow through the chambers and valves of your heart and to show the strength of your heart muscle.

Your doctor also may order two newer tests along with stress testing if more information is needed about how well your heart works. These new tests are magnetic resonance imaging (MRI) and positron emission tomography (PET) scanning of the heart. MRI shows detailed images of the structures and beating of your heart, which may help your doctor better assess if parts of your heart are weak or damaged. PET scanning shows the level of chemical activity in different areas of your heart. This can help your doctor determine if enough blood is flowing to the areas of your heart. A PET scan can show decreased blood flow caused by disease or damaged muscles that may not be detected by other scanning methods.

Chapter 32

Electroencephalograms (EEGs)

Electroencephalography (EEG) records brain waves, but it doesn't read minds or measure IQs. Instead, it's used to detect the level of electrical activity in the brain. Your brain cells communicate by electrical impulses, and an EEG measures and records these electrical impulses to detect anything abnormal.

An EEG measures primarily grey matter or higher brain function. The largest part of the brain is comprised of the cerebrum, which is split into right and left hemispheres. The cerebrum controls voluntary actions, thought, speech, and memory. In humans, the cerebrum comprises most of the brain, while in other mammals it's relatively small. This allows us to perform much more complicated actions than other species can.

The outer layer of the cerebrum, called the cerebral cortex, is responsible for most higher brain functions such as thought, reasoning, memory, and voluntary muscle movement. The cerebral cortex is mostly made up of neurons, which are nerve cells that carry messages throughout the body. In turn, the activity of the cerebral cortex is regulated by two structures that are deeper in the brain: the thalamus, which is located in the center of the brain and carries signals from

"EEG (Electroencephalography)," September 2007, reprinted with permission from www.kidshealth.org. Copyright © 2007 The Nemours Foundation. This information was provided by KidsHealth, one of the largest resources online for medically reviewed health information written for parents, kids, and teens. For more articles like this one, visit www.KidsHealth.org, or www.TeensHealth.org.

the sensory organs to the brain, and the reticular activating system, which sends signals to tell us to go to sleep and to wake us up.

The electrical activity of all these structures is the primary focus of the EEG.

How is an EEG done?

The procedure is not painful in any way. A technician arranges the electrodes, usually a dozen, at specific sites on the child's head, fixing the electrodes in place with sticky paste. The patient must remain still and lie down while the EEG is taken. Motion can interfere with the EEG—sometimes this might be difficult for an awake child, but it's necessary to record an accurate EEG. However, the patient can't be sedated to achieve stillness because the sedative can cause an inaccurate reading. Natural sleep EEGs, however, can be very helpful.

In the past, the electrodes transmitted the electrical signal by wires to a receiver and amplifier, and the results were recorded on a continuous roll of paper. These days, it's possible to send these signals wirelessly to a computer, where they can be stored in the computer's memory or on a disk. Technological advances have allowed for more expanded EEG testing and the combination of EEG testing with video monitoring of seizure activity.

Through a surgical procedure, wireless transmission also allows the placing of electrodes within the skull, or even within the brain itself, to precisely identify the location of any areas of unstable electrical impulses. These areas are known as seizure foci.

Why are EEGs done?

EEGs help in the diagnosis and management of:

- Seizure disorders. The EEG is the key test in diagnosing, pinpointing, and managing certain areas of unstable electrical impulses in the brain that cause epilepsy (in other words, the EEG tries to find the seizure foci). EEGs can identify other very rare seizure syndromes, and are also used to judge the effectiveness of anti-convulsion therapy, which is used in the treatment of seizure disorders.

- Encephalopathies. An encephalopathy is any disease that alters brain function, such as Parkinson disease or cerebral palsy. Encephalopathies can be caused by kidney, liver, or respiratory failure, or chemical imbalance in the blood (called metabolic encephalopathy), low blood sugar (hypoglycemia), or drug over-doses. Others may be due to infection and other causes of brain inflammation (encephalitis), or due to the effects of injured neurons (this case is very rare).

- Stupor and coma. Stupor is defined as reduced or slowed responsiveness, and coma is defined as unresponsiveness (not waking up, or if appearing awake, then not reacting to stimuli). Although EEGs may record the lack of electrical activity in some comatose patients, which can be used as evidence of brain death, in many other instances EEGs turn up treatable conditions like otherwise undetected seizures disorders or chemical imbalances. EEGs may also uncover signs of an otherwise unexpected good prognosis, like otherwise undetectable responses to stimuli, or evidence of normal sleep patterns.

In the past, EEGs played a bigger roll than they do now in the diagnosis of brain injury due to strokes and in the diagnosis and identification of brain tumors. Computer-assisted techniques such as CT-scans (an x-ray image of the body, also called a CAT scan); MRIs (magnetic resonance imaging, which uses radio waves and magnetic fields to produce and image); and PET scans (positron emission tomography, which uses a radioactive tracer that is injected into the body to help form a picture), have taken over most of the tasks of diagnosing these conditions, since they tend to be more sensitive and specific in the diagnosis of strokes and tumors and are simpler to do and easier to interpret than EEGs.

How long will it take to get results?

EEGs are read (analyzed and interpreted) by specially trained electroencephalographers, almost always neurologists. How long the analysis and interpretation takes depends on how long the EEG record itself is, the frequency and complexity of the potential abnormality being sought, and the availability of a competent interpreter. Since records can be transmitted now by telephone or internet, even complex EEGs are now usually read and interpreted within a day or two, sometimes at sites far distant from where they're performed. Emergency EEGs done on coma patients are often simple to read, and may be available within an hour of the record's completion.

Chapter 33

Electromyography and Nerve Conduction Velocities

Diagnosis of neuromuscular disease hinges on a doctor's ability to identify a specific defect of neuromuscular function. Sometimes, a doctor can infer this functional defect—and the disease associated with it—by giving a physical exam, doing a blood test, or looking at the anatomy of nerves and muscles.

But other times, the doctor may have to directly evaluate the functions of nerves and muscles and the connections between them by using two complementary techniques—nerve conduction velocity testing (NCVs) and electromyography (EMGs).

Action Potentials

Both NCV and EMG rely on the fact that the activity of nerves and muscles produces electrical signals called action potentials. A nerve is actually a bundle of axons, cables that conduct action potentials from one end of a nerve cell (or neuron) to the other.

In motor neurons (neurons that connect to muscle), these action potentials travel toward the muscle, where they cause release of a chemical called acetylcholine. Acetylcholine opens tiny pores in the muscle, and the flow of sodium and potassium ions through these pores creates action potentials in the muscle, leading to contraction.

"Simply Stated ... Electromyography and Nerve Conduction Velocities," reprinted by permission of the Muscular Dystrophy Association of the United States, © 2000. Reviewed by David A. Cooke, M.D., June 2008.

In NCV and EMG, these tiny electrical events are amplified electronically, then visualized on a TV-like monitor called an oscilloscope and even heard using audio equipment.

NCV and Axons

NCV measures action potentials conducted by axons, so doctors use it for diagnosing diseases that primarily affect nerve function, such as different forms of Charcot-Marie-Tooth disease (CMT).

It's done by placing surface electrodes (similar to those used for electrocardiograms) on the skin at various points over a nerve. One electrode delivers a mild electrical shock to the nerve, stimulating it to generate an action potential. The other electrodes record the action potential as it's conducted through the nerve.

Doctors often use NCV to determine the speed of nerve conduction (hence, its name). Conduction speed is influenced by a coating around axons, called myelin. Myelin insulates each axon and normally forces action potentials to "jump" quickly from one end of the axon to the other. If the myelin breaks down (as in CMT1), the action potential travels more slowly.

NCV also can measure the strength of the action potential in the nerve, which is proportional to the number of axons that contribute to it. If axons degenerate (as in amyotrophic lateral sclerosis [ALS]) or become clogged with debris (as in CMT2), the action potential becomes smaller.

EMG and Muscle

An electromyogram measures the action potentials produced by muscles and is, therefore, useful for diagnosing diseases that primarily affect muscle function, including the muscular dystrophies. Also, some EMG data can reveal defects in nerve function.

In EMG, the doctor inserts a needle-like electrode into a muscle. The electrode records action potentials that occur when the muscle is at rest and during voluntary contractions directed by the doctor.

While a healthy muscle appears quiet at rest, spontaneous action potentials are seen in damaged muscles or muscles that have lost input from nerve cells (as in ALS or myasthenia gravis). During voluntary contraction, dystrophic (wasted) muscles show very small action potentials, and myotonic (stiff) muscles show prolonged trains of action potentials. Altered patterns of muscle action potentials can indicate defects in nerve function.

A Little Discomfort

Though NCVs and EMGs are valuable tools for doctors, they can be distressing for patients. Some people find the electric shocks of the NCV or the needle penetration of the EMG uncomfortable or even painful. Young children might struggle during the tests, making it difficult for doctors to carefully monitor nerve and muscle activity. To ease discomfort, topical anesthetic can be applied to the skin—but it won't prevent muscle pain during the EMG. Sometimes sedating medications are needed to keep a child calm.

Partly because of these factors, NCVs and EMGs are generally used when it's not possible to gather the right information from other diagnostic tests. Muscle biopsy (excising and examining muscle tissue) can reveal hallmark anatomical features of some neuromuscular diseases, making EMG and NCV unnecessary. Genetic tests are now available for diagnosing some diseases, and in those cases, EMG and NCV usually can be bypassed.

Nonetheless, NCV and EMG remain the gold standards for evaluating the function of nerve and muscle. So, when a doctor suspects that a patient has a neuromuscular disease that isn't clearly associated with anatomical or genetic defects (like some types of CMT or myasthenia gravis), NCV and EMG are among the most valuable diagnostic tools.

Chapter 34

Endoscopic Tests

Chapter Contents

Section 34.1

Upper Endoscopy

What is upper endoscopy?

Upper endoscopy (also known as gastroscopy, EGD, or esophago-gastroduodenoscopy) is a procedure that enables your surgeon to examine the lining of the esophagus (swallowing tube), stomach, and duodenum (first portion of the small intestine). A bendable, lighted tube about the thickness of your little finger is placed through your mouth and into the stomach and duodenum.

Why is an upper endoscopy performed?

Upper endoscopy is performed to evaluate symptoms of persistent upper abdominal pain, nausea, vomiting, difficulty swallowing, or heartburn. It is an excellent method for finding the cause of bleeding from the upper gastrointestinal tract. It can be used to evaluate the esophagus or stomach after major surgery. It is more accurate than x-rays for detecting inflammation, ulcers, or tumors of the esophagus, stomach, and duodenum. Upper endoscopy can detect early cancer and can distinguish between cancerous and noncancerous conditions by performing biopsies of suspicious areas. Biopsies are taken by using a specialized instrument to sample tissue. These samples are then sent to the laboratory to be analyzed. A biopsy is taken for many reasons and does not mean that cancer is suspected.

A variety of instruments can be passed through the endoscope that allows the surgeon to treat many abnormalities with little or no discomfort. Your surgeon can stretch narrowed areas, remove polyps, remove swallowed objects, or treat upper gastrointestinal bleeding. Safe and effective control of bleeding has reduced the need for transfusions and surgery in many patients.

What preparation is required?

The stomach should be completely empty. You should have nothing to eat or drink for approximately eight hours before the examination. Your surgeon will be more specific about the time to begin fasting depending on the time of day that your test is scheduled.

Medication may need to be adjusted or avoided. It is best to inform your surgeon of all your current medications as well as allergies to medications a few days prior to the examination. Most medications can be continued as usual. Medication use such as aspirin, vitamin E, nonsteroidal anti-inflammatories, blood thinners, and insulin should be discussed with your surgeon prior to the examination. It is essential that you alert your surgeon if you require antibiotics prior to undergoing dental procedures, since you may also require antibiotics prior to gastroscopy.

Also, if you have any major diseases, such as heart or lung disease that may require special attention during the procedure, discuss this with your surgeon.

You will most likely be sedated during the procedure and an arrangement to have someone drive you home afterward is imperative. Sedatives will affect your judgment and reflexes for the rest of the day. You should not drive or operate machinery until the next day.

What can be expected during the upper endoscopy?

You may have your throat sprayed with a local anesthetic before the test begins and given medication through a vein to help you relax during the examination. You will be laid on your side or back in a comfortable position as the endoscope is gently passed through your mouth and into your esophagus, stomach, and duodenum. Air is introduced into your stomach during the procedure to allow a better view of the stomach lining. The procedure usually lasts 15–60 minutes. The endoscope does not interfere with your breathing. Most patients fall asleep during the procedure; a few find it only slightly uncomfortable.

What happens after upper endoscopy?

You will be monitored in the endoscopy area for one to two hours until the effects of the sedatives have worn off. Your throat may be a little sore for a day or two. You may feel bloated immediately after the procedure because of the air that is introduced into your stomach during the examination. You will be able to resume your diet and take your routine medication after you leave the endoscopy area, unless otherwise instructed. Your surgeon will usually inform you of your test results on the day of the procedure, unless biopsy samples were taken. These results take several days to return. If you do not remember what your surgeon told you about the examination or follow up instructions, call your surgeon's office to find out what you were supposed to do.

What complications can occur?

Gastroscopy and biopsy are generally safe when performed by surgeons who have had special training and are experienced in these endoscopic procedures. Complications are rare, however, they can occur. They include bleeding from the site of a biopsy or polypectomy and a tear (perforation) through the lining of the intestinal wall. Blood transfusions are rarely required. A reaction to the sedatives can occur. Irritation to the vein that medications were given is uncommon, but may cause a tender lump lasting a few weeks. Warm, moist towels will help relieve this discomfort.

It is important for you to recognize the early signs of possible complications and to contact your surgeon if you notice symptoms of difficulty swallowing, worsening throat pain, chest pains, severe abdominal pain, fevers, chills, or rectal bleeding of more than one-half cup.

Section 34.2

Colonoscopy

What is a colonoscopy?

Colonoscopy is a procedure that enables your surgeon to examine the lining of the rectum and colon. It is usually done in the hospital or an endoscopic procedure room. A soft, bendable tube about the thickness of the index finger is gently inserted into the anus and advanced into the rectum and the colon.

Why is a colonoscopy performed?

A colonoscopy is usually done 1) as part of a routine screening for cancer, 2) in patients with known polyps or previous polyp removal, 3) before or after some surgeries, 4) to evaluate a change in bowel habits or bleeding, or 5) to evaluate changes in the lining of the colon known as inflammatory disorders.

What preparation is required?

The rectum and colon must be completely emptied of stool for the procedure to be performed. In general, preparation consists of consumption of a special cleansing solution or several days of clear liquids, laxatives and enemas prior to the examination. Your surgeon or his staff will give you instructions regarding the cleansing routine to be used.

Follow your surgeon's instructions carefully. If you do not complete the preparation, it may be unsafe to perform the colonoscopy and the procedure may have to be rescheduled. If you are unable to take the preparation, contact your surgeon.

Most medications can be continued as usual. Medication use such as aspirin, vitamin E, nonsteroidal anti-inflammatories, blood thinners, and insulin should be discussed with your surgeon prior to the examination as well as any other medication you might be taking. It is essential that you alert your surgeon if you require antibiotics prior to undergoing dental procedures, since you may also require antibiotics prior to colonoscopy.

You will most likely be sedated during the procedure and an arrangement to have someone drive you home afterward is imperative. Sedatives will affect your judgment and reflexes for the rest of the day. You should not drive or operate machinery until the next day.

What can be expected during colonoscopy?

The procedure is usually well tolerated, but there is often a feeling of pressure, gassiness, bloating, or cramping at various times during the procedure. Your surgeon will give you medication through a vein to help you relax and better tolerate any discomfort that you may experience. You will be lying on your side or your back while the colonoscope is advanced through the large intestine. The lining of the colon is examined carefully while inserting and withdrawing the instrument. The procedure usually lasts for 15 to 60 minutes. In rare instances the entire colon cannot be visualized and your surgeon could request a barium enema.

What if colonoscopy shows an abnormality?

If your surgeon sees an area that needs more detailed evaluation, a biopsy may be obtained and submitted to a laboratory for analysis. Placing a special instrument through the colonoscope to sample the lining of the colon does this. Polyps are generally removed. The majority of polyps are benign (noncancerous), but your surgeon cannot always tell by the appearance alone. They can be removed by burning (fulgurating) or by a wire loop (snare). It may take your surgeon more than one sitting to do this if there are numerous polyps or they are very large. Sites of bleeding can be identified and controlled by injecting certain medications or coagulating (burning) the bleeding vessels. Biopsies do not imply cancer, however, removal of a colonic polyp is an important means of preventing colorectal cancer.

What happens after colonoscopy?

Your surgeon will explain the results to you after your procedure or at your follow up visit. You may have some mild cramping or bloating from the air that was placed into the colon during the examination. This should quickly improve with the passage of the gas. You should be able to eat normally the same day and resume your normal activities after leaving the hospital. Do not drive or operate machinery until the next day, as the sedatives given will impair your reflexes.

If you have been given medication during the procedure, you will be observed until most of the effects of the sedation have worn off (one to two hours). You will need someone to drive you home after the procedure. If you do not remember what your surgeon told you about the examination or follow up instructions. Call your surgeon's office that day or the next to find out what you were supposed to do.

If polyps were found during your procedure, you will need to have a repeat colonoscopy. Your surgeon will decide on the frequency of your colonoscopy exams.

What complications can occur?

Colonoscopy and biopsy are safe when performed by surgeons who have had special training and are experienced in these endoscopic procedures. Complications are rare, however, they can occur. They include bleeding from the site of a biopsy or polypectomy and a tear (perforation) through the lining of the bowel wall. Should this occur, it may be necessary for your surgeon to perform abdominal surgery to repair the intestinal tear. Blood transfusions are rarely required. A reaction to the sedatives can occur. Irritation to the vein that medications were given is uncommon, but may cause a tender lump lasting a few weeks. Warm, moist towels will help relieve this discomfort.

It is important to contact your surgeon if you notice symptoms of severe abdominal pain, fevers, chills, or rectal bleeding of more than one-half cup. Bleeding can occur up to several days after a biopsy.

Section 34.3

Flexible Sigmoidoscopy

"Flexible Sigmoidoscopy" is reprinted with permission from the Society of American Gastrointestinal Endoscopic Surgeons (SAGES), © 2004. For additional information, contact SAGE, 11300 West Olympic Boulevard, Suite 600, Los Angeles, CA 90064, 310-437-0544, or visit www.sages.org.

What is flexible sigmoidoscopy?

Flexible sigmoidoscopy is a procedure that enables your surgeon to examine the lining of the rectum and lower colon (bowel). It is usually done in the surgeon's office or a procedure room, but occasionally may be done in the hospital. A lubricated soft, bendable tube about the thickness of the index finger is gently inserted into the anus (rectal opening) and moved into the rectum and the lower part of the colon.

Why is flexible sigmoidoscopy performed?

Flexible sigmoidoscopy is often done as part of a routine screening for cancer for patients over 50 years old, before some surgeries, or to evaluate the causes of symptoms (such as diarrhea, bleeding, colitis, changes in bowel habits and, changes in stool form or color). Flexible sigmoidoscopy is also used as a screening tool for patients whose families have a history of colorectal cancer.

What preparation is required?

The rectum and lower colon must be completely emptied of stool for the procedure to be performed. One or two enemas prior to the procedure is all that is necessary, but laxatives or dietary modifications may be recommended by your surgeon in certain instances. Your surgeon or his/her staff will give you instructions regarding the cleansing routine to be used. If the area to be examined is not clear of stool the surgeon will not be able to perform an effective examination. Be sure to follow your surgeon's preparation instructions.

Most of your medications can be continued as usual. However, the use of medication such as aspirin, vitamin E, nonsteroidal anti-inflammatories, and blood thinners should be discussed with your surgeon prior to the examination. It is essential that you alert your surgeon if you require antibiotics prior to undergoing dental procedures, since you may also require antibiotics prior to sigmoidoscopy.

What can be expected during flexible sigmoidoscopy?

You will be awake during the procedure. Occasionally, the surgeon may give you some light sedation. The procedure is well tolerated and rarely causes discomfort. The inside of the colon has few nerve endings; therefore, it is unusual to feel the scope moving within the body. Air is injected to distend or widen the passage. This may cause a feeling of pressure, gassiness, bloating, or cramping during the procedure. You will lie on your side while the sigmoidoscope is advanced through the rectum and lower colon. The lining of the intestine is examined carefully. The procedure usually lasts for five to fifteen minutes. If there is extreme discomfort, you should tell your surgeon and the procedure will be terminated.

What happens after flexible sigmoidoscopy?

Your surgeon will explain the results to you and discuss any findings. You may have some mild cramping or bloating from the air that was placed into the colon during the examination. This should quickly improve with the passage of gas. You should be able to eat and resume normal activities after leaving the surgeon's office or hospital. If your surgeon sees an area that needs more detailed evaluation during the procedure, a biopsy may be obtained and submitted to a laboratory for analysis. This is done by placing a special instrument through the sigmoidoscope to extract a tiny sample of the lining of the colon. This procedure is painless. If polyps or growths are found, your surgeon will usually request that you have a colonoscopy, which is a complete endoscopic examination of the entire colon. A colonoscopy is more suitable to remove polyps and enables the surgeon to check the remaining colon for any other polyps or lesions.

What complications can occur?

Flexible sigmoidoscopy and biopsy are safe when performed by surgeons with appropriate training and experience in endoscopic procedures. Complications are rare, however, they can occur. They include bleeding from the site of a biopsy or a perforation, which is a tear through the lining of the bowel wall. It is important to contact your surgeon if you notice symptoms of severe abdominal pain, abdominal distension, nausea, fevers, chill, or rectal bleeding equal to more than half a cup. Bleeding can occur up to several days after a biopsy.

Section 34.4

Endoscopic Retrograde Cholangiopancreatography (ERCP)

"ERCP (Endoscopic Retrograde Cholangio-Pancreatography)" is reprinted with permission from the Society of American Gastrointestinal Endoscopic Surgeons (SAGES), © 2004. For additional information, contact SAGE, 11300 West Olympic Boulevard, Suite 600, Los Angeles, CA 90064, 310-437-0544, or visit www.sages.org.

What is endoscopic retrograde cholangiopancreatography (ERCP)?

ERCP is a procedure that enables your surgeon to examine the pancreatic and bile ducts. A bendable, lighted tube (endoscope) about the thickness of your index finger is placed through your mouth and into your stomach and top part of the small intestine (duodenum). In the duodenum a small opening is identified (ampulla) and a small plastic tube (cannula) is passed through the endoscope and into this opening. Dye (contrast material) is injected and x-rays are taken to study the ducts of the pancreas and liver.

Why is an ERCP performed?

ERCP is most commonly performed to diagnose conditions of the pancreas or bile ducts, and is also used to treat those conditions. It is used to evaluate symptoms suggestive of disease in these organs, or to further clarify abnormal results from blood tests or imaging tests such as ultrasound or computed tomography (CT) scan. The most common reasons to do ERCP include abdominal pain, weight loss, jaundice, or an ultrasound or CT scan that shows stones or a mass in these organs.

ERCP may be used before or after gallbladder surgery to assist in the performance of that operation. Bile duct stones can be diagnosed and removed with an ERCP. Tumors, both cancerous and noncancerous, can be diagnosed and then treated with indwelling plastic tubes that are used to bypass a blockage of the bile duct. Complications from gallbladder surgery can also sometimes be diagnosed and treated with ERCP.

In patients with suspected or known pancreatic disease, ERCP will help determine the need for surgery or the best type of surgical procedure to be performed. Occasionally, pancreatic stones can be removed by ERCP.

What preparation is required?

Your stomach must be empty, so you should not eat or drink anything for approximately eight hours before the examination. Your surgeon will be more specific about the time to begin fasting depending on the time of day that your test is scheduled.

Your current medications may need to be adjusted or avoided. Most medications can be continued as usual. Medication use such as aspirin, vitamin E, nonsteroidal anti-inflammatories, blood thinners, and insulin should be discussed with your surgeon prior to the examination as well as any other medication you might be taking. It is therefore best to inform your surgeon of any allergies to medications, iodine, or shellfish. It is essential that you alert your surgeon if you require antibiotics prior to undergoing dental procedures, since you may also require antibiotics prior to ERCP.

Also, if you have any major diseases, such as heart or lung disease that may require special attention during the procedure, discuss this with your surgeon.

To make the examination comfortable, you will be sedated during the procedure, and, therefore, you will need someone to drive you home afterward. Sedatives will affect your judgment and reflexes for the rest of the day, so you should not drive or operate machinery until the next day.

What can be expected during the ERCP?

Your throat will be sprayed with a local anesthetic before the test begins to numb your throat and prevent gagging. You will be given medication intravenously to help you relax during the examination. While you are lying in a comfortable position on an x-ray table, an

443

endoscope will be gently passed through your mouth, down your esophagus, and into your stomach and duodenum. The procedure usually lasts about an hour. The endoscope does not interfere with your breathing. Most patients fall asleep during the procedure or find it only slightly uncomfortable. You may feel temporarily bloated during and after the procedure due to the air used to inflate the duodenum. As x-ray contrast material is injected into the pancreatic or bile ducts, you may feel some minor discomfort.

What happens after ERCP?

You will be monitored in the endoscopy area for one to two hours until the effects of the sedatives have worn off. Your throat may be a little sore for a day or two. You will be able to resume your diet and take your routine medication after you leave the endoscopy area, unless otherwise instructed.

Your surgeon will usually inform you of your test results on the day of the procedure. Biopsy results take several days to return, and you should make arrangements with your surgeon to get these results. The effects of sedation may make you forget what you were instructed after the procedure. Call your surgeon's office for the results.

What complications can occur?

ERCP is safe when performed by surgeons who have had specific training and are experienced in this specialized endoscopic procedure. Complications are rare, however, they can occur. Pancreatitis due to irritation of the pancreatic duct by the x-ray contrast material or cannula is the most common complication. A reaction to the sedatives can occur. Irritation to the vein in which medications were given is uncommon, but may cause a tender lump lasting a few weeks. Warm moist towels will help relieve this discomfort.

If your ERCP included a therapeutic procedure such as removal of stones or placement of a stent (drain), there are additional small risks of bleeding or perforation (making a hole in the intestine). Blood transfusions are rarely required. It is important for you to recognize the early signs of possible complications and to contact your surgeon if you notice symptoms of severe abdominal pain, fever, chills, vomiting, or rectal bleeding.

Section 34.5

Capsule Endoscopy

What is capsule endoscopy?

Capsule endoscopy lets your doctor examine the lining of the middle part of your gastrointestinal tract, which includes the three portions of the small intestine (duodenum, jejunum, ileum). Your doctor will use a pill sized video capsule called an endoscope, which has its own lens and light source and will view the images on a video monitor. You might hear your doctor or other medical staff refer to capsule endoscopy as small bowel endoscopy, capsule enteroscopy, or wireless endoscopy.

Why is capsule endoscopy done?

Capsule endoscopy helps your doctor evaluate the small intestine. This part of the bowel cannot be reached by traditional upper endoscopy or by colonoscopy. The most common reason for doing capsule endoscopy is to search for a cause of bleeding from the small intestine. It may also be useful for detecting polyps, inflammatory bowel disease (Crohn disease), ulcers, and tumors of the small intestine.

As is the case with most new diagnostic procedures, not all insurance companies are currently reimbursing for this procedure. You may need to check with your own insurance company to ensure that this is a covered benefit.

How should I prepare for the procedure?

An empty stomach allows for the best and safest examination, so you should have nothing to eat or drink, including water, for approximately twelve hours before the examination. Your doctor will tell you when to start fasting.

Tell your doctor in advance about any medications you take including iron, aspirin, bismuth subsalicylate products, and other "over-the-counter" medications. You might need to adjust your usual dose prior to the examination.

Discuss any allergies to medications as well as medical conditions, such as swallowing disorders and heart or lung disease.

Tell your doctor of the presence of a pacemaker, previous abdominal surgery, or previous history of obstructions in the bowel, inflammatory bowel disease, or adhesions.

What can I expect during capsule endoscopy?

Your doctor will prepare you for the examination by applying a sensor device to your abdomen with adhesive sleeves (similar to tape). The capsule endoscope is swallowed and passes naturally through your digestive tract while transmitting video images to a data recorder worn on your belt for approximately eight hours. At the end of the procedure you will return to the office and the data recorder is removed so that images of your small bowel can be put on a computer screen for physician review.

What happens after capsule endoscopy?

You will be able to drink clear liquids after two hours and eat a light meal after four hours following the capsule ingestion, unless your doctor instructs you otherwise. You will have to avoid vigorous physical activity such as running or jumping during the study. Your doctor generally can tell you the test results within the week following the procedure; however, the results of some tests might take longer.

What are the possible complications of capsule endoscopy?

Although complications can occur, they are rare when doctors who are specially trained and experienced in this procedure, such as members of the American Society for Gastrointestinal Endoscopy, perform the test. Potential risks include complications from obstruction. This usually relates to a stricture (narrowing) of the intestine from inflammation, prior surgery, or tumor. It's important to recognize early signs of possible complications. If you have evidence of obstruction, such as unusual bloating, pain, and/or vomiting, call your doctor immediately. Also, if you develop a fever after the test, have trouble swallowing, or experience increasing chest pain, tell your doctor immediately. Be careful not to prematurely disconnect the system as this may result in loss of image acquisition.

Section 34.6

Endoscopic Ultrasonography (EUS)

You've been referred to have an endoscopic ultrasonography, or EUS, which will help your doctor, evaluate or treat your condition. This section will give you a basic understanding of the procedure—how it is performed, how it can help, and what side effects you might experience. It can't answer all of your questions, since a lot depends on the individual patient and the doctor. Please ask your doctor about anything you don't understand. Endoscopists are highly trained specialists who welcome your questions regarding their credentials, training, and experience.

What is EUS?

EUS allows your doctor to examine the lining and the walls of your upper and lower gastrointestinal tract. The upper tract is the esophagus, stomach, and duodenum; the lower tract includes your colon and rectum. EUS is also used to study internal organs that lie next to the gastrointestinal tract, such as the gall bladder and pancreas.

Your endoscopist will use a thin, flexible tube called an endoscope. Your doctor will pass the endoscope through your mouth or anus to the area to be examined. Your doctor then will turn on the ultrasound component to produce sound waves that create visual images of the digestive tract.

Why is EUS done?

EUS provides your doctor more detailed pictures of your digestive tract anatomy. Your doctor can use EUS to diagnose the cause of conditions such as abdominal pain or abnormal weight loss. Or, if your doctor has ruled out certain conditions, EUS can confirm your diagnosis and give you a clean bill of health.

EUS is also used to evaluate an abnormality, such as a growth, that was detected at a prior endoscopy or by x-ray. EUS provides a detailed picture of the growth, which can help your doctor determine its nature and decide upon the best treatment.

In addition, EUS can be used to diagnose diseases of the pancreas, bile duct, and gallbladder when other tests are inconclusive.

Why is EUS used for patients with cancer?

EUS helps your doctor determine the extent of certain cancers of the digestive and respiratory systems. EUS allows your doctor to accurately assess the cancer's depth and whether it has spread to adjacent lymph glands or nearby vital structures such as major blood vessels. In some patients, EUS can be used to obtain tissue samples to help your doctor determine the proper treatment.

How should I prepare for EUS?

For EUS of the upper gastrointestinal tract, you should have nothing to eat or drink, not even water, usually six hours before the examination. Your doctor will tell you when to start this fasting.

For EUS of the rectum or colon, your doctor will instruct you to either consume a large volume of a special cleansing solution or to follow a clear liquid diet combined with laxatives or enemas prior to the examination. The procedure might have to be rescheduled if you don't follow your doctor's instructions carefully.

What about my current medications or allergies?

Tell your doctor in advance of the procedure about all medications that you're taking and about any allergies you have to medication. He or she will tell you whether or not you can continue to take your medication as usual before the EUS examination. In general, you can safely take aspirin and nonsteroidal anti-inflammatories (Motrin, Advil, Aleve, etc.) before an EUS examination, but it's always best to discuss their use with your doctor. Check with your doctor about which medications you should take the morning of the EUS examination, and take essential medication with only a small cup of water.

If you have an allergy to latex you should inform your doctor prior to your test. Patients with latex allergies often require special equipment and may not be able to have an EUS examination.

Do I need to take antibiotics?

Antibiotics aren't generally required before or after EUS examinations. But tell your doctor if you take antibiotics before dental procedures.

If your doctor feels you need antibiotics, antibiotics might be ordered during the EUS examination or after the procedure to help prevent an infection. Your doctor might prescribe antibiotics if you're having specialized EUS procedures, such as to drain a fluid collection or a cyst using EUS guidance. Again, tell your doctor about any allergies to medications.

Should I arrange for help after the examination?

If you received sedatives, you won't be allowed to drive after the procedure, even if you don't feel tired. You should arrange for a ride home. You should also plan to have someone stay with you at home after the examination, because the sedatives could affect your judgment and reflexes for the rest of the day.

What can I expect during EUS?

Practices vary among doctors, but for an EUS examination of the upper gastrointestinal tract, your endoscopist might spray your throat with a local anesthetic before the test begins. Most often you will receive sedatives intravenously to help you relax. You will most likely begin by lying on your left side. After you receive sedatives, your endoscopist will pass the ultrasound endoscope through your mouth, esophagus, and stomach into the duodenum. The instrument does not interfere with your ability to breathe. The actual examination generally takes between 15 to 45 minutes. Most patients consider it only slightly uncomfortable, and many fall asleep during it.

An EUS examination of the lower gastrointestinal tract can often be performed safely and comfortably without medications, but you will probably receive a sedative if the examination will be prolonged or if the doctor will examine a significant distance into the colon. You will start by lying on your left side with your back toward the doctor. Most EUS examinations of the lower gastrointestinal tract last from 10 to 30 minutes.

What happens after EUS?

If you received sedatives, you will be monitored in the recovery area until most of the sedative medication's effects have worn off. If you had an upper EUS, your throat might be sore. You might feel bloated because of the air and water that were introduced during the examination. You'll be able to eat after you leave the procedure area, unless you're instructed otherwise.

Your doctor generally can inform you of the results of the procedure that day, but the results of some tests will take longer.

What are the possible complications of EUS?

Although complications can occur, they are rare when doctors with specialized training and experience perform the EUS examination. Bleeding might occur at a biopsy site, but it's usually minimal and rarely requires follow-up. You might have a sore throat for a day or more. Nonprescription anesthetic-type throat lozenges and painkillers help relieve the sore throat. Other potential, but uncommon, risks of EUS include a reaction to the sedatives used; backwash of stomach contents into your lungs; infection; and complications from heart or lung diseases. One major, but very uncommon, complication of EUS is perforation. This is a tear through the lining of the intestine that might require surgery to repair.

The possibility of complications increases slightly if a deep needle aspiration is performed during the EUS examination. These risks must be balanced against the potential benefits of the procedure and the risks of alternative approaches to the condition.

Additional Questions

If you have any questions about your need for EUS, alternative approaches to your problem, the cost of the procedure, methods of billing, or insurance coverage, do not hesitate to speak to your doctor or doctor's office staff about it.

Section 34.7

Cystoscopy and Ureteroscopy

National Kidney and Urologic Diseases Information Clearinghouse, NIH Pub. 06-4800, November 2005.

When you have a urinary problem, your doctor may use a cystoscope to see inside your bladder and urethra. The urethra is the tube that carries urine from the bladder to the outside of the body. The cystoscope has lenses like a telescope or microscope. These lenses let the doctor focus on the inner surfaces of the urinary tract. Some cystoscopes use optical fibers (flexible glass fibers) that carry an image from the tip of the instrument to a viewing piece at the other end. The cystoscope is as thin as a pencil and has a light at the tip. Many cystoscopes have extra tubes to guide other instruments for procedures to treat urinary problems.

Your doctor may recommend cystoscopy for any of the following conditions:

- Frequent urinary tract infections
- Blood in your urine (hematuria)
- Loss of bladder control (incontinence) or overactive bladder
- Unusual cells found in urine sample
- Need for a bladder catheter
- Painful urination, chronic pelvic pain, or interstitial cystitis
- Urinary blockage such as prostate enlargement, stricture, or narrowing of the urinary tract
- Stone in the urinary tract
- Unusual growth, polyp, tumor, or cancer

If you have a stone lodged in your ureter or have an area that needs more study in your ureter, your doctor may recommend an ureteroscopy, usually with general or regional anesthesia. The ureter is the tube that carries urine from the kidney to the bladder. The ureteroscope is a special, very thin instrument used to look directly at and visualize

451

the inside of the ureter. Some ureteroscopes are flexible like a small, very long straw. Others are more rigid and firm. Through the uretero-scope, the doctor can see the stone. The doctor can then move the stone, either by removing it with a small basket at the end of a wire inserted through an extra tube in the ureteroscope or by extending a flexible fiber that carries a laser beam to break the stone into smaller pieces that can then pass out of the body in your urine. How and what the doctor will do is determined by the location, size, and composition of the stone. The doctor may leave a stent, a flexible tube that keeps the ureter open for drainage after the procedure.

Preparation

Ask your doctor about any special instructions. In most cases, you will be able to eat normally and return to normal activities after the test.

Since any medical procedure has a small risk of injury, you will need to sign a consent form before the test. Do not hesitate to ask your doctor about any concerns you might have.

You may be asked to give a urine sample before the test to check for infection. Avoid urinating for an hour before this part of the test.

You will wear a hospital gown for the examination, and the lower part of your body will be covered with a sterile drape. In most cases, you will lie on your back with your knees raised and apart. A nurse or technician will clean the area around your urethral opening and apply a local anesthetic.

If you are going to have a ureteroscopy, you may receive a spinal or general anesthetic. If you know this is the case, you will want to arrange a ride home after the test.

Test Procedures

The doctor will gently insert the tip of the cystoscope into your ure-thra and slowly glide it up into the bladder. Relaxing your pelvic muscles will help make this part of the test easier. A sterile liquid (water or saline) will flow through the cystoscope to slowly fill your bladder and stretch it so that the doctor has a better view of the bladder wall.

As your bladder reaches capacity, you will feel some discomfort and the urge to urinate. You will be able to empty your bladder as soon as the examination is over.

The time from insertion of the cystoscope to removal may be only a few minutes, or it may be longer if the doctor finds a stone and decides to remove it. Taking a biopsy (a small tissue sample for examination under a microscope) will also make the procedure last longer. In most cases, the entire examination, including preparation, will take about 15 to 20 minutes.

After the Test

You may have a mild burning feeling when you urinate, and you may see small amounts of blood in your urine. These problems should not last more than 24 hours. Tell your doctor if bleeding or pain is severe or if problems last more than a couple of days.

To relieve discomfort, drink two 8-ounce glasses of water each hour for two hours. Ask your doctor if you can take a warm bath to relieve the burning feeling. If not, you may be able to hold a warm, damp washcloth over the urethral opening.

Your doctor may give you an antibiotic to take for one or two days to prevent an infection. If you have signs of infection—including pain, chills, or fever—call your doctor.

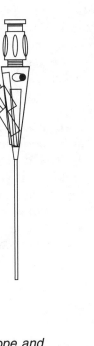

Figure 34.1. Rigid Cystoscope and
Semirigid Ureteroscope

Section 34.8

Nasal Endoscopy

"An Introduction to Nasal Endoscopy," by Martin J. Citardi, M.D.
© 2008 American Rhinologic Society. Reprinted with permission.

The Nasal Telescope

The nasal telescope is an optical instrument for examining the nose. This examination is known as diagnostic nasal endoscopy. Because the telescope is so slender (only 2.7–4.0 mm in diameter), it may be passed easily through the nostril to examine the nasal passages and the sinuses. In some nasal telescopes, the view is straight ahead from the tip of the instrument; in other telescopes, the view is at an angle from the tip of the telescope. These 'angled' telescopes can be used to see around corners—much like a child's toy periscope. The standard nasal examination is quite limited; however, nasal endoscopy provides a detailed examination of both the nasal cavity and sinuses. Also, nasal telescopes are also used during surgical procedures in the office and operating room.

Nasal Endoscopy Room

Nasal endoscopy is commonly performed in the office of otorhinolaryngologists (ENT doctors). The ENT doctor can look directly through the telescope. Alternatively, a medical video camera can be attached to the telescope, and then the images are viewed on a special video monitor as shown here. The examination may be recorded on a VCR, or a digital image archive (like a digital camera) may be used. If a patient wishes, he or she may view the images from his or her own examination.

Nasal Endoscopy

Patients tolerate nasal endoscopy very well. Many ENT doctors will apply a topical nasal decongestant and numbing medicine to the lining of the nose by a nasal spray prior to endoscopy. Often, the examination can be completed without any special medicines at all.

Nasal Instruments

These instruments are designed to be used in the nose and sinuses during nasal endoscopy. They may be used both in the operating room and in the office.

Frontal Sinus Instruments

These instruments are also designed to be used during nasal endoscopy both in the operating room and in the office. Note that the instruments are curved. Because the instruments are bent, it is possible to reach around corners. These instruments are used with the 'angled' telescopes.

More Frontal Sinus Instruments

These instruments are for procedures aimed at the frontal sinus (located in the forehead). Because the frontal sinus is located above the nose, the instruments are curved, so that they can reach the entrance to the sinus while the instruments are passed through the nose. Endoscopic frontal sinus surgery is very complicated, since the anatomy of this region is so complex.

Nasal Endoscopy in the Operating Room

Since the early 1980s, endoscopic sinus surgery has become a common method for the treatment of surgical treatment of sinus infections that do not improve with antibiotic treatment. Some surgeons prefer to look directly through the telescope, while other surgeons (shown here) will use a medical video camera that sends a TV picture to a video monitor. The reference frame is used for computer-aided surgery (described below). It is important to remember that endoscopic sinus surgery is a challenging and demanding surgical procedure.

Computer-Aided Sinus Surgery

Recently, computer-aided surgery (CAS) systems have been introduced into sinus surgery. This technology allows a surgeon to directly localize specific points seen during endoscopy with the CT scans that have been obtained prior to surgery. CAS provides important anatomic information—as a result, CAS probably decreases the risks of surgery and may improve the results of surgery.

455

Section 34.9

Bronchoscopy

From the *Diseases and Conditions Index*, National Heart
Lung and Blood Institute (www.nhlbi.nih.gov), January 2008.

What is bronchoscopy?

Bronchoscopy is a procedure used to look inside the lungs' airways, called the bronchi and bronchioles. The airways carry air from the trachea, or windpipe, to the lungs.

During the procedure, your doctor passes a thin, flexible tube called a bronchoscope through your nose (or sometimes your mouth), down your throat, and into the airways. If you have a breathing tube, the bronchoscope can be passed through it to your airways.

At the bronchoscope's tip are a light and a mini-camera, so the doctor can see your windpipe and airways. You will be given medicine to make you relaxed and sleepy during the procedure.

If there's a lot of bleeding in your lungs or a large object stuck in your throat, your doctor may use a bronchoscope with a rigid tube. The rigid tube, which is passed through the mouth, is wider. This allows your doctor to see inside it more easily, treat bleeding, and remove stuck objects.

A rigid bronchoscopy is usually done in a hospital operating room while you're under general anesthesia. Anesthesia is used so you will sleep through the procedure and not feel any pain.

Overview

- Bronchoscopy is usually done to find the cause of a lung problem. Your doctor may take samples of mucus or tissue from your lungs during the procedure to test in a lab.

- Bronchoscopy may show a tumor, signs of an infection, excess mucus in the airways, the site of bleeding, or something blocking the airway, like a piece of food.

- Sometimes bronchoscopy is used to treat lung problems. It may be done to insert a stent in an airway. An airway stent is a small tube that holds the airway open. It's used when a tumor or other condition blocks an airway.

- In children, the procedure is most often used to remove something blocking the airway. In some cases, it's used to find out what's causing a cough that has lasted for at least a few weeks.

Outlook

- Bronchoscopy is usually a safe procedure. You may be hoarse and have a sore throat after the procedure. There's a slight risk of minor bleeding or developing a fever or pneumonia.

- A rare but more serious risk is a pneumothorax, or collapsed lung. In this condition, air collects in the space around the lungs, which causes them to collapse. This problem is easily treated.

- Scientists are studying new methods of bronchoscopy, including virtual bronchoscopy. This is a kind of computed tomography (CT) scan. A CT scan uses special x-ray equipment to take clear, detailed pictures of the inside of your body. During the scan, you lie on a table that slides through the center of a tunnel-shaped x-ray machine. X-ray tubes in the scanner rotate around you and take pictures of your lungs.

- Virtual bronchoscopy is still not used often.

Who needs bronchoscopy?

The most common reason why your doctor may decide to do a bronchoscopy is if you have an abnormal chest x-ray or computed tomography (CT) scan. These tests may show a tumor, a collapsed lung, or signs of an infection.

A chest x-ray takes a picture of the heart and lungs. A CT scan uses special x-ray equipment to take pictures of the inside of your body.

Other reasons for bronchoscopy include if you're coughing up blood or if you have a cough that has lasted more than a few weeks.

The procedure also can be done to remove something that's stuck in an airway (like a piece of food), to place medicine in the lung to treat a lung problem, or to insert a stent (small tube) in an airway to hold it open when a tumor or other condition causes a blockage.

Bronchoscopy also can be used to check for swelling in the upper airways and vocal cords of people who were burned around the throat area or inhaled smoke from a fire.

In children, the procedure is most often used to remove something blocking an airway. In some cases, it's used to find out what's causing a cough that has lasted for at least a few weeks.

What should I expect before a bronchoscopy?

Your doctor will do the bronchoscopy in a special clinic or in the hospital. To prepare for the procedure, tell your doctor what medicines you're taking, including prescription and over-the-counter medicines. It's helpful to give your doctor a list of the medicines you take, about any previous bleeding problems; and about any allergies to medicines or latex.

Arrange for someone to drive you home from the clinic or hospital. The medicine you'll receive before the procedure will make you sleepy.

Avoid eating or drinking for four to eight hours before the procedure. Your doctor will let you know the right amount of time.

What should I expect during a bronchoscopy?

Your doctor will do the procedure in an exam room at a special clinic or in the hospital. The bronchoscopy itself usually lasts about 30 minutes. But the entire procedure, including preparation and recovery time, takes about four hours.

Your doctor will give you medicine through an intravenous (IV) line in your bloodstream or by mouth to make you sleepy and relaxed.

Your doctor also will squirt or spray a liquid medicine into your nose and throat to make them numb. This helps prevent coughing and gagging when the bronchoscope (long, thin tube) is inserted.

Then, your doctor will insert the bronchoscope through your nose or mouth and into your airways. As the tube enters your mouth, you may gag a little. Once it enters your throat, that feeling will go away.

Your doctor will look at your vocal cords and airways through the bronchoscope (which has a light and a mini-camera at its tip).

During the procedure, your doctor may take a sample of lung fluid or tissue for further testing. A chest x-ray may be used to help find the exact area to take the sample.

Samples can be taken through the following methods:

- **Bronchoalveolar lavage:** The doctor passes a small amount of salt water (a saline solution) through the bronchoscope and into part of your lung and then suctions it back out. The fluid picks up cells and bacteria from the airway, which your doctor can study.

- **Transbronchial lung biopsy:** The doctor inserts forceps into the bronchoscope and takes a small sample of tissue from inside the lung.

- **Transbronchial needle aspiration:** The doctor inserts a needle into the bronchoscope and removes cells from the lymph nodes in your lungs. These nodes are small, bean-shaped masses. They trap bacteria and cancer cells and help fight infection.

You may feel short of breath during bronchoscopy, but enough air is getting to your lungs. Your doctor will check your oxygen level. If the level drops, you'll be given oxygen.

If there's a lot of bleeding in your lungs or a large object stuck in your throat, your doctor may use a bronchoscope with a rigid tube. The rigid tube, which is passed through the mouth, is wider. This allows your doctor to see inside it more easily, treat bleeding, and remove stuck objects.

A rigid bronchoscopy is usually done in a hospital operating room while you're under general anesthesia. Anesthesia is used so you will sleep through the procedure and not feel any pain.

After the procedure is done, your doctor will remove the bronchoscope.

What should I expect after a bronchoscopy?

After bronchoscopy, you'll need to stay at the clinic or hospital for up to a few hours. If your doctor uses a bronchoscope with a rigid tube, there's a longer recovery time. While you're at the hospital or clinic:

- you may have a chest x-ray if your doctor took a sample of tissue from your lung. This test will check for a pneumothorax and bleeding. A pneumothorax is a condition in which air or gas collects in the space around the lungs. This can cause the lung(s) to collapse. The condition is easily treated.

- a health care provider will check your breathing and blood pressure.

- you can't eat or drink until the numbness in your throat wears off. This takes one to two hours.

After recovery, you'll need to have someone take you home. You'll be too sleepy to drive.

If samples of tissue or fluid were taken during the procedure, they'll be tested in a lab. Ask your doctor when you'll receive the lab results.

What is recovery and recuperation like?

Ask your doctor when you can return to your normal activities, such as driving, working, and physical activity. For the first few days, you may have a sore throat, cough, and hoarseness. Call your doctor right away if you develop a fever, have chest pain, have trouble breathing, or cough up more than a few tablespoons of blood.

What does bronchoscopy show?

Bronchoscopy may show a tumor, signs of an infection, excess mucus in the airways, the site of bleeding, or something blocking your airway.

Your doctor will use the procedure results to decide how to treat any lung problems that were found. Other tests may be needed.

What are the risks of bronchoscopy?

Bronchoscopy is usually a safe procedure. However, there's small risk for problems. The risks include the following:

- A drop in your oxygen level during the procedure. The doctor will give you oxygen if this happens.

- A slight risk of minor bleeding and developing a fever or pneumonia.

A rare but more serious side effect is a pneumothorax. A pneumothorax is a condition in which air or gas collects in the space around the lungs. This can cause the lung(s) to collapse.

This condition is easily treated and may go away on its own. If it interferes with breathing, a tube may need to be placed in the space around the lungs to remove the air.

A chest x-ray may be done after bronchoscopy to check for problems.

Chapter 35

Laparoscopy

Patients may be referred to surgeons because of an undiagnosed abdominal problem. If your surgeon has recommended a diagnostic laparoscopy, this information will:

- help you understand what laparoscopy is,

- describe how laparoscopy helps to find out what the problem is, and

- explain what complications can occur with the procedure.

What is diagnostic laparoscopy?

A laparoscope is a telescope designed for medical use. It is connected to a high intensity light and a high-resolution television camera so that the surgeon can see what is happening inside of you. The laparoscope is put into the abdominal cavity through a hollow tube and the image of the inside of your abdomen is seen on the television screen. In most cases, this procedure (operation) will be able to diagnose or help discover what the abdominal problem is.

"Diagnostic Laparoscopy" is reprinted with permission from the Society of American Gastrointestinal Endoscopic Surgeons (SAGES), © 2004. For additional information, contact SAGE, 11300 West Olympic Boulevard, Suite 600, Los Angeles, CA 90064, 310-437-0544, or visit www.sages.org.

Why is diagnostic laparoscopy performed?

1. **Abdominal pain:** Laparoscopy has a role in the diagnosis of both acute and chronic abdominal pain. There are many causes of abdominal pain. Some of these causes include appendicitis, adhesions or intra-abdominal scar tissue, pelvic infections, endometriosis, abdominal bleeding, and, less frequently, cancer. It is used in patients with irritable bowel disease to exclude other causes of abdominal pain. Surgeons can often diagnose the cause of the abdominal pain and, during the same procedure, correct the problem.

2. **Abdominal mass:** A patient may have a lump (mass or tumor), which can be felt by the doctor, the patient, or seen on an x-ray. Most masses require a definitive diagnosis before appropriate therapy or treatment can be recommended. Laparoscopy is one of the techniques available to your physician to look directly at the mass and obtain tissue to discover the diagnosis.

3. **Ascites:** The presence of fluid in the abdominal cavity is called ascites. Sometimes the cause of this fluid accumulation cannot be found without looking into the abdominal cavity, which can often be accomplished with laparoscopy.

4. **Liver disease:** Non-invasive x-ray imaging techniques (sonogram, computed tomography (CT) scan, and magnetic resonance imaging (MRI)) may discover a mass inside or on the surface of the liver. If the non-invasive x-ray cannot give your physician enough information, a liver biopsy may be needed to establish the diagnosis. Diagnostic laparoscopy is one of the safest and most accurate ways to obtain tissue for diagnosis. In other words, it is an accurate way to collect a biopsy to sample the liver or mass without actually opening the abdomen.

5. **"Second look" procedure or cancer staging:** Your doctor may need information regarding the status of a previously treated disease, such as cancer. This may occur after treatment with some forms of chemotherapy or before more chemotherapy is started. Also, information may be provided by diagnostic laparoscopy before planning a formal exploration of the abdomen, chemotherapy, or radiation therapy.

6. **Other:** There are other reasons to undergo a diagnostic laparoscopy, which cannot all be listed here. This should be reviewed and discussed with your surgeon.

What tests are necessary before laparoscopy?

Ultrasound may be ordered by your doctor as a non-invasive diagnostic test. In many cases, information is provided which will allow your surgeon to have a better understanding of the problem inside your abdomen. This test is not painful, is very safe, and can improve the effectiveness of the diagnostic laparoscopy.

CT scan is an x-ray that uses computers to visualize the intra-abdominal contents. In certain circumstances, it is accurate in making the diagnosis of abdominal disease. It will allow your surgeon to have a "road map" of the inside of your abdomen. A radiologist may use a CT scan to place a needle inside your abdomen. This is known as a CT guided needle biopsy. This will often be done before a diagnostic laparoscopy to decide if laparoscopy is appropriate for your condition.

MRI uses magnets, x-rays, and computers to view the inside of the abdominal cavity. It is not required for most abdominal problems, but may be necessary for some.

Routine blood test analysis, urinalysis, and possible chest x-ray or electrocardiogram may be needed before diagnostic laparoscopy. Your physician will decide which tests are necessary and will review the results of those tests, which have already been performed.

What type of anesthesia is used?

Diagnostic laparoscopy is performed either under local anesthesia with sedation or with general anesthesia. With your help, your surgeon and an anesthesiologist will decide on a method of anesthesia to perform safe and successful surgery.

Local anesthesia can be injected into the skin of the abdominal wall to completely numb the area and allow safe placement of a laparoscope. Most patients feel a short-lived "bee sting" that lasts a second or two. Small doses of intravenous sedation are given at the same time allowing the patient to experience what is known as "twilight" sleep in which patients are arousable but asleep. Once an adequate depth of sleep is reached and local anesthesia administered, gas is placed into the abdominal cavity. This is called a pneumoperitoneum. The patient may experience a bloated feeling. The gas is removed at the end of the operation. The two most common gases used are nitrous oxide ("laughing gas") or carbon dioxide. There is very little risk of ill-effects of the gas.

General anesthesia is given to those patients who are not candidates for "twilight" sleep or who want to be completely asleep. General anesthesia may be preferable in patients who are young, who cannot lie still on the operating table, or have a medical condition that is safer to perform in this manner. Some patients end up having a general anesthesia even though they prefer local anesthesia with sedation, as the appropriate anesthesia for laparoscopy differs from patient to patient.

What preparation is required?

- After your surgeon reviews with you the potential risks and benefits of the operation, you will need to provide written consent for surgery.

- It is acceptable to shower the night before or morning of the operation.

- Most diagnostic laparoscopy procedures are performed as an outpatient; meaning you will go home the same day the procedure was performed.

- You should have nothing to eat or drink for six to eight hours before the procedure.

- Standard blood, urine, or x-ray testing may be required before your operative procedure. This will depend on your age and medical conditions.

- It is acceptable to shower the night before or morning of the operation. Report to the hospital at the correct time, which is usually one to two hours earlier than your scheduled surgery.

- If you take medication on a daily basis, discuss this with your surgeon prior to surgery as you may need to take some or all of the medication on the day of surgery with a sip of water. If you take aspirin, vitamin E, blood thinners, or arthritis medication, discuss this with your surgeon so they can be stopped at the proper time before your surgery.

- You will need to ask your surgeon or his/her office staff what specifically is required in preparation for your surgery.

You will most likely be sedated during the procedure and an arrangement to have someone drive you home afterward is imperative. Sedatives will affect your judgment and reflexes for the rest of the day. You should not drive or operate machinery until the next day.

What can be expected during diagnostic laparoscopy?

- The surgery is performed under anesthesia, so that the patient will not feel pain during the procedure.

- A cannula (a narrow tube-like instrument) is placed into the abdominal cavity in the upper abdomen or flank just below the ribs.

- A laparoscope (a tiny telescope) connected to a special camera is inserted through the cannula. This gives the surgeon a magnified view of the patient's internal organs on a television screen.

- Other cannulas are inserted which allow your surgeon to see the internal organs and make a decision on the proper diagnosis or treatment.

- After the surgeon completes the operation, the small incisions are closed with absorbable sutures or with surgical tapes.

What should I expect after the operation?

Following the operation, you will be transferred to the recovery room, where you will be monitored carefully until all the sedatives and anesthetics have worn off. Even though you may feel fully awake, the effects of any anesthetic may persist for several hours. Once you are able to walk and get out of bed unassisted, you may be discharged. Because the effects of anesthesia can linger for many hours, it is necessary to have someone accompany you to the office or hospital and drive you home after the procedure.

You can expect some soreness around any incision site; this is normal. Your pain should improve daily even though you may need to take a pain reliever. Your surgeon will instruct you on the use of pain relievers and may give you a prescription for pain medication.

Most patients are able to shower the day after surgery and begin all normal activities within a week. Your surgeon can answer any specific restrictions that apply to you.

You should call and schedule a follow-up appointment within two weeks after your procedure.

What complications can occur?

Any procedure may have complications associated with it. The most frequent complications of any operation are bleeding and infection. There is a small risk of other complications that include, but are not limited to, injury to the abdominal organs, intestines, urinary bladder, or blood vessels. If you suffer with ascites, this ascites may leak from one of the operative sites, temporarily, before stopping.

In a small number of patients the laparoscopic method cannot be performed. The decision to perform the open procedure is a judgment decision made by your surgeon either before or during the actual operation. When the surgeon feels that it is safest to convert the laparoscopic procedure to an open one, this is not a complication, but rather sound surgical judgment. The decision to convert to an open procedure is strictly based on patient safety.

When to Call Your Doctor

Be sure to call your surgeon or physician if you develop any of the following:

- Fever above 101 degrees F (39 C)
- Drainage from or redness any of your incisions
- Continued nausea or vomiting
- Increasing abdominal swelling
- Bleeding
- Chills
- Persistent cough or shortness of breath
- Inability to urinate
- Pain not controlled by medication

Chapter 36

Holter and Event Monitors

What are Holter and event monitors?

Holter and event monitors are medical devices that record the heart's electrical activity. Doctors most often use these monitors to diagnose arrhythmias. These are problems with the speed or rhythm of the heartbeat. During an arrhythmia, the heart can beat too fast, too slow, or irregularly.

Holter and event monitors also are used to detect silent myocardial ischemia. In this condition, not enough oxygen-rich blood reaches the heart muscle. "Silent" means that no symptoms occur.

These monitors also can check whether treatments for arrhythmia and silent myocardial ischemia are working.

This chapter focuses on using Holter and event monitors to diagnose problems with the heart's speed or rhythm.

Holter and event monitors are similar to an EKG (electrocardiogram). An EKG is a simple test that detects and records the heart's electrical activity. It's the most common test for diagnosing a heart rhythm problem.

However, a standard EKG only records the heartbeat for a few seconds. It won't detect heart rhythm problems that don't occur during the test.

Holter and event monitors are small, portable devices. You can wear one while you do your normal daily activities. This allows the monitor to record your heart for a longer time than an EKG.

National Heart Lung and Blood Institute, December 2007.

Some people have heart rhythm problems that only occur during certain activities, such as sleep or physical exertion. Using a Holter or event monitor increases the chance of recording these problems.

Although similar, Holter and event monitors aren't the same. A Holter monitor records your heart's electrical activity the entire time you're wearing it. An event monitor only records your heart's electrical activity at certain times while you're wearing it.

What are the different types of Holter and event monitors?

Holter monitors: Holter monitors are sometimes called continuous EKGs (electrocardiograms). This is because Holter monitors record the heart rhythm continuously for 24 to 48 hours.

A Holter monitor is about the size of a large deck of cards. You can clip it to a belt or carry it in a pocket. Wires connect the device to sensors (called electrodes) that are stuck to your chest using sticky patches. These sensors pick up your heart's electrical signals, and the monitor records your heart's rhythm.

Wireless Holter monitors: Wireless Holter monitors have a longer recording time than standard Holter monitors. The wireless version records your heart's electrical activity for a preset amount of time.

These monitors are called wireless because they use a cell phone to send the data to your doctor's office. This happens automatically at certain times. These monitors still have wires that connect the device to the sensors stuck to your chest.

You can use a wireless Holter monitor for days or even weeks until signs or symptoms of a heart rhythm problem occur. These monitors usually are used to detect heart rhythm problems that don't occur often.

Although wireless Holter monitors work for longer periods, they have a down side. You must remember to write down the time of symptoms, so your doctor can match it to the heart rhythm recording. Also, the batteries in the wireless monitor must be changed every one to two days.

Event monitors: Event monitors are similar to Holter monitors. You wear one while you do your normal daily activities. Most event monitors have wires that connect the device to sensors that are stuck to your chest using sticky patches.

Unlike Holter monitors though, event monitors don't continuously record the heart's electrical activity. They only record when symptoms occur. For many event monitors, you need to start the monitor when you feel symptoms.

Event monitors tend to be smaller than Holter monitors because they don't need to store as much data.

Different types of event monitors work in slightly different ways. Your doctor will explain how to use the monitor before you start wearing it.

Postevent recorders: Postevent recorders are among the smallest event monitors. You can wear a postevent recorder like a wristwatch or carry it in your pocket. The pocket version is about the size of a thick credit card. These recorders don't have wires that connect the device to chest sensors.

When you feel a symptom, you start the recorder. A postevent recorder only records what happens after you start it. It may miss a heart rhythm problem that occurs before and during the onset of symptoms. Also, it may be hard to start the monitor when a symptom is in progress.

In some cases, this missing data would have helped your doctor diagnose the heart rhythm problem.

Presymptom memory loop recorders: Presymptom memory loop recorders are the size of a small cell phone. They're also called continuous loop event recorders.

You can clip this event monitor to your belt or carry it in your pocket. Wires connect the device to sensors on your chest.

These recorders are always recording and erasing data. When you feel a symptom, you push a button on the device. The normal erase process stops. The recording will show a few minutes of the data from before, during, and after the symptom.

In some cases, this makes it possible for your doctor to see very brief changes in your heart's rhythm.

Autodetect recorders: Autodetect recorders are about the size of the palm of your hand. Wires connect the device to sensors on your chest.

You don't need to start an autodetect recorder during symptoms. These recorders detect abnormal heart rhythms and automatically record and send the data to your doctor's office.

Implantable loop recorders: You may need an implantable loop recorder if other event monitors can't provide enough data. Implantable loop recorders are about the size of a pack of gum. This type of event monitor is inserted under the skin on your chest. No wires or chest sensors are used.

The device records either when you activate it or automatically when symptoms occur. It depends on how your doctor programs it. Devices may differ, so your doctor will tell you how to use it. In some cases, a special card is held close to the recorder to start it.

What other names are used for Holter and event monitors?

- Ambulatory EKG (electrocardiogram)

- Continuous EKG

- EKG event monitors

- Episodic monitors

- Mobile cardiac outpatient telemetry systems. This is another name for autodetect recorders.

- Thirty-day event recorders

- Transtelephonic event monitors. These are monitors that require the patient to send the collected data to a doctor's office. This is done using a telephone.

Who needs a Holter or event monitor?

You may need a Holter or event monitor if your doctor suspects you have an arrhythmia. This is a problem with the speed or rhythm of your heartbeat. Holter or event monitors are most often used to detect arrhythmias in people who have the following symptoms:

- Fainted or sometimes feel dizzy. A monitor may be used if causes other than a heart rhythm problem have been ruled out.

- Palpitations that recur with no known cause. Palpitations are the feeling that your heart is pounding, racing, fluttering, or beating unevenly.

People who are being treated for a heart rhythm problem also may need to use a Holter or event monitor. These monitors can show how treatment is working.

In some people, heart rhythm problems only occur during certain events, such as sleep or physical exertion. Holter and event monitors record the heart rhythm while a person does his or her normal daily routine. This allows the doctor to see how the heart responds to different daily activities, which helps diagnose the problem.

Holter and event monitors also are used for elderly people who may have trouble getting to and from clinics.

What should I expect before using a Holter or event monitor?

Your doctor will do a physical exam before giving you a Holter or event monitor. He or she will perform the following tasks:

- Check your pulse to find out how fast your heart is beating and measure your blood pressure

- Listen to the rate and rhythm of your heart

- Check for swelling in your legs or feet. This could be a sign of an enlarged heart or heart failure, which may cause arrhythmias (problems with the speed or rhythm of the heartbeat).

- Look for signs of other diseases (such as thyroid disease) that could be causing heart rhythm problems

You may have an EKG (electrocardiogram) test before your doctor sends you home with a Holter or event monitor. An EKG detects and records the electrical activity of the heart for a few seconds. It shows how fast the heart is beating and its rhythm (steady or irregular). It also records the strength and timing of electrical signals as they pass through each part of the heart.

A standard EKG won't detect heart rhythm problems that don't happen during the test. For this reason, your doctor may give you a Holter or event monitor. These monitors are portable. You can wear one while doing your normal daily activities. This increases the chance of recording symptoms that only occur once in a while.

Your doctor will explain how to wear and use the Holter or event monitor. Usually, you will leave the office wearing it.

Each type of monitor is slightly different, but most have sensors (called electrodes) that are attached to the skin on your chest with sticky patches. It's important that the sensors have good contact with your skin. Poor contact can result in poor results.

Oil, too much sweat, and hair can keep the patches from sticking to your skin. You may need to shave the area on your chest where your doctor will attach each patch. You will need to clean the area with a special prep pad that the doctor will provide.

You may need to use a small amount of special paste or gel to make the patches stick to your skin better. Some patches come with paste or gel on them.

What should I expect when using a Holter or event monitor?

Your experience while using a Holter or event monitor depends on the type of monitor you have. However, most monitors have some factors in common.

Recording the heart's electrical activity: All monitors record the heart's electrical activity. So, it's important to maintain a clear signal between the sensors (electrodes) and the recording device.

In most cases, the sensors are attached to your chest with sticky patches. Wires connect the sensors to the monitor. You usually can clip the monitor to your belt or carry it in your pocket. (Postevent and implantable loop recorders don't have chest sensors.)

A good stick between the patches and your skin helps provide a clear signal. Poor contact leads to a poor recording, which is hard for your doctor to read.

Oil, too much sweat, and hair can keep the patches from sticking to your skin. You may need to shave the area where your doctor will attach each patch. You will need to clean the area with a special prep pad that your doctor provides.

You may need to use a small amount of special paste or gel to make the patches stick to your skin better. Some patches come with paste or gel on them.

Too much movement can pull the patches away from the skin or create "noise" on the rhythm strip. A rhythm strip is a graph showing the pattern of the heartbeat. Noise looks like a lot of jagged lines and makes it hard for the doctor to see the real rhythm of the heart.

When you have a symptom, stop what you're doing. This way you can be sure that the recording shows the heart's activity rather than your movement.

Your doctor will tell you whether you need to adjust your activity level during the testing period. If you exercise, choose a cool location to avoid sweating too much. This will help the patches stay sticky.

Other everyday items also can disrupt the signal between the sensors and the monitor. These items include magnets, metal detectors, microwave ovens, and electric blankets, toothbrushes, and razors. Avoid using these items. Also avoid areas with high voltage.

Cell phones and iPods may interfere with the signal if they're too close to the monitor. When using any electronic device, try to keep it at least six inches away from the monitor.

Keeping a diary: When using a Holter or event monitor, you need to keep a diary of your symptoms and activities. Write down when symptoms occur, what they are, and what you were doing at the time.

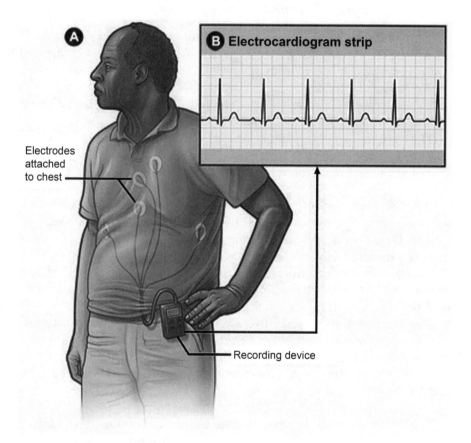

Figure 36.1. Holter or Event Monitor. This drawing illustrates how a Holter or event monitor attaches to a patient. In this example, the monitor is clipped to the patient's belt and electrodes are attached to his chest. Figure B shows an electrocardiogram strip, which maps the data from the Holter or event monitor.

The most common symptoms of heart rhythm problems include palpitations (this is the feeling that your heart is pounding, racing, fluttering, or beating unevenly) and fainting or feeling dizzy.

It's important to note the time symptoms occur, because your doctor matches the data with the information in your diary. This allows your doctor to see whether certain activities trigger changes in your heart rate and rhythm.

You also should include details in your diary about when you take any medicine or if you feel stress at certain times during the test.

What to Expect with Specific Monitors

Holter Monitor: The Holter monitor is about the size of a large deck of cards. You wear it for 24 to 48 hours. When the test is complete, you return the device to your doctor's office. The results are stored on the device.

You can't get the monitor wet, so you won't be able to bathe or shower. You can take a sponge bath if needed.

The recording period for a standard Holter monitor may be too short to capture a heart rhythm problem. If this is the case, you may need a wireless Holter monitor.

Wireless Holter Monitors: Wireless Holter monitors can record for a longer time than standard Holter monitors. A wireless monitor records for a preset amount of time. It then automatically sends data from the monitor to your doctor's office.

These monitors are called wireless because they use a cell phone to send the data to your doctor's office. They still have wires that connect the device to the sensors stuck to your chest.

You can use a wireless Holter monitor for days or even weeks until signs or symptoms of a heart rhythm problem occur.

The batteries in the wireless monitor must be changed every one to two days. You will need to detach the sensors to shower or bathe and then reattach them.

Event Monitors: Event monitors are slightly smaller than Holter monitors. Event monitors record heart rhythm problems when you activate them. They can be worn for weeks or until symptoms occur.

Most event monitors are worn like Holter monitors—clipped to a belt or carried in a pocket. When you have symptoms, you simply push a button to start recording.

Postevent Recorders: Postevent recorders may be worn like a wristwatch or carried in a pocket. The pocket version is about the size of a thick credit card. These recorders don't have wires that connect the device to chest sensors.

To start the recorder when you feel a symptom, you hold it to your chest. To start the wristwatch version, you touch a button on the side of the watch.

You send the stored data to your doctor's office using a telephone. Your doctor will explain how to use the monitor before you leave the office.

Autodetect Recorders: Autodetect recorders are about the size of the palm of your hand. Wires connect the device to sensors on your chest.

You don't need to start an autodetect recorder. This type of monitor automatically starts recording when it detects an abnormal heart rhythm. It then sends the data to your doctor's office.

Implantable Loop Recorders: Implantable loop recorders are about the size of a pack of gum. This type of event monitor is inserted under the skin on your chest. No chest sensors are used.

The device records either when you activate it or automatically when symptoms occur. It depends on how your doctor programs it. Devices may differ, so your doctor will tell you how to use it. In some cases, a special card is held close to the recorder to start it.

What should I expect after using a Holter or event monitor?

After you're finished using a Holter or event monitor, you return it to your doctor's office or the place you got it from.

If you were using an implantable loop recorder, you will need to have it removed. Your doctor will discuss the procedure with you.

Your doctor will tell you when to expect the results. Once your doctor has reviewed the recordings, he or she will discuss the results with you.

What does a Holter or event monitor show?

A Holter or event monitor may show what's causing symptoms of an arrhythmia. This is problem with the speed or rhythm of the heartbeat.

Holter and event monitors also can show whether a heart rhythm problem is harmless or whether it needs treatment. Treatment is needed if the problem causes serious symptoms or increases your chance for complications.

Serious symptoms may include dizziness, chest pain, and fainting. Complications may include heart failure, stroke, or sudden cardiac arrest.

If the symptoms of your heart rhythm problem occur often, a Holter or event monitor has a good chance of capturing them. You may not have symptoms while using a monitor. Even so, your doctor may learn more about your heart rhythm from the test results.

Sometimes, these monitors can't help doctors diagnose heart rhythm problems. If this happens, talk to your doctor about other steps you can take.

One option may be to try a different type of monitor. The wireless Holter monitor and the implantable loop recorder have longer recording periods. This may allow the monitor to get the data that your doctor needs to make a diagnosis.

What are the risks from using a Holter or event monitor?

The sticky patches used to attach the sensors (electrodes) to your chest have a small risk of skin irritation. You also may have an allergic reaction the paste or gel that's sometimes used to attach the patches. The irritation will go away once the patches are removed.

If you're using an implantable loop recorder, you may get an infection or have pain where the device is placed under the skin. You may be given medicine to treat these complications.

Chapter 37

Sleep Studies

What are sleep studies?

Sleep studies allow doctors to measure how much and how well you sleep. They also help show whether you have sleep problems and how severe they are.

Sleep studies are important because untreated sleep disorders can increase your risk for high blood pressure, heart attack, stroke, and other medical conditions. People usually aren't aware of their breathing and movements while sleeping. They may never think to talk to their doctors about sleep- and health-related issues that may be linked to sleep problems.

Doctors can diagnose and treat sleep disorders. Talk to your doctor if you feel tired or very sleepy while at work or school most days of the week. You also may want to talk to your doctor if you often have trouble falling or staying asleep, or if you wake up too early and aren't able to get back to sleep. These are common signs of a sleep disorder.

Doctors can diagnose some sleep disorders by asking questions about your sleep schedule and habits and by getting information from sleep partners or parents. To diagnose other sleep disorders, doctors also use the results from sleep studies and other medical tests.

Sleep studies can help doctors diagnose problems such as the following:

• Sleep-related breathing disorders (such as sleep apnea)

National Heart Lung and Blood Institute, October 2007.

- Sleep-related seizure disorders
- Parasomnias (such as sleepwalking)
- Narcolepsy
- Insomnia
- Circadian rhythm disorders

What are the different types of sleep studies?

Four common sleep studies are used to help diagnose sleep-related problems: polysomnogram, or PSG; multiple sleep latency test, or MSLT; maintenance of wakefulness test, or MWT; and actigraphy.

Polysomnogram: A PSG is usually done while you stay overnight at a sleep center. A PSG records brain activity, eye movements, heart rate, and blood pressure.

It also records the amount of oxygen in your blood, how much air is moving through your nose while you breathe, and chest movements that show whether you're making an effort to breathe. In some cases, breathing sounds, including snoring, also are recorded.

PSG results are used to help diagnose the following disorders:

- Insomnia
- Sleep-related breathing disorders (such as sleep apnea)
- Narcolepsy (PSG and MSLT results will be reviewed together)
- Sleep-related seizure disorders
- Parasomnias (such as sleepwalking)

Your doctor also may use a PSG to find the right setting for you on a continuous positive airway pressure (CPAP) machine. CPAP is the most common treatment for sleep apnea.

A CPAP machine uses a small pump to gently supply air to your nose or mouth through a special mask. The right setting involves adding just enough extra air to create mild pressure that keeps your airways open while you sleep.

If your doctor thinks that you have sleep apnea, he or she may schedule a split-night sleep study. During the first half of the night, your sleep will be checked without a CPAP machine. This will show if you have sleep apnea and how severe it is.

If the PSG shows signs that you have sleep apnea, you will use a CPAP machine during the second half of the split-night study. A technician checks your breathing using the PSG and adjusts the flow of air through the CPAP mask to find the correct setting for you.

A PSG also helps doctors adjust CPAP settings after weight loss or gain, recheck your sleep if symptoms return despite treatment with CPAP, or find out how well surgery has worked to correct a sleep-related breathing problem.

Multiple sleep latency test: This daytime sleep study measures how sleepy you are. It's typically done the day after a PSG. You relax in a quiet room for about 30 minutes while a technician checks your brain activity.

The MSLT records whether you fall asleep during the test and what types and stages of sleep you're having. Sleep has two basic types: rapid eye movement (REM) and non-REM. REM sleep and non-REM sleep occur in patterns throughout the night.

The types and stages of sleep can help your doctor diagnose sleep disorders such as narcolepsy, idiopathic hypersomnia, and circadian rhythm disorders.

The test is repeated three or four times throughout the day. This is because your ability to fall asleep also changes throughout the day.

Maintenance of wakefulness test: This daytime sleep study measures your ability to stay awake and alert. It's usually done the day after a PSG and takes most of the day.

Results may be used to show whether your inability to stay awake is a public or personal safety concern or to check your response to treatment.

Actigraphy: This sleep study is done while you go about your normal daily routine. It doesn't require an overnight stay at the sleep clinic.

The Actigraph is a simple device that's usually worn like a wrist-watch. The doctor may ask you to wear the device for several days—except when bathing or swimming.

This test gives your doctor a better idea about your sleep habits, such as when you sleep or nap and whether the lights are on while you sleep.

Who needs a sleep study?

If you often feel very tired during the day—even though you spent enough time in bed to be well rested—talk to your doctor. This is a common sign of a sleep disorder. A number of sleep disorders can disrupt your sleep, leaving you sleepy during the day.

Other common signs of sleep disorders include the following:

- It takes you more than 30 minutes to fall asleep at night

- You awaken often during the night and then have trouble falling back to sleep, or you awaken too early in the morning

- You feel sleepy during the day and fall asleep within five minutes if you have an opportunity to nap, or you fall asleep at inappropriate times during the day

- Your bed partner claims you snore loudly, snort, gasp, or make choking sounds while you sleep, or your partner notices your breathing stops for short periods

- You have creeping, tingling, or crawling feelings in your legs that are relieved by moving or massaging them, especially in the evening and when you try to fall asleep

- You have vivid, dreamlike experiences while falling asleep or dozing

- You have episodes of sudden muscle weakness when you're angry, fearful, or when you laugh

- You feel as though you can't move when you first wake up

- Your bed partner notes that your legs or arms jerk often during sleep

- You regularly feel the need to use stimulants to stay awake during the day

Describe your signs and symptoms to your doctor. It's important to note how tired you feel and whether your signs and symptoms affect your daily routine. Early signs of sleep disorders aren't easy to detect during routine visits. There are no blood tests for sleep disorders, and the doctor isn't watching you sleep.

If you've had a sleep disorder for a long time, it may be hard for you to notice its impact on your daily routine.

Your doctor can decide whether you need a sleep study. A sleep study allows your doctor to observe sleep patterns and to diagnose a sleep disorder, which can then be treated.

Certain medical conditions have been linked to sleep disorders. These include heart failure, coronary artery disease, obesity, diabetes, high blood pressure, and stroke or transient ischemic attack (TIA, or "mini-stroke"). If you have one of these conditions, talk with your doctor about whether it would be helpful to have a sleep study.

What should I expect before a sleep study?

Before a sleep study, your doctor may ask you about your sleep habits and whether you feel well rested and alert during the day.

You may be asked to keep a sleep diary or sleep log. You will record information such as when you went to bed, when you woke up, how many times you woke up during the night, and more.

What to bring with you: Depending on what type of sleep study you're having, you may need to bring these items:

- Notes from your sleep diary or sleep log. These may be helpful to your doctor.
- Pajamas and a toothbrush for overnight sleep studies.
- A comfortable pillow.
- A book or something to do between testing periods if you're having a multiple sleep latency test or a maintenance of wakefulness test (MWT).

How to prepare: You may need to stop or limit the use of tobacco, caffeine, and stimulants before having a sleep study. Your doctor may ask you about alcohol, medicines, or other substances that you take and about allergies that you have.

You may routinely take medicine that affects your sleep patterns. If so, a sleep specialist will help you plan how to take it during and possibly before the test.

You should try to sleep well the night before you have an MWT, because you will have to try to stay awake during this test. If you're being tested as a requirement for a transportation- or safety-related job, you may be asked to take a drug-screening test.

What should I expect during a sleep study?

Sleep studies are painless. Parents can go with their children to a sleep study.

The polysomnogram (PSG), multiple sleep latency test (MSLT), and maintenance of wakefulness test (MWT) are usually done at a sleep center. The room the sleep study is done in may look like a hotel room. A technician makes the room comfortable for you and sets the temperature to your liking.

Most of your contact at the sleep center will be with nurses or technicians. You can ask them any questions that you may have about the sleep study.

During a polysomnogram: Sticky patches called sensors are placed on your scalp, face, chest, limbs, and a finger. While you sleep, these devices record your brain activity, eye movements, heart rate and rhythm, blood pressure, and the amount of oxygen in your blood.

Elastic belts are placed around your chest and abdomen. They measure chest movements and the strength and duration of each exhaled breath.

Wires attached to the sensors transmit the data to a computer in the next room. The wires are very thin and flexible and are bundled together to minimize discomfort. You will be able to roll in any direction.

A technician in another room monitors the recordings as you sleep. He or she fixes any problems with the recordings that occur.

The technician also helps keep you comfortable and disconnects the equipment if you need to go to the bathroom.

When it's time for you to sleep, the room will be dark and quiet.

If you show signs of sleep apnea, you may have a split-night sleep study. During the first half of the night, the technician records your sleep patterns. At the start of the second half of the night, he or she wakes you to fit a continuous positive airway pressure (CPAP) mask over your nose and mouth.

The mask is connected to a small machine that gently blows air through the mask. This creates mild pressure that keeps your airways open while you sleep.

The technician checks how you sleep with the CPAP machine. He or she adjusts the flow of air through the mask to find the setting that's right for you.

At the end of the PSG, the technician helps you out of bed and removes the sensors. If you're having a daytime sleep study, such as an MSLT, some of the sensors may be left on for that test.

During a multiple sleep latency test: The MSLT is a daytime sleep study that's usually done after a PSG. Sensors on your scalp, face, and chin usually are used for this test. These sensors record brain activity. They show various stages of sleep and how long it takes you to fall asleep. Sometimes your breathing also is checked during an MSLT.

A technician in another room watches these recordings as you sleep. He or she fixes any problems with the recordings that occur.

Starting an hour and a half to three hours after you wake from the PSG, you're asked to relax in a quiet room for about 30 minutes. The test is repeated three or four times throughout the day. This is because your ability to fall asleep changes throughout the day.

You get two-hour breaks between tests. You need to stay awake during the breaks.

The MSLT records whether you fall asleep during the test and what types and stages of sleep you have. Sleep has two basic types: rapid eye movement (REM) and non-REM. Non-REM sleep has four distinct stages. REM sleep and the four stages of non-REM sleep occur in patterns throughout the night.

The types and stages of sleep can help your doctor diagnose a sleep disorder such as narcolepsy, idiopathic hypersomnia, or a circadian rhythm disorder.

During a maintenance of wakefulness test: This sleep study occurs during the day. It's usually done after a PSG and takes most of the day. Sensors on your scalp, face, and chin are used to measure when you're awake or asleep.

You sit quietly on a bed in a comfortable position and look straight ahead. Then, you simply try to stay awake for a period of time.

An MWT typically includes four trials lasting about 40 minutes each. If you fall asleep, the technician will wake you after about 90 seconds. There are usually two-hour breaks between trials. During these breaks, you can read, or watch television.

If you're being tested as a requirement for a transportation- or safety-related job, you may need a drug-screening test before the MWT.

During an Actigraph test: You don't have to go to a sleep center for this study. The Actigraph is a small device that's usually worn like a wristwatch. You can go about your normal daily routine while you wear it. You remove it while swimming or bathing.

The Actigraph measures your sleep-wake behavior over three to seven days. Results give your doctor a better idea about your sleep habits, such as when you sleep or nap and whether the lights are on while you sleep.

You may be asked to keep a sleep diary while you wear the Actigraph.

What should I expect after a sleep study?

Once the sensors are removed after a polysomnogram, multiple sleep latency test, or maintenance of wakefulness test, you can go home. If you used an Actigraph to measure your sleep-wake behavior, you return it to your doctor's office.

You won't receive a diagnosis right away. Your primary care doctor or sleep specialist will review the results of your sleep study or sleep studies. He or she will use your medical history, your sleep history, and the test results to make a diagnosis.

It may take a couple of weeks to get the results of your sleep study. Usually, your doctor, nurse, or sleep specialist will explain the test results and work with you and your family to develop a treatment plan.

What do sleep studies show?

Sleep studies allow doctors to watch sleep patterns and note sleep-related problems that patients don't know or can't describe during routine office visits. These studies are needed to diagnose certain sleep disorders, such as narcolepsy and sleep apnea.

After the sleep study, your doctor will get the results. The results will include information that the sleep technician records about sleep and wake times, sleep stages, abnormal breathing, the amount of oxygen in your blood, and any movement during sleep.

Your doctor will use your sleep study results and your medical and sleep histories to make a diagnosis and create a treatment plan.

If you have sleep apnea, your doctor also may use a PSG to find the right setting for you on a continuous positive airway pressure (CPAP) machine. A CPAP machine uses a small pump to gently supply air to your nose or mouth through a special mask. The right setting involves adding just enough extra air to create mild pressure that keeps your airways open while you sleep.

For sleep-related breathing disorders, such as sleep apnea, technicians use a PSG to record the number of abnormal breathing events. These include either pauses in breathing or dips in the level of oxygen in your blood.

In adults, when the number of events is ten or more per hour, treatment may be needed. Children who have one to three events per hour also may need treatment.

Results from a multiple sleep latency test: MSLT results are used to help diagnose narcolepsy, idiopathic hypersomnia, and circadian rhythm disorders.

For narcolepsy, technicians study how quickly you fall asleep. The MSLT also shows how long it takes you to reach different types and stages of sleep. Sleep has two basic types: rapid eye movement (REM) and non-REM. Non-REM sleep has four distinct stages. REM sleep and the four stages of non-REM sleep occur in patterns throughout the night.

People who fall asleep in less than five minutes or quickly reach REM sleep may need treatment for a sleep disorder.

Results from a maintenance of wakefulness test: Maintenance of wakefulness test (MWT) results may be used to show whether your inability to stay awake is a public or personal safety concern. This study also is used to show how well treatment is working.

Results from an Actigraph test: Actigraph results give your doctor a better idea about your sleep habits, such as when you sleep or nap and whether the lights are on while you sleep. This study also is used to help diagnose circadian rhythm disorders.

What are the risks of sleep studies?

Sleep studies are painless. There is a small risk of skin irritation from the sensors. The irritation will go away once the sensors are removed.

Although the risks of sleep studies are minimal, these studies take time (at least several hours). If you're having a daytime sleep study, bring a book or something to entertain yourself with during the test.

Chapter 38

Stress Testing

What is stress testing?

Stress testing provides your doctor with information about how your heart works during physical stress. Some heart problems are easier to diagnose when your heart is working hard and beating fast. During a stress test, you exercise (walk or run on a treadmill or pedal a bicycle) or are given a medicine to make your heart work harder while heart tests are performed.

During these tests, your heart is monitored using images or through dime-sized electrodes attached to your chest, arms, or legs. You may be asked to breathe into a special tube during the test. This will allow your doctor to see how well you're breathing.

You may have arthritis or another medical problem that prevents you from exercising during a stress test. If so, your doctor can give you a medicine that makes your heart work harder, as it would if you were exercising. This is called a pharmacological stress test.

Doctors usually use stress testing to help diagnose coronary artery disease (CAD) or to see how serious this disease is in those who are known to have it. It's sometimes used to assess other problems such as heart valve abnormalities or heart failure.

CAD occurs when the arteries that supply blood to the heart muscle (the coronary arteries) become hardened and narrowed with a material called plaque (plak). Plaque is made up of fat, cholesterol, calcium, and

---

National Heart Lung and Blood Institute, September 2007.

other substances found in the blood. Plaque builds up on the insides of the arteries, narrowing them and restricting blood flow to your heart.

You may not have any signs or symptoms of CAD when your heart is at rest. But when your heart has to work harder during exercise, it needs more blood and oxygen, and narrowed arteries aren't able to supply enough blood for your heart to work well. Thus, the signs and symptoms may occur only during exercise.

A stress test can detect the following indications that your heart may not be getting enough blood during exercise.

- Abnormal changes in your heart rate or blood pressure
- Symptoms such as shortness of breath or chest pain
- Abnormal changes in your heart rhythm or the electrical activity of your heart

During the stress test, if you can't exercise for as long as what's considered normal for someone your age, it may be a sign that not enough blood is flowing to your heart. But other factors besides CAD can prevent you from exercising long enough (for example, lung diseases, anemia, or poor general fitness).

Stress testing using imaging: Some stress tests take pictures of the heart when you exercise and when you're at rest. These imaging stress tests can show how well blood is flowing in the different parts of your heart or how well your heart squeezes out blood when it beats.

One type of imaging stress test involves echocardiography, which is a test that uses sound waves to create a moving picture of your heart. An echocardiogram stress test can show how well your heart's chambers and valves are working when your heart is under stress. The test can identify areas of poor blood flow to your heart, dead heart muscle tissue, and areas of the heart muscle wall that aren't contracting normally. These areas may have been damaged during a heart attack or may be getting too little blood.

Other imaging stress tests use a radioactive dye to create images of the blood flow to your heart. The dye is injected into your bloodstream before pictures are taken of your heart. The pictures show how much of the dye has reached various parts of your heart during exercise and at rest.

Tests that use a radioactive dye include a thallium or sestamibi stress test and a positron emission tomography (PET) stress test. The amount of radiation in the dye is safe and not a danger to you or those around you. However, if you're pregnant, you shouldn't have this test because of risks it might pose to your unborn child.

Some doctors may use magnetic resonance imaging (MRI) to take pictures of the heart when it's working hard. This test doesn't use a radioactive dye or sound waves. Instead, it uses radio waves and magnetic fields to create images that show blood flow in the heart and whether all parts of the heart wall are contracting strongly.

Imaging stress tests tend to be more accurate at detecting CAD than standard (nonimaging) stress tests.

An imaging stress test may be done first if you:

- Can't exercise for enough time to get your heart working its hardest. (Medical problems, such as arthritis or leg arteries clogged by plaque, may prevent you from exercising enough.)

- Have abnormal heartbeats or other problems that will cause a standard exercise stress test to be inaccurate.

- Are a woman. Standard stress tests are less accurate in women than in men. If you're a woman and live far from a testing facility, your doctor may want you to skip a standard stress test and get an imaging stress test instead. That way, you don't have to make a second trip for the imaging stress test if there are any questions about the results from the standard stress test.

Other Names for Stress Testing

- Exercise test
- Treadmill test
- Exercise echocardiogram or exercise stress echo
- Thallium stress test
- Sestamibi stress test
- Stress EKG
- Myocardial perfusion imaging
- Pharmacological stress test
- MRI stress test
- PET stress test
- Nuclear stress test

Who needs stress testing?

You may need a stress test if you've had chest pains, shortness of breath, or other symptoms of limited blood flow to your heart. Imaging stress tests are particularly helpful in showing whether you have coronary artery disease (CAD) or a problem with one of the valves in your heart. (Heart valves are like doors that let blood flow between the heart's chambers and into the heart's arteries. So, like CAD, faulty heart valves can limit the amount of blood reaching your heart.)

If you've been diagnosed with CAD or recently had a heart attack, you may need stress testing to see whether you can tolerate an exercise program. The testing also can show whether treatments designed to improve blood flow in the heart's arteries are necessary and likely to help you. These treatments include angioplasty (with or without stents) and coronary artery bypass grafting. After having one of these treatments, your doctor may want you to have a stress test to see how well the treatment relieves your signs or symptoms of CAD.

You also may need a stress test if, during exercise, you feel faint, get a rapid heartbeat or a fluttering feeling in your chest, or have other symptoms of an arrhythmia (an irregular heartbeat). The stress test can detect an arrhythmia and show whether you need medicine or a pacemaker or implantable cardioverter defibrillator (ICD) to correct irregular heartbeats. It also can reveal the effectiveness of such devices.

You may need a stress test even if you don't have chest pain when you exercise, but just get short of breath. The test can help show whether a heart problem, rather than a lung problem or being out of shape, is causing your breathing problems. For such testing, you breathe into a special tube so a technician can measure the gases you breathe out.

Breathing into the special tube and monitoring of the heart as part of a stress test also is done to assess fitness before a heart transplant. Your doctor also may use this monitoring to figure out the best exercise plan for you after recovery from a heart attack.

Stress testing isn't routinely done to screen people for CAD. Usually you have to have symptoms of CAD before a doctor will recommend that you have a stress test. But your doctor may want to use a stress test to screen for CAD if you have diabetes, which increases your risk for developing CAD.

What should I expect before stress testing?

Standard stress testing can often be done in a doctor's office. But imaging stress testing is usually done at a hospital. Be sure to wear athletic or other shoes in which you can exercise comfortably. You may be asked to wear comfortable clothes in which you can easily exercise, or you may be given a gown to wear during the test.

Your doctor may ask you not to eat or drink anything but water for a short time before the test. If you're diabetic, ask your doctor whether you need to adjust your medicines on the day of your test.

For some stress tests, you can't drink coffee or other caffeinated drinks for a day before the test. Certain over-the-counter or prescribed medicines also may interfere with some stress tests. Ask your doctor whether you can take all your medicines as usual and whether you need to avoid certain drinks or foods.

If you use an inhaler for asthma or other breathing problems, bring it to the test and be sure to let the doctor know that you use it.

What should I expect during stress testing?

During all types of stress testing, a technician will always be with you to closely monitor your health status.

Before you start the "stress" part of a stress test, a technician will put small sticky patches called electrodes on the skin of your chest, arms, and legs. To help an electrode stick to the skin, the technician may have to shave a patch of hair where the electrode will be attached.

The electrodes are connected to a machine that records the electrical activity of your heart. This recording, which is called an EKG (electrocardiogram), shows how fast your heart is beating and the heart's rhythm (steady or irregular). The machine also records the strength and timing of electrical signals as they pass through each part of your heart.

The technician will put a blood pressure cuff on your arm to monitor your blood pressure during the stress test. (The cuff will feel tight on your arm when it expands every few minutes.) In addition, you may be asked to breathe into a special tube so the gases you breathe out can be monitored.

After these preparations, you will exercise on a treadmill or stationary bicycle. If such exercise poses a problem for you, you may instead turn a crank with your arms. During the test, the exercise level will get harder. But you can stop whenever you feel the exercise is too much for you.

If you can't exercise, a technician will inject a medicine into a vein in your arm or hand. This medicine will increase the flow of blood through the coronary arteries or make your heart beat faster, as would exercise. This results in your heart working harder, so the stress test can be performed. The medicine may make you flushed and anxious, but the effects disappear as soon as the test is over. The medicine may also give you a headache.

While you're exercising or receiving medicine to make your heart work harder, the technician will ask you frequently how you're feeling. You should tell him or her if you feel chest pain, shortness of

491

breath, or dizzy. The exercise or medicine infusion will continue until you reach a target heart rate, or until you experience symptoms such as the following:

- Feel moderate to severe chest pain

- Get too out of breath to continue

- Develop abnormally high or low blood pressure or an arrhythmia (an abnormal heartbeat)

- Become dizzy

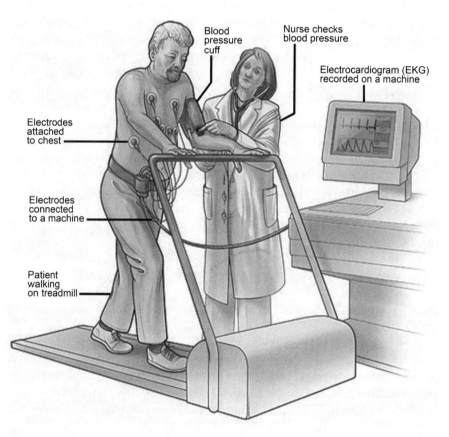

Figure 38.1. Stress Testing. Electrodes are attached to the patient's chest and connected to an EKG (electrocardiogram) machine. The EKG records the heart's electrical activity. A blood pressure cuff is used to record the patient's blood pressure while he walks on a treadmill.

The technician will continue to monitor your heart functions and blood pressure for a short time after you stop exercising or stop receiving the stress-creating medicine. The "stress" part of a stress test (when you're exercising or given a medicine that makes your heart work hard) usually lasts only about 15 minutes or less. But there is preparation time before the test and monitoring time afterward. Both extend the total test time to about an hour for a standard stress test, and up to three hours or more for some imaging stress tests.

Exercise stress echocardiogram test: For an exercise stress echocardiogram test, the technician will take pictures of your heart using echocardiography before you exercise and after you finish. A sonographer (a person who specializes in using ultrasound techniques) will apply a gel to your chest and then will briefly put a wand-like device (called a transducer) against your chest and move it around. The transducer sends and receives high-pitched sounds that you usually can't hear. The echoes from the sound waves are converted into moving pictures of your heart on a screen.

You may be asked to lie on your side on an examining table for this test. Some stress echocardiogram tests also use a dye to improve imaging. This dye is injected into your bloodstream while the test occurs.

Sestamibi stress test or other imaging stress test involving radioactive dye: For a sestamibi or other imaging stress test that uses a radioactive dye, the technician will inject a small amount of the dye (such as sestamibi) into your bloodstream via a needle placed in a vein of your arm or hand. You're usually given the dye about a half-hour before you start exercising or are given a medicine that makes your heart work hard. The amount of radiation in the dye is safe and not a danger to you or those around you. However, if you're pregnant, you shouldn't have this test because of risks it might pose to your unborn child.

Pictures will be taken of your heart at least two times—when it's at rest and when it's working its hardest. For such imaging, you will lie down on a table and a special camera or scanner that can see the dye in your bloodstream will take pictures of your heart. Some pictures may not be taken until you lie quietly for a few hours after exercising or receiving the stress-creating medicine. Some patients may even be asked to return in a day or so for more pictures to be taken.

Magnetic resonance imaging stress test: A magnetic resonance imaging (MRI) stress test may use a medicine rather than exercise

493

to get your heart to work harder. But some facilities have you exercise on a specially made bicycle or treadmill that allows you to exercise while lying on your back. For this test, you will be put inside a tunnel-like MRI machine that takes pictures of your heart when it's working hard and when your body is at rest.

What should I expect after stress testing?

After stress testing, you're able to return to normal activities. If you had a test that involved radioactive dye, your doctor may ask you to drink plenty of fluids to flush it out of your body. You also shouldn't have certain other imaging tests until the dye is no longer in your body. Your doctor can advise you about this.

What does stress testing show?

Stress testing provides your doctor with information about how your heart works during physical stress (exercise) and how healthy your heart is. Standard exercise stress testing uses an EKG (electrocardiogram) to monitor changes in the electrical activity of your heart. Imaging stress tests take pictures of the blood flow to different parts of your heart.

Both types of stress testing are used to look for signs that your heart isn't getting enough blood flow during exercise. Abnormal results on stress testing may be due to coronary artery disease (CAD), but also can be due to other factors such as a lack of physical fitness.

If you have a standard exercise stress test and the results are normal, no further testing or treatment may be needed. But if your standard exercise stress test results are abnormal, or if you're physically unable to exercise, your doctor may want you to have an imaging stress test or undergo other testing. Even if your standard exercise stress test results are normal, your doctor may want you to have an imaging stress test if you continue having symptoms (such as shortness of breath or chest pain).

Standard exercise stress testing isn't equally accurate in men and women. Normal results from a standard exercise stress test usually accurately rule out CAD in both men and women. But a standard exercise stress test can show abnormal results even when the patient doesn't have CAD (these results are called false positives). False positive exercise stress tests happen more often in women than in men.

Imaging stress tests are more accurate than standard exercise stress tests (in men and women) because they directly show how well blood is flowing in heart muscle and reveal parts of the heart that aren't contracting strongly. But imaging stress tests are much more expensive than standard exercise stress tests.

Imaging stress tests can show the parts of the heart not getting enough blood, as well as dead tissue in the heart, where no blood flows. (A heart attack can cause some tissue in the heart to die.) If your imaging stress test suggests significant CAD, your doctor may want you to have more testing or treatment.

What are the risks of stress testing?

There's little risk of being seriously harmed from any type of stress testing. The chance of these tests causing a heart attack or death is about one in 5,000. More common but less serious side effects linked to stress testing include:

- **Arrhythmia** (an irregular heartbeat): This often will go away quickly once you're at rest. But if it persists, you may need to go to the hospital and be monitored or get treatment.

- **Low blood pressure**, which can cause you to feel dizzy or faint: This will go away once your heart stops working hard; it doesn't usually require treatment.

- **Jitteriness or discomfort** while getting medicine to make your heart work harder (you will be given medicine if you can't exercise): These side effects usually disappear shortly after you stop getting the medicine, but in some cases may last a few hours.

Chapter 39

Urodynamic Testing

If you have a problem with urine leakage or blocked urine flow, your doctor or nurse may be able to help. One of the tools they may use to evaluate the cause of your symptoms is urodynamic testing.

Several muscles, organs, and nerves are involved in collecting, storing, and releasing urine. The kidneys form urine by filtering wastes and extra water from the bloodstream. The ureters are tubes that carry urine from the kidneys to the bladder. Normally urine flows in one direction. If urine backs up toward the kidneys, infections and kidney damage can occur.

The bladder, a hollow muscular organ shaped like a balloon, sits in the pelvis and is held in place by ligaments attached to other organs and to the pelvic bones. The bladder stores urine until you are ready to empty it. It swells into a round shape when it is full and gets smaller as it empties. A healthy bladder can hold up to 16 ounces (2 cups) of urine comfortably. How frequently it fills depends on how much excess water your body is trying to get rid of.

The bladder opens into the urethra, the tube that allows urine to pass outside the body. Circular muscles called sphincters close tightly to keep urine from leaking. The involuntary leakage of urine is called incontinence.

Nerves in the bladder tell you when it is time to empty your bladder. When the bladder begins to fill with urine, you may notice a feeling

National Kidney and Urologic Diseases Information Clearinghouse (NKUDIC), November 2006.

that you need to urinate. The sensation becomes stronger as the bladder continues to fill and reaches its limit. At that point, nerves in the bladder send a message to the brain, and your urge to urinate intensifies.

When you are ready to urinate, the brain signals the sphincter muscles to relax. At the same time, the brain signals the bladder muscles to squeeze, thus allowing urine to flow through the urethra. When these signals occur in the correct order, normal urination occurs.

Problems in the urinary system can be caused by aging, illness, or injury. The muscles in and around your bladder and urethra tend to become weaker with age. Weak bladder muscles may result in your not being able to empty your bladder completely, leaving you at a higher risk for urinary tract infections. Weak muscles of the sphincters and pelvis can lead to urinary incontinence because the sphincter muscles cannot remain tight enough to hold urine in the bladder, or the bladder does not have enough support from the pelvic muscles to stay in its proper position.

Urodynamics is a study that assesses how the bladder and urethra are performing their job of storing and releasing urine. Urodynamic tests help your doctor or nurse see how well your bladder and sphincter muscles work and can help explain symptoms such as the following:

- incontinence
- frequent urination
- sudden, strong urges to urinate
- problems starting a urine stream
- painful urination
- problems emptying your bladder completely
- recurrent urinary tract infections

These tests may be as simple as urinating behind a curtain while a doctor or nurse listens or more complicated, involving imaging equipment that films urination and pressure monitors that record the pressures of the bladder and urethra.

Seeing Your Doctor or Nurse

The first step in solving a urinary problem is to talk with your doctor or nurse. He or she should ask you about your general medical history, including any major illnesses or surgeries. You should talk about the medicines you take, both prescription and nonprescription, because they might be part of the problem. You should talk about how much fluid you drink a day and whether you use alcohol or caffeine. Give as many details as you can about the problem and when it started. The doctor or nurse may ask you to keep a voiding diary, which is a record of fluid intake and trips to the bathroom, plus any episodes of leakage.

If leakage is the problem, the doctor or nurse may ask you to do a pad test. This test is a simple way to measure how much urine leaks out. You will be given a number of absorbent pads and plastic bags of a standard weight. You will be told to wear the pad for one or two hours while in the clinic or to wear a series of pads at home during a specific period of time. The pads are collected and sealed in a plastic bag. Your health care team will then weigh the bags to see how much urine has been caught in the pad. A simpler but less precise method is to change pads as often as you need to and keep track of how many pads you use in a day.

A physical exam will also be performed to rule out other causes of urinary problems. This exam usually includes an assessment of the nerves in the lower part of your body. It will also include a pelvic exam in women to assess the pelvic muscles and the other pelvic organs. In men, a rectal exam is given to assess the prostate. Your doctor will also want to check your urine for evidence of infection or blood.

Preparing for the Test

If the doctor or nurse recommends bladder testing, usually no special preparations are needed, but make sure you understand any instructions you do receive. Depending on the test, you may be asked to come with a full bladder or an empty one. Also, ask whether you should change your diet or skip your regular medicines and for how long.

Taking the Test

Any procedure designed to provide information about a bladder problem can be called a urodynamic test. The type of test you take depends on your problem.

Most urodynamic testing focuses on the bladder's ability to empty steadily and completely. It can also show whether the bladder is having abnormal contractions that cause leakage. Your doctor will want to know whether you have difficulty starting a urine stream, how hard you have to strain to maintain it, whether the stream is interrupted, and whether any urine is left in your bladder when you are done. The remaining urine is called the postvoid residual. Urodynamic tests can range from simple observation to precise measurement using sophisticated instruments.

Uroflowmetry (Measurement of Urine Speed and Volume)

A uroflowmeter automatically measures the amount of urine and the flow rate—that is, how fast the urine comes out. You may be asked to urinate privately into a toilet that contains a collection device and scale. This equipment creates a graph that shows changes in flow rate from second to second so the doctor or nurse can see the peak flow rate and how many seconds it took to get there. Results of this test will be abnormal if the bladder muscle is weak or urine flow is obstructed.

Your doctor or nurse can also get some idea of your bladder function by using a stopwatch to time you as you urinate into a graduated container. The volume of urine is divided by the time to see what your average flow rate is. For example, 330 milliliters (mL) of urine in 30 seconds means that your average flow rate is 11 mL per second.

Measurement of Postvoid Residual

After you have finished, you may still have some urine, usually only an ounce or two, remaining in your bladder. To measure this postvoid residual, the doctor or nurse may use a catheter, a thin tube that can be gently glided into the urethra. He or she can also measure the postvoid residual with ultrasound equipment that uses harmless sound waves to create a picture of the bladder. A postvoid residual of more than 200 mL, about half a pint, is a clear sign of a problem. Even 100 mL, about half a cup, requires further evaluation. However, the amount of postvoid residual can be different each time you urinate.

Cystometry (Measurement of Bladder Pressure)

A cystometrogram (CMG) measures how much your bladder can hold, how much pressure builds up inside your bladder as it stores urine, and how full it is when you feel the urge to urinate. The doctor or nurse will use a catheter to empty your bladder completely. Then a special, smaller catheter will be placed in the bladder. This catheter has a pressure-measuring device called a manometer. Another catheter may be placed in the rectum to record pressure there as well.

Your bladder will be filled slowly with warm water. During this time you will be asked how your bladder feels and when you feel the need to urinate. The volume of water and the bladder pressure will be recorded. You may be asked to cough or strain during this procedure. Involuntary bladder contractions can be identified.

Measurement of Leak Point Pressure

While your bladder is being filled for the CMG, it may suddenly contract and squeeze some water out without warning. The manometer will record the pressure at the point when the leakage occurred. This reading may provide information about the kind of bladder problem you have. You may also be asked to apply abdominal pressure to the bladder by coughing, shifting position, or trying to exhale while holding your nose and mouth. These actions help the doctor or nurse evaluate your sphincter muscles.

Pressure Flow Study

After the CMG, you will be asked to empty your bladder. The catheter can measure the bladder pressures required to urinate and the flow rate a given pressure generates. This pressure flow study helps to identify bladder outlet obstruction that men may experience with prostate enlargement. Bladder outlet obstruction is less common in women but can occur with a fallen bladder or rarely after a surgical procedure for urinary incontinence. Most catheters can be used for both CMG and pressure flow studies.

Electromyography (Measurement of Nerve Impulses)

If your doctor or nurse thinks that your urinary problem is related to nerve or muscle damage, you may be given an electromyography. This test measures the muscle activity in and around the urethral sphincter by using special sensors. The sensors are placed on the skin near the urethra and rectum or they are located on the urethral or rectal catheter. Muscle activity is recorded on a machine. The patterns of the impulses will show whether the messages sent to the bladder and urethra are coordinated correctly.

Video Urodynamics

Urodynamic tests may be performed with or without equipment to take pictures of the bladder during filling and emptying. The imaging equipment may use x-rays or sound waves. If x-ray equipment is used, the bladder will be filled with a contrast medium that will show up on the x-ray instead of the warm water. The pictures and videos show the size and shape of the urinary tract and help your doctor or nurse understand your problem.

After the Test

You may have mild discomfort for a few hours after these tests when you urinate. Drinking an 8-ounce glass of water each half-hour for two hours should help. Ask your doctor whether you can take a warm bath. If not, you may be able to hold a warm, damp washcloth over the urethral opening to relieve the discomfort.

Your doctor may give you an antibiotic to take for one or two days to prevent an infection. If you have signs of infection—including pain, chills, or fever—call your doctor at once.

Getting the Results

Results for simple tests can be discussed with your doctor or nurse immediately after the test. Results of other tests may take a few days. You will have the chance to ask questions about the results and possible treatments for your problem.

Chapter 40

Pulmonary Function Tests

What Are Lung Function Tests?

Lung function tests measure the size of your lungs, how much air you can breathe in and out, how fast you can breathe air out, and how well your lungs deliver oxygen to your blood. These tests also are called pulmonary function tests.

Lung function tests are used to look for the cause of breathing problems (like shortness of breath). These tests are used to check for conditions such as asthma, lung tissue scarring, sarcoidosis, and chronic obstructive pulmonary disease (COPD).

Lung function tests also are used to see how well treatments for breathing problems, such as asthma medicines, are working. The tests may be used to check on whether a condition, such lung tissue scarring, is getting worse.

Overview

Lung function tests measure:

- how much air you can take into your lungs. This amount is compared to that of other people your age, height, and sex. This allows your doctor to see whether you're in the normal range.

"Lung Function Tests," from the *Diseases and Conditions Index*, National Heart Lung and Blood Institute, February 2008.

- how much air you can blow out of your lungs and how fast you can do it.

- how well your lungs deliver oxygen to your blood.

- how strong your breathing muscles are.

Breathing Tests

The breathing tests most often used are the following:

- **Spirometry:** This test measures how much air you can breathe in and out. It also measures how fast you can blow air out.

- **Peak flow meter:** This meter is a small, hand-held device that's sometimes used by people who have asthma. The meter helps track their breathing.

- **Lung volume measurement:** This test, in addition to spirometry, measures how much air you have left in your lungs after you breathe out completely.

- **Lung diffusing capacity:** This test measures how well oxygen passes from your lungs to your bloodstream.

These tests may not show what's causing breathing problems. Other tests, such as a cardiopulmonary exercise test, also may be done. This test measures how well your lungs and heart work while you exercise on a treadmill or bicycle.

Tests to Measure Oxygen Level

Pulse oximetry and arterial blood gas are two tests used to measure the oxygen level in the blood. They're also called blood oxygen tests.

Pulse oximetry measures blood oxygen levels using a special light. During an arterial blood gas test, your doctor inserts a small needle into an artery, usually in your wrist, and takes a sample of blood. The oxygen level of the blood sample is then checked.

Outlook

Lung function tests usually are painless and rarely cause side effects. You may feel some discomfort during the arterial blood gas test when the needle is inserted into the artery.

Types of Lung Function Tests

Breathing Tests

Spirometry: Spirometry measures how much air you breathe in and out and how fast you blow it out. This is measured in two ways: peak expiratory flow rate (PEFR) and forced expiratory volume in one second (FEV1). PEFR refers to the amount of air you can blow air out as quickly as possible. FEV1 refers to the amount of air you can blow out in one second.

During the test, a technician will ask you to take a deep breath in and then blow as hard as you can into a tube connected to a small machine. Your doctor may have you inhale a medicine that helps open your airways. He or she will want to see whether the medicine changes or improves the test results.

Spirometry is done to look for diseases and conditions that affect how much air you can breathe in, such as sarcoidosis or lung tissue scarring. It's also done to look for diseases that affect how fast you can breathe air out, like asthma and COPD (chronic obstructive pulmonary disease).

Peak flow meter: A peak flow meter is a small, hand-held device that you blow into. It shows how well air moves out of your lungs. People who have asthma sometimes use this device. It helps them (and their doctors) check their breathing. A peak flow meter can be used at home or in a doctor's office.

Lung volume measurement: This test measures the size of your lungs and how much air you can breathe in and out. During the test, you sit inside a glass booth and breathe into a tube that's hooked to a computer.

Sometimes you breathe in nitrogen or helium gas and then blow it out. The gas you breathe out is then measured to test how much air your lungs can hold.

The test can help diagnose lung tissue scarring or a stiff or weak chest wall.

Lung diffusion capacity: This test measures how well oxygen passes from your lungs to your bloodstream. During this test, you breathe in a gas through a tube. You hold your breath for a brief moment and then blow the gas out.

Abnormal test results may suggest loss of lung tissue, emphysema (a type of COPD), very bad scarring, or problems with blood flow through the body's arteries.

Tests to Measure Oxygen Level

Pulse oximetry and arterial blood gas tests show how much oxygen is in your blood. During pulse oximetry, a small light is placed over your fingertip, earlobe, or toe to measure the oxygen. This test is painless and no needles are used.

During an arterial blood gas test, your doctor inserts a small needle into an artery, usually in your wrist. He or she takes a sample of blood. The oxygen level of the blood is checked in a lab.

Testing in Infants and Young Children

Spirometry and other measures of lung function usually can be done in children older than six years, if they can follow directions well. Spirometry may be tried in children as young as five years. However, technicians who have special training with young children may need to do the testing.

Instead of spirometry, a growing number of medical centers measure respiratory system resistance. This is another way to test lung function in young children.

The child wears nose clips and has his or her cheeks supported with an adult's hands. The child breathes in and out quietly on a mouthpiece, while the technician measures changes in pressure at the mouth. During these lung function tests, parents can help comfort their children and encourage them to cooperate.

Very young children (younger than two years) may need an infant lung function test. This requires special equipment and medical staff. This type of test is only available at a few centers. The doctor gives the child medicine to help him or her sleep through the test.

A technician places a mask over your child's nose and mouth and a vest around your child's chest. The mask and vest are attached to a lung function machine. The machine gently pushes air into your child's lungs through the mask. As your child exhales, the vest slightly squeezes his or her chest. This helps push more air out of the lungs. The exhaled air is then measured.

In children younger than five years, the doctor likely will use signs and symptoms, medical history, and a physical exam to diagnose lung problems.

Pulse oximetry and arterial blood gas tests may be used for children of all ages.

Other Names for Lung Function Tests

- Lung diffusion testing; also called diffusing capacity and diffusing capacity of the lung for carbon monoxide, or DLCO

- Pulmonary function tests, or PFTs

Arterial blood gas tests also are called blood gas analyses, or ABGs.

Who Needs Lung Function Tests?

People who have breathing problems, such as shortness of breath, may need lung function tests. These tests help find the cause of breathing problems. They're used to check for conditions such as asthma, lung tissue scarring, sarcoidosis, and COPD (chronic obstructive pulmonary disease).

Lung function tests also are used to see how well treatments for breathing problems, such as asthma medicines, are working.

Diagnosing Lung Conditions

Your doctor will diagnose a lung condition based on your medical history, a physical exam, and test results.

Medical History

Your doctor will ask you questions, such as:

- Do you ever feel like you can't get enough air?

- Does your chest feel tight sometimes?

- Do you have periods of coughing or wheezing (a whistling sound when you breathe)?

- Do you ever have chest pain?

- Can you walk or run as fast as other people your age?

Your doctor also will ask if you or anyone in your family has ever:

- had asthma and/or allergies;

- had heart disease;

- smoked;

- traveled to places where you may have been exposed to tuberculosis; or

- had a job that exposed you to dust, fumes, or particles (like asbestos).

Physical Exam

Your doctor will measure your heart rate, breathing rate, and blood pressure. He or she also will listen to your heart and lungs with a stethoscope and feel your abdomen and limbs.

Your doctor will look for signs of heart or lung disease, or another disease that could cause your symptoms.

Lung and Heart Tests

Based on your medical history and physical exam, your doctor will decide what tests you need. A chest x-ray usually is the first test done to find the cause of breathing problems. This test takes pictures of the organs and structures inside your chest.

Your doctor may do lung function tests to find out even more about how well your lungs work.

Your doctor also may do tests to check your heart, such as an EKG (electrocardiogram) or a stress test. An EKG detects and records your heart's electrical activity. A stress test shows how well your heart works during physical activity.

What to Expect before Lung Function Tests

If you take breathing medicines, your doctor may ask you to stop them for a short time before spirometry, a lung volume measurement test, or a lung diffusion capacity test.

No special preparation is needed before pulse oximetry and arterial blood gas tests. If you're being treated with oxygen, your doctor may ask you to stop using it for a short time before the tests. This is done to check your blood oxygen level without the added oxygen.

What to Expect during Lung Function Tests

Breathing Tests

Spirometry tests may be done in your doctor's office or in a special lung function lab. Your doctor may ask you to use a peak flow meter in the office and suggest that you also do the test at home. The lung volume measurement and lung diffusion capacity tests are done in a special lab or clinic.

For the lung volume measurement and lung diffusion capacity tests, you sit in a chair next to a machine that measures your breathing. For spirometry, you sit or stand next to the machine.

Before the tests, a technician places soft clips on your nose. This allows you to breathe only through a tube that's attached to the testing machine. The technician will tell you how to breathe into the tube. For example, you may be asked to breathe normally, slowly, or rapidly.

The deep breathing done in some of the tests may make you feel short of breath, dizzy, or lightheaded, or it may make you cough.

Spirometry: In this test, you take a deep breath and then exhale as fast and as hard as you can into the tube. With spirometry, your doctor may give you a medicine that helps open your airways. Your doctor will want to see whether it changes or improves the test results.

Peak flow meter: In this test, you take a deep breath and then exhale as fast and as hard as you can into a small, hand-held device that's connected to a mouthpiece.

Lung volume measurement: For this test, you sit in a clear glass booth and breathe through the tube attached to the testing machine. The changes in pressure inside the booth are measured to show how much air you can breathe into your lungs.

Sometimes you breathe in nitrogen or helium gas and then breathe it out. The gas that you exhale is then measured.

Lung diffusion capacity: During this test, you breathe in gas through the tube, hold your breath for 10 seconds, and then rapidly blow it out. The gas contains a small amount of carbon monoxide, which won't harm you.

Tests to Measure Oxygen Level

Pulse oximetry is done in a doctor's office or hospital. Arterial blood gas tests are done in a lab or hospital.

Pulse oximetry: During this test, a small light is placed over your fingertip, earlobe, or toe using a clip or flexible tape. It's then attached to a cable that leads to a small machine called an oximeter. The oximeter shows the amount of oxygen in your blood. This test is painless and no needles are used.

Arterial blood gas: During this test, your doctor or technician inserts a small needle into an artery, usually in your wrist, and takes a sample of blood. You may feel some discomfort when the needle is inserted. The oxygen level of the blood sample is then checked in a lab.

After the needle is removed, you may feel mild pressure or throbbing at the needle site. Applying pressure to the area for five to ten minutes should stop the bleeding. You will be given a small bandage to lace on the area.

What to Expect after Lung Function Tests

You can return to your normal activities and restart your medicines after lung function tests. Talk to your doctor about when you'll get the test results.

What Do Lung Function Tests Show?

Breathing Tests

Spirometry: Spirometry can show whether you have:

- blockage (obstruction) in your airways. This may be a sign of asthma, COPD (chronic obstructive pulmonary disease), or another obstructive lung condition.

- smaller than normal lungs (restriction). This may be a sign of heart failure, damage or scarring of the lung tissues, or another restrictive lung condition.

Peak flow meter: A peak flow meter shows the fastest rate at which you can blow air out of your lungs. People who have asthma use this device to help track their breathing.

Lung volume measurement: This test shows the size of your lungs. Abnormal test results may show that you have lung tissue scarring or a stiff chest wall.

Lung diffusion capacity: This test can show a problem with oxygen moving from your lungs into your bloodstream. This may be a sign of loss of lung tissue, emphysema (a type of COPD), or problems with blood flow through the body's arteries.

Tests to Measure Oxygen Level

Pulse oximetry and arterial blood gas tests measure the oxygen level in your blood. These tests show how well your lungs are taking in oxygen and moving it into the bloodstream. A low level of oxygen in the blood may be a sign of a lung or heart condition.

What Are the Risks of Lung Function Tests?

Breathing Tests

Spirometry, peak flow meter, lung volume measurement, and lung diffusion capacity tests usually are safe. These tests rarely cause problems.

Tests to Measure Oxygen Level

Pulse oximetry has no risks. Side effects from arterial blood gas tests are rare.

Part Six

In-Home and Self-Ordered Medical Tests

Chapter 41

What You Should Know about Home-Use Medical Tests

Chapter Contents

Section 41.1

Advantages and Limitations
of Home Health Care Tests

What is home health care testing?

Diagnostic testing (that is, laboratory tests) in the home in which
the consumer performs his/her own test(s).

What are some examples of the types of kits available for home use?

- Ovulation Detection Test
- Pregnancy Test
- Cholesterol Test
- Fecal Occult Blood Test
- Blood Glucose Testing Kit
- Urinary Tract Infection Screening Test
- Skin Growth Monitoring

Do I need a doctor's prescription before I can perform a home health care test?

No, these kits can be purchased over the counter and are most commonly found in supermarkets and drugstores.

How much will a home health care test cost me?

Prices will vary depending on the type of test purchased. Average
prices for some of these tests are:

- Pregnancy Test—$12.00
- Ovulation Detection Test—$21.00

- Cholesterol Test—$20
- Glucose Monitoring Instrument—$30–$100
- Glucose Test Strips—$30.00

You will need to consult your individual insurance carrier to determine if these costs are covered.

What are some advantages of home health care testing?

1. Allows individuals to monitor a disease that has already been detected (for example, monitoring glucose levels in diabetic patients).

2. Allows consumers to detect certain conditions in the privacy of their home. Note: All positive test results should be reported to your health care practitioner.

3. Allows consumers to get instant results (for example, you're the first to know you're pregnant).

4. Some products are inexpensive and easy to use.

What are some of the limitations of a home test kit?

1. Many tests require the consumer to obtain a blood sample.

2. Consumers may be embarrassed to disclose their test results (for example positive HIV test) and a positive test must be followed up.

3. May get a false positive test—what this means is that something other than what you're testing for made the test result positive. There should always be a follow-up test performed by a qualified health care practitioner to confirm the initial positive result.

4. A negative test result may occur even when disease is present.

When should I perform a home test before seeing my health care practitioner?

The decision to perform a home test is best made after the consumer determines why it is they want the information. Is it because:

1. You are health conscious and want to monitor a particular constituent (for example, cholesterol)?

2. You have been diagnosed with a disease and want to monitor a particular constituent (for example, glucose)?

3. Or, do you suspect you're pregnant and want to be the first to know?

Regardless of what the reason is for performing a home test, any result you obtain should be brought to the attention of your health care provider.

What should I look for when purchasing a home health care test?

1. Review the test steps on the package in order to insure that you will be able to collect the sample and follow the directions. It is very important to follow the package instructions exactly as they are written. This includes how the sample is collected, how the sample is applied to the testing device and adhering to the timing of the test to insure useful results.

2. Look to see if a number is listed in the event you have any questions about how to use the product or what to do after obtaining the results.

Note: If you're going to perform a home test for the first time, it would be advisable to call the company if there is anything in the directions you are unclear about (for example, how do I perform a fingerstick?). It's also important to read the package insert carefully in order to determine if there are any foods you are eating or medications you are taking that may interfere with the accuracy of your test results.

Important Considerations

1. Using a home test to monitor the presence of certain substances (for example, glucose) that will result in the self-administration of medication (for example, insulin) should be conducted under the guidance of a qualified health care practitioner.

2. The presence of a negative test result (for example, negative pregnancy test/negative glucose test) when there are clinical indications (for example late menstruation/symptoms of diabetes)

that contradict the test result should be reported to your health care practitioner.

3. A positive test result should always be reported to your health care practitioner so that the result can be confirmed by a qualified laboratory.

Section 41.2

Direct-to-Consumer Tests: Just What the Doctor Didn't Order

Lenexa, Kansas, resident Garry Porter, 52, ponders the results of his recent self-ordered full-body scan. You've heard the expression "the customer is always right." This notion is being tested in the world of health care, where consumers can now order a battery of health tests without a doctor's consultation.

The gain to patients is dubious. Cholesterol tests, computerized tomography scans, prostate-specific antigen tests, and sexually transmitted infections (STI) screens are all available—at a price—regardless of whether a person would benefit from such testing. One pharmacy chain even offers coupons in its store flyers for discounted osteoporosis screening.

Family physicians are taking notice.

"Sometimes knowing more is doing worse," said American Academy of Family Physicians (AAFP) Board Chair Richard Roberts, M.D., J.D., of Madison, Wisconsin, who has taken the lead for the Academy in responding to inquiries about these tests. "What people really need is the ongoing relationship with a physician they trust who can help them put the pieces of the health care puzzle together."

Do the tests empower patients? Do they cause unnecessary concern? Do they falsely reassure patients? Do they drive up costs?

"Yes," said Roberts. "All of the above."

Playing on Fears

Roberts said he approves of the tests "to the extent that the tests prompt people to engage the system. But that's not how they are being used." The way he sees it, consumers are being given a false promise that submitting to testing somehow confers good health on the person tested.

Of course, some tests are useful, Roberts said.

"There are clearly some tests that have been helpful—home glucose testing, for instance. That said, there are lots of instances where tests are being used inappropriately and are not proved to improve people's health," he said.

On a recent weekday, Alan Klaus, 53, arrived at his local pharmacy in Kansas City, Montana, to get his cholesterol screened. The convenience appealed to him. Within five minutes, he was seated with a tube in his arm to have blood drawn for a cholesterol test. "My wife is a nurse, and she told me I should do this," he said. At the suggestion of the pharmacy representative, Klaus also agreed to have a prostate specific antigen (PSA) test.

The problem, said Roberts, is that cholesterol levels are only a minute factor in assessing a person's risk for heart disease. "Total cholesterol is only one small piece of the puzzle. For a pharmacist to say, 'Oh, your cholesterol is normal,' may give the patient false reassurance," he said.

Then there's the PSA test that Klaus was offered. Roberts contends that the PSA test is one example of a test that has not been shown to improve people's health. Furthermore, suspicious findings may come back that warrant further, more invasive tests.

Striking a Balance

Other family physicians worry about the profit motive in making the tests available.

"Anytime you market directly to consumers—whether diagnostic tests or medications—you have to strike a balance between the positive values of giving patients more information about their health options and empowering them to request or even demand some health services that might benefit them, versus the negative values of driving up costs, misinforming the public so that private industry can make a profit, and so forth," said Howard Brody, M.D., Ph.D., professor of family practice and philosophy and former director of the Center for Ethics in the Humanities at Michigan State University, Lansing.

But Emily Essex, director of advertising and sales promotion for InterFit Health, a national health screening group based in Houston, said the direct testing is giving patients ownership of their health. InterFit is an outfit that provides the medical staff—phlebotomists and medical assistants—who administer screenings at chain stores.

Max Bouja, M.D., dean of the medical school at the University of Texas, Houston, is InterFit's corporate medical director. The organization has a medical advisory board, and there's a medical director in each state in which InterFit provides testing at corporations or in retail venues. Laurie Lee, president of InterFit, said, "We're not functioning in a vacuum. We're functioning under medical directors."

Essex said, "Our main objective is to help people take charge of their health. We give them the ability to take care of themselves in a more appropriate way and read their own results."

Physicians should not feel threatened by patients' direct access to the tests, she said. "Because we provide this service, they can have more time with their patients."

See Your Doctor?

Patients whose test results indicate intervention is imperative are contacted directly by an InterFit nurse or doctor and encouraged to see their own physician, said Essex. With slightly or significantly out-of-range results, patients' reports are stamped with an advisory note to consult their personal physician. However, there is no mechanism to ensure that patients follow through, she conceded.

What Theodore Ganiats, M.D., of La Jolla, California, finds worrisome is the accuracy of these tests. "All direct-to-consumer tests will have a certain number of false-positive results," said Ganiats, immediate past chair of the Commission on Clinical Policies and Research. "What are the patient and physician to do if the consumer test is positive? Retest in the doctor's office? What if the two results disagree? What is the appropriate management strategy?

"Unfortunately, this is rarely worked out in advance, so both the patient and physician move forward guessing what is the best management path."

But false-positive and false-negative results are only part of the problem, said Roberts. "The real danger is that these tests undermine and erode the doctor-patient relationship."

Full-Body Scans

At the extreme end of the direct-to-consumer health test trend is the availability of body scans—ranging from scans of specific organ systems to full-body scans.

Scare tactics abound. The brochure of one imaging center warned, "Heart attacks happen every day, even in apparently healthy people," and went on to list those who were at risk: men over age 35, women over age 40. A fairly broad range.

Roberts took issue with a June 24 [2002] *Wall Street Journal* article titled "Don't Let Your Doctor Keep You From Getting a Body Scan," in which the writer asserted, "the medical establishment has a vested interest in keeping patients out of scanning centers."

"That's laughable," said Roberts. "These tests generate more visits to the doctor.

"If you're doing the tests to avoid the doctor, you're going to need to see the doctor (to confirm the results) eventually anyway. Either me or the undertaker."

Section 41.3

Be Cautious about Buying Medical Test Kits Online

"Buying Diagnostic Tests from the Internet: Buyer Beware!" Center for Devices and Radiological Health, U.S. Food and Drug Administration (FDA), October 2001. Reviewed by David A. Cooke, M.D., June 2008.

"Sally" was afraid that she had been exposed to HIV. She didn't want to buy a test in the local pharmacy because someone she knew might see her. She didn't want to go to a clinic for the same reason. So, like many other consumers, Sally decided to purchase her HIV test from an internet source. She took the test and was distraught to find that the result was positive. After several agonizing weeks, she went to her doctor who did a confirmatory test with a more sophisticated testing method—and the result was negative. Sally did not have HIV.

The test she purchased from the internet had not been approved or cleared by the Food and Drug Administration (FDA), so it did not include the required labeling for a confirmatory test and counseling after a positive result.

Tests such as Sally bought are called in vitro diagnostic (IVD for short) tests. They use a sample of blood, urine, or other specimen taken from the human body. A doctor uses IVD tests along with a physical examination and a medical history to get a picture of a patient's health status. Rarely does one IVD test provide a diagnosis.

Although many quality IVD tests are being sold over the internet, other tests sold online may not work or be harmful. Some tests are illegal, that is, being sold without clearance or approval by the FDA. Examples of some types of IVD tests available from the internet include the following:

- Pregnancy
- Hepatitis
- Fertility
- Cholesterol
- Drugs of abuse
- Blood sugar
- HIV
- Antibodies to silicone

While some of the above tests are approved or cleared for sale directly to the consumer (called over-the-counter or OTC), most IVD tests are not. FDA has cleared or approved many tests for use in a doctor's office or for professional use only, but internet marketers are selling them OTC or for unapproved uses.

Misleading advertising is another problem. Ads promise in-home results, but most IVD tests should be followed with a second, more sophisticated laboratory test to confirm the results. For example, tests to detect prostate cancer, called PSA (prostate surface antigen) test, are for screening only and should be used in conjunction with a rectal exam performed by a doctor. Elevated PSA test results often are further evaluated using additional tests such free PSAs or complexed PSA.

Internet sources also heavily advertise tests for detecting the presence of drugs such as marijuana, nicotine, amphetamine, and methamphetamine in children and employees. Again, to be sure of their accuracy, the positive results for these tests must be confirmed by additional laboratory tests. Another example of false advertising is claiming that disposable supplies, such as test strips for blood glucose monitors, will work in "any meter."

So what precautions can a consumer take? If you think that you have a medical condition or disease, see your doctor or healthcare professional. Don't try to diagnose yourself with questionable products obtained over the internet. If you still want to buy an IVD test over the internet, how can you tell if it is a legitimate product? First, ask if FDA has cleared or approved the product for use at home. Second, be wary if you see that any of these conditions apply to the test:

- Claims to diagnose more than one illness, for example, cancer, arthritis, and anemia

- Is made in a country other than the United States. If so, check to see if FDA has cleared or approved the test for use at home.

- Is made by only one laboratory and sold directly to the public. This is a "home-brew" test and is not intended for OTC sale.

The following general precautions apply to any healthcare purchase on the internet:

- Don't be fooled by a professional-looking website. Anyone can hire a webpage designer to create an appealing site.

- Avoid websites with only a post office number and no telephone number.

- Avoid websites that use the words "new cure" or "miracle cure."

- Avoid products with impressive-sounding terminology that can hide bad science.

- Avoid products that claim the government, medical profession, or research scientists have conspired to suppress the product.

- Beware of claims that the test complies with all regulatory agencies.

- Beware of tests labeled for export only. This usually means that the test is not cleared or approved for sale in the U.S.

Although FDA's resources are limited, the agency is taking action against internet websites with misleading marketing or unsafe products. FDA has sent warning letters that demand the owners of these websites stop selling medical devices until they can prove FDA has cleared or approved the devices for sale. In a warning letter, FDA typically requests that the firm send to FDA (by a certain date) a description of the corrective action that it plans to take. FDA is working with the Federal Trade Commission (FTC) whose laws allow it to quickly regulate practices that are unfair and deceptive (see http://www.ftc .gov). FDA also sends information about deceptive companies to the National Consumer League's Fraud Information Center.

If you have questions or complaints about a particular medical device or website, you can call FDA at 888-INFO-FDA (888-463-6332) or your local FDA district office. They will be able to tell you if FDA has cleared or approved the medical device in question. Finally, if you want to purchase an IVD test promising a diagnosis for treatment of a serious illness, talk to your healthcare provider before using it to find out if additional tests will be needed.

You can report false claims to the Federal Trade Commission (FTC) at 877-FTC-HELP (382-4357); TDD at 202-32602501; by mail to Consumer Response Center, FTC, Washington, DC 20850. Report to the Food and Drug Administration's (FDA) MedWatch program at 800-FDA-1088 or at www.fda.gov/medwatch.

Chapter 42

Home-Use Tests for Cholesterol

What does this test do?

This is a home-use test kit to measure total cholesterol.

What is cholesterol?

Cholesterol is a fat (lipid) in your blood. High-density lipoprotein (HDL) ("good" cholesterol) helps protect your heart, but low-density lipoprotein (LDL) ("bad" cholesterol) can clog the arteries of your heart. Some cholesterol tests also measure triglycerides, another type of fat in the blood.

What type of test is this?

This is a quantitative test—you find out the amount of total cholesterol present in your sample.

Why should you do this test?

You should do this test to find out if you have high total cholesterol. High cholesterol increases your risk of heart disease. When the blood vessels of your heart become clogged by cholesterol, your heart does not receive enough oxygen. This can cause heart disease.

"Home-Use Tests: Cholesterol," U.S. Food and Drug Administration, Center for Devices and Radiological Health, February 2003.

How often should you test for cholesterol?

If you are more than 20 years old, you should test your cholesterol about every five years. If your doctor has you on a special diet or drugs to control your cholesterol, you may need to check your cholesterol more frequently. Follow your doctor's recommendations about how often you test your cholesterol.

What should your cholesterol levels be?

Your total cholesterol level should be 200 mg/dL or less, according to recommendations in the National Cholesterol Education Program (NCEP) Third Adult Treatment Panel (ATP III). You should try to keep your LDL values less than 100 mg/dL, your HDL values greater or equal to 40 mg/dL, and your triglyceride values less than 150 mg/dL.

How accurate is this test?

This test is about as accurate as the test your doctor uses, but you must follow the directions carefully.

Total cholesterol tests vary in accuracy from brand to brand. Information about the test's accuracy is printed on its package. Tests that say they are "traceable" to a program of the Centers for Disease Control and Prevention (CDC) may be more accurate than others.

What do you do if your test shows high cholesterol?

Talk to your doctor if your test shows that your cholesterol is higher than 200 mg/dL. Many things can cause high cholesterol levels including diet, exercise, and other factors. Your doctor may want you to test your cholesterol again.

How do you do this test?

You prick your finger with a lancet to get a drop of blood. Then put the drop of blood on a piece paper that contains special chemicals. The paper will change color depending on how much cholesterol is in your blood. Some testing kits use a small machine to tell you how much cholesterol there is in the sample.

Are there home tests for HDL cholesterol ("good" cholesterol)?

Yes, FDA has cleared home tests for HDL cholesterol.

Are there home tests for triglycerides?

Yes, FDA has cleared home tests for triglycerides.

Where can you get more information about cholesterol and cholesterol testing?

- Centers for Disease Control (CDC): Cholesterol Fact Sheet which is available online at http://www.cdc.gov/dhdsp/library/fs_cholesterol.htm.

- National Institutes of Health (NIH) National Cholesterol Education Program which has information available online at http://www.nhlbi.nih.gov/about/ncep/index.htm.

- Lab Tests Online from the American Association for Clinical Chemistry (AACC) which as information available online at http://labtestsonline.org/understanding/analytes/cholesterol/glance.html.

Chapter 43

Home-Use Tests for Fecal Occult Blood

What does this test do?

This is a home-use test kit to measure the presence of hidden (occult) blood in your stool (feces).

What is fecal occult blood?

Fecal occult blood is blood in your feces that you cannot see in your stool or on your toilet paper after you use the toilet.

What type of test is this?

This is a qualitative test—you find out whether or not you have occult blood in your feces, not how much is present.

Why should you do this test?

You should do this test, because blood in your feces may be an early sign of a digestive condition, for example abnormal growths (polyps) or cancer in your colon.

How often should you test for fecal occult blood?

The American Cancer Society recommends that you test for fecal occult blood every year after you turn 50. Some doctors suggest that

"Home-Use Tests: Fecal Occult Blood," U.S. Food and Drug Administration, Center for Devices and Radiological Health, February 2003.

you start testing at age 40, if your family is thought to be at increased risk. Follow your doctor's recommendations about how often you test for fecal occult blood.

How accurate is this test?

This test is about as accurate as the test your doctor uses, but you must follow the directions carefully. For accurate results, you must prepare properly for the test and get a good stool sample.

Does a positive test mean you have hidden blood in your stool?

A positive result means that the test has detected blood. This does not mean you have tested positive for cancer or any other illness. False positive results may be caused by diet or medications. Further testing and examinations should be performed by the physician to determine the exact cause and source of the occult blood in the stool.

If the test results are negative, can you be sure that you do not have a bowel condition?

No. You could still have bowel condition that you should know about. You should use this test again in a year.

How do you do this test?

There are several different methods for detecting hidden blood in the stool.

In one method, you collect stool samples and smear them onto paper cards in a holder. You then either send these cards to a laboratory for testing or test them at home. If you test them at home, you add a special solution from your test kit to the paper cards to see if they change color. If the paper cards change color, it means there was blood in the stool.

In another method, you put special paper in the toilet after a bowel movement. If the special paper changes color, it indicates there was blood in the toilet.

You will need to test your feces from three separate bowel movements. These bowel movements should be three in a row, closely spaced in time to minimize the time you need to be on the special diet. This is necessary because if you have polyps, they may not bleed all the time. You improve your chances of catching any bleeding if you sample three different bowel movements.

Unless you use the method where you put a test solution into the toilet, it is best to catch your feces before it enters the toilet. You can do this by holding a piece of toilet paper in your hand. After you catch it, cut it apart in two places with the little wooden stick you get in the kit. Take a little bit of the feces from each place where you cut it apart and put these bits on one place in the cardboard in the kit. You use the second and third spots on the cardboard for other bowel movements.

What interferes with this test?

To get good results with this test, you have to follow the instructions. You may find it difficult because you need to things you do not ordinarily do.

Because the test is for blood, any source of blood will give a positive test. Blood from another source, like bleeding hemorrhoids or your menstrual period will interfere with the test, so you won't be able to tell what made the test positive.

Pay attention to your diet before the test:

- Eat a high fiber diet, such as one that has cereals and breads with bran.

- Cook your fruits and vegetables well.

- Don't eat raw turnips, radishes, broccoli, or horseradish. These foods can make it look like you have hidden blood when you don't.

- Don't eat red meat. (You may eat poultry or fish). Red meat in your diet can make it look like you have hidden blood when you don't.

Avoid the following drugs for the seven days before the test—they can make it look like you have hidden blood when you don't:

- Aspirin

- Anti-inflammatory drugs, such as Motrin

Don't take vitamin C supplements for the seven days before the test. Then can prevent the test from detecting your hidden blood.

Where can you get more information about polyps, colon cancer, and fecal occult blood testing?

- MEDLINEplus Health Information: Colonic diseases which is available online at http://www.nlm.nih.gov/medlineplus/colonicdiseases.html.

Chapter 44

Home-Use Tests for Managing Diabetes

Glucose

What does this test do?

This is a home-use test kit to measure blood sugar (glucose) in your blood.

What is glucose?

Glucose is blood sugar that your body uses as a source of energy. Unless you have diabetes, you body regulates the amount of glucose in your blood. People with diabetes have poorly controlled blood glucose.

What type of test is this?

This is a quantitative test—you find out the amount of glucose present in your sample.

Why should you do this test?

You should do this test if you have diabetes and you need to monitor your blood sugar (glucose) levels. You can use the results to help

"Home-Use Tests: Glucose," U.S. Food and Drug Administration (FDA), Center for Devices and Radiological Health, February 2003; and "FDA Clears Home Glycated Hemoglobin Test for Diabetics," FDA, December 2002. Revised by David A. Cooke, M.D., June 20, 2008.

you determine your daily adjustments in treatment, know if you have dangerously high or low levels of glucose, and understand how your diet and exercise change your glucose levels.

The Diabetes Control and Complications Trial (1993) showed that good glucose control using home monitors led to fewer complications.

How often should you test your glucose?

Follow your doctor's recommendations about how often you test your glucose. You may need to test yourself several times each day to determine adjustments in your treatment.

What should your glucose levels be?

For a healthy, nondiabetic person, your fasting blood glucose level (after not eating for eight to ten hours) should be lower than 126 mg/dL. For a nondiabetic, your blood glucose level immediately after eating should be lower than 200 mg/dL.

For diabetic patients, the targets will depend upon the patient. In most cases, however, doctors like to see blood sugars between 90 and 140 mg/dL most of the time.

How accurate is this test?

The accuracy of this test depends on many factors including the following:

- The quality of your meter
- The quality of your test strips
- How well you are trained to do the test
- Your hematocrit (the amount of red blood cells in the blood). If you have a high hematocrit, you may test low for blood glucose. Or, if you have a low hematocrit, you may test high for glucose. If you know your hematocrit is low or high, discuss with your health care provider how it may affect your glucose testing.
- Interfering substances (some substances, such as vitamin C and uric acid, may interfere with your glucose testing). Check the package insert for your meter and test strips to find out what substances may affect the testing accuracy.
- Altitude, temperature, and humidity (high altitude, low and high temperatures, and humidity can cause unpredictable effects

on glucose results). Check the meter and test strip package inserts for more information. Store and handle the meter and strips according to instructions.

How do you do this test?

Before you self-monitor your blood glucose, you must read and understand the instructions for your meter. In general, you prick your finger with a lancet to get a drop of blood. Place the blood on a disposable "test strip" that is coated with chemicals that react with glucose. Then place the test strip in your meter. Some meters measure the amount of electricity that passes through the test strip. Others measure how much light reflects from it. In the U.S. meters report results in milligrams of glucose per deciliter of blood or mg/dl.

You can get information about your meter and test strips from several different sources including the toll free number in the user manual or the manufacturer's website. If you have an urgent problem, always contact your healthcare provider or a local emergency room for advice.

How do you choose a glucose meter?

You can purchase more than 25 different types of meters. They differ in several ways:

- amount of blood needed for each test
- how easy it is to use
- pain associated with using the product
- accuracy
- testing speed
- overall size
- ability to store test results in memory
- cost of the meter
- cost of the test strips used
- doctor's recommendation
- technical support provided by the manufacturer
- special features such as automatic timing, multiple strip or lancet cartridges, error codes, large display screen, or spoken instructions or results

Talk to your health care practitioner about glucose meters and how to use them.

How do I compare my home test glucose values with the laboratory values?

Most home blood glucose meters in the U.S. measure glucose in whole blood. Most lab tests, in contrast, measure glucose in plasma. Plasma is blood without the cells. A lab test of your blood glucose will be about 10–15% higher than the value given by your meter. Look at the instructions for your meter to find out if it gives its results as "whole blood" or "plasma equivalent." Many meters now sold give values that are "plasma equivalent," which means they can be compared more directly to lab test values.

Should you use generic or "third party" test strips?

You may choose test strips that are made by a different company than the one that made meter. Sometimes, generic test strips are cheaper. If you choose generic test strips make sure the generic strips will work with your meter. Check the label of the test strips to make sure they will work with the make and model of your meter. Just because the generic test strip looks like it will work does not mean that it will work. Also, watch for inconsistent results. If you get poor results, try strips made or recommended by the maker of your meter until you again get consistent results.

How can you check your meter's performance?

1. **Use liquid control solution:** a) every time you open a new container of test strips; b) occasionally as you use the container of test strips; c) whenever you get unusual results. You test a drop of these solutions just like you test a drop of your blood. The value you get should match that written on the liquid control solution bottle.

2. **Use electronic checks:** Every time you turn on your meter, it does an electronic check. If it detects a problem it will give you an error code. Look in your owner's manual to see what the error codes mean and how to fix the problem.

3. **Compare your meter with a laboratory meter:** Take your meter with you to your next appointment with your health care

provider. Ask your provider to watch your technique to make sure you are using the meter correctly. Ask your healthcare provider have your blood tested with a routine laboratory method. If the values you obtain on your glucose meter match the laboratory values, then your meter is working well and you are using good technique.

What should you do if your meter malfunctions?

If your meter malfunctions, you should tell your health care professional and the company that made your meter and strips.

Can you test blood glucose from sites other than your fingers?

Some new meters allow you to test blood from the base of your thumb, upper arm, forearm, thigh, or calf. If your glucose changes rapidly, these other sites may not give you accurate results. You should probably use your fingers to get your blood for testing if any of the following applies:

- You have just taken insulin
- You think your blood sugar is low
- You are not aware of symptoms when you become hypoglycemic
- The site results do not agree with the way you feel
- You have just eaten
- You have just exercised
- You are ill
- You are under stress

Can you test blood glucose without a needle stick?

Researchers have been trying to find ways to test glucose without finger sticks, but none are available yet.

Some new methods may make it easier for some people to monitor their glucose levels between finger sticks:

- Cygnus GlucoWatch Automatic Glucose Biographer (information available online at http://www.fda.gov/cdrh/mda/docs/p990026 .html) and

- MiniMed Continuous Glucose Monitoring System (CGMS) (information available online at http://www.fda.gov/cdrh/pdf/p980022b .pdf).

Several reports in the literature describe methods where you shine a beam of light on the skin and interpret the way the glucose under the skin responds to the light. The Food and Drug Administration (FDA) has not yet approved any of these methods.

Where can you get more information about glucose and glucose testing?

- FDA Diabetes Information (available online at http://www.fda .gov/diabetes)

- National Institute of Diabetes and Digestive and Kidney Diseases, Information on Diabetes (available online at http:// diabetes.niddk.nih.gov)

- American Association for Clinical Chemistry Lab Tests Online: Glucose Tests (available online at http://www.labtestsonline.org/ understanding/analytes/glucose/glance.html)

Glucose Meter Test Results: Useful Tips to Increase Accuracy and Reduce Errors

Have you ever wondered why you got a bad glucose meter test result when there is nothing obvious wrong with your meter, your test strips are new, and you've been running glucose tests for years? The simple answer is that glucose meters are not perfect, and neither are the people who use them. Here are some tips to help you get the most accurate results from your glucose meter.

- Follow the user instructions about sample size. Repeat the test if you have any doubt that enough blood was added. If there is insufficient blood on the test strip, the meter may not be able to read the glucose level accurately. Although many meters are designed to alert you when the sample size is too small, some meters detect only large errors. There have been cases where meters have displayed glucose levels that were less than half the actual levels without displaying error messages.

- Insert the test strip completely into the meter guides. When a test strip is not fully inserted into the meter, the meter cannot read the entire strip area. Many meters are designed to detect strip placement errors and will not provide a result. But, just as described above, many meters detect only large problems. There have been cases where meters have displayed glucose levels that were significantly higher or lower than the actual levels when there was only a small error in strip placement.

- Keep the meter clean. Even small amounts of blood, grease, or dirt on a meter's lens can alter the reading.

- Check the test strip package to make sure the strips are compatible with your meter. Test strips are not always interchangeable, and meters cannot always detect incompatible strips. Test strips that look alike may have different chemical coatings. Small variations in strip dimensions can also affect results.

- Check the expiration date on the test strips. As a test strip ages, its chemical coating breaks down. If the strip is used after this time, it may give inaccurate results.

- Enter the correct calibration code from the outside of the strip bottle each time you run a test (if applicable). Results can vary significantly between manufactured lots of reagent strips; the calibration codes help the meter compensate for these variations.

- Run quality control as directed. Running quality control is typically the only way to know when test strips have gone bad. Test strips do not always last until the expiration date on the bottle. This may be because the manufacturer has over-estimated the dating or because the cap was not replaced promptly after use.

- Check the results from your meter against laboratory results as often as possible. Over time, test systems can drift apart. Since results from either test system maybe used to treat your patients, it is important for the systems to remain synchronized.

- Question results that are not consistent with physical symptoms. If a test result seems wrong, have a blood sample tested by the main laboratory. There may be many reasons why a test result is incorrect. In addition to the items above, some physiological conditions such as dehydration, hyperosmolarity, high hematocrit, or shock may significantly affect test results.

541

Common Problems with the Use of Glucose Meters

Diabetes care has come a long way since the introduction of insulin and the first oral anti-hyperglycemic medicines. Life span and quality of life have improved for majority of affected individuals. Even better, a large part of diabetic care formerly performed in hospital clinics can now be managed at home with use of well designed home based glucose meters, a telephone, and a good patient-doctor relationship.

The Office of In Vitro Diagnostics (OIVD) is charged with the job of evaluating many devices, including glucose meters. OIVD helps these meters come to the public market. Another of its tasks is the continuous evaluation of the same devices for long term safety and effectiveness not just of the devices, but of how the devices are used.

OIVD is taking this opportunity to provide some friendly tips in Point of Care glucose testing inspired by some comments we have received from manufactures and users of these devices.

Causes of false results may be patient/sample based or user/device based. Some common problems and their effects on meter glucose readings are listed in Table 44.1.

The advantage of Point of Care testing is eliminated if proper technique is not followed. In addition to the above recommendations, laboratory professionals must remember to wash hands and change gloves between patients. Also, clean the surface of the meter if blood gets on it. This "each time, every time" approach helps protect both the patient and the health care worker from blood borne agents like HIV and HCV.

All operators, from patients to non-lab health care workers to medical technologists and physicians, should be thoroughly familiar with any device prior to using it. The best way to do this is to read the package insert and user manual carefully before using a device for the first time. It sounds simple, and it is. If you have any questions, ask someone who is familiar with the device. Another option is calling the customer service telephone number located on most package inserts. The people on the other end are there to help. Another good tip is to re-read the package insert every few months. It is a good practice and their may be changes.

Next, watch an experienced laboratory professional, doctor, nurse, or diabetic educator perform the test. Then perform the test in front of someone who has experience in using the glucose meter and instructing others on its performance. Ask for tips.

Specific problems come up from time to time including glucose readings that don't make sense. For example you might feel fine when the glucose meter reading is obviously too high or too low. Remember, the best way to resolve any questionable result, and the best sample from any sick patient, is still a venous blood sample tested at a central lab. Even then any result that does not fit the clinical picture needs to be investigated and, at a minimum, repeated.

Table 44.1. Common problems that affect meter glucose readings.

Problem	Result	Recommendation
Sensor strips not fully inserted into meter	False low	Always be sure strip is fully inserted in meter
Patient sample site (for example the fingertip) is contaminated with sugar	False high	Always clean test site before sampling
Not enough blood applied to strip	False low	Repeat test with a new sample
Batteries low on power	Error codes	Change batteries and repeat sample collection
Test strips/Controls solutions stored at temperature extremes	False high/low	Store kit according to directions
Patient is dehydrated	False high	Stat venous sample on main lab analyzer
Patient in shock	False low	Stat venous sample on main lab analyzer
Squeezing fingertip too hard because blood is not flowing	False low	Repeat test with a new sample from a new stick
Sites other than fingertips	High/low	results from alternative sites may not match finger stick results
Test strip/"Control" solution vial cracked	False high/low	Always inspect package for cracks, leaks, etc.
Anemia/decrease hematocrit	False high	Venous sample on main lab analyzer
Polycythemia/increased hematocrit	False low	Venous sample on main lab analyzer

Home Glycated Hemoglobin Test for Diabetics

The Food and Drug Administration (FDA) has cleared the first over-the-counter test that measures glycated hemoglobin in people with diabetes to help monitor how well they are managing their disease (glycemic control).

The test, called Metrika A1c Now, is currently available by prescription only. Over-the-counter status means that the test can now be purchased without a prescription and used at home, with results on the spot, making it readily available to people with diabetes.

Diabetes is a chronic disease in which blood glucose (sugar) levels are too high. Abnormally high levels of glucose can damage the small and large blood vessels, leading to blindness, kidney disease, amputation of limbs, stroke, and heart disease.

Glycated hemoglobin is a unique substance created as a result of interaction between hemoglobin and glucose.

The level of glycated hemoglobin provides information on the average level of glucose in the body over a 90 to 120 day period of time.

The glycated hemoglobin test should be performed two to four times a year to monitor long-term control over blood glucose levels. Glycated hemoglobin tests provide information to complement that obtained from daily finger stick blood glucose tests that measure glucose at a single point in time.

To perform the Metrika A1c Now test, the patient takes a blood sample from his finger with a lancet and places it in a monitor. The monitor displays test results in eight minutes. Unlike some other products, there is no need to send the sample back to the physician to get results. The patient gets the results on the spot.

FDA cleared the test for non-prescription use based on a clinical study conducted by the manufacturer, Metrika, Inc., of Sunnyvale, California The study compared test results obtained by lay users of the device to test results obtained by medical professionals. In the study, 286 patients—271 diabetics and 15 non-diabetics—used the test without physician supervision.

The results were comparable to those obtained by medical professionals.

The Metrika A1c Now test has been certified by the National Glycohemoglobin Standardization Program, an independent certification body.

About 17 million Americans have diabetes. Many of them may find the new home glycated hemoglobin test helpful.

Chapter 45

Home-Use for Prothrombin Time (PT)

What does this test do?

This is a home-use test kit to measure how long it takes for your blood to clot.

What type of test is this?

This is a quantitative test—you find out the length of time it takes your blood to clot.

Why should you do this test?

If you take blood-thinning drugs such as Coumadin or warfarin, you may need to test you blood regularly to make sure it clots properly. Doctors often prescribe these drugs to prevent blood clots in patients who have artificial heart valves, irregular heart beats or inherited clotting tendencies. Your doctor will prescribe this test for you if you need to do it.

How often should you do this test?

You should follow your doctor's instructions about how often you do this test. Your doctor may ask you to use the results to adjust the

"Home-Use Tests: Prothrombin Time," U.S. Food and Drug Administration, Center for Devices and Radiological Health, February 2003.

amount of drugs you to take to control your blood clotting. Never change the drugs you take without your doctor's permission.

How do you do this test?

You prick your finger with a lancet to get a drop of blood. Place the drop of blood on a test strip or cartridge, and insert it into your test meter. Your meter will measure how long it takes for the blood to form a clot and how much anticoagulant effect there is.

How can you make sure your meter works properly?

Your meter has some built-in features that allow it to test itself and detect problems in its operation. Your meter comes with sample solutions to use instead of your blood to assure that it is working properly. Look in your meter's operator manual to see how to check on its accuracy.

Take your meter with you to your doctor's office. Have your doctor watch you do your testing. Your doctor may want to take a sample of your blood and compare the clotting time of that sample with the time your meter gives. If the value you get matches your doctor's value, that you will know your meter is working well and that you are doing the test correctly.

Where can you get more information about blood clotting and measuring prothrombin time?

- MEDLINEplus Health Information Medical Encyclopedia: Prothrombin (available online at http://www.nlm.nih.gov/medlineplus/ency/article/003652.htm)

- American Association for Clinical Chemistry Lab Tests Online: Prothrombin Time (available online at http://www.labtestsonline.org/understanding/analytes/pt/glance.html)

Chapter 46

Home Pregnancy Tests

How do pregnancy tests work?

Pregnancy tests look for a special hormone in the urine or blood that is only there when a woman is pregnant. This hormone, human chorionic gonadotropin (hCG), can also be called the pregnancy hormone.

The pregnancy hormone, hCG, is made in your body when a fertilized egg implants in the uterus. This usually happens about six days after conception. But studies show that the embryo doesn't implant until later in some women. The amount of hCG increases drastically with each passing day you are pregnant.

Many home pregnancy tests claim they can tell if you're pregnant on the day you expect your period. But a recent study shows that most don't give accurate results this early in pregnancy. Waiting one week after a missed period will usually give a more accurate answer.

What's the difference between pregnancy tests that check urine and those that test blood? Which one is better?

There are two types of pregnancy tests. One tests the blood for the pregnancy hormone, hCG. The other checks the urine for this hormone. You can do a urine test at home with a home pregnancy test. You need to see a doctor to have blood tests.

"Pregnancy Tests," National Women's Health Information Center, March 2006.

These days, most women first use home pregnancy tests (HPT) to find out if they are pregnant. HPTs are inexpensive, private, and easy to use. Urine tests will be able to tell if you're pregnant about two weeks after ovulation. Some more sensitive urine tests claim that they can tell if you are pregnant as early as one day after a missed period.

If a HPT says you are pregnant, you should call your doctor right away. You doctor can use a more sensitive test along with a pelvic exam to tell for sure if you're pregnant. Seeing your doctor early on in your pregnancy will help you and your baby stay healthy.

Doctors use two types of blood tests to check for pregnancy. Blood tests can pick up hCG earlier in a pregnancy than urine tests can. Blood tests can tell if you are pregnant about six to eight days after you ovulate (or release an egg from an ovary). A quantitative blood test (or the beta hCG test) measures the exact amount of hCG in your blood. So it can find even tiny amounts of hCG. This makes it very accurate. Qualitative hCG blood tests just check to see if the pregnancy hormone is present or not. So it gives a yes or no answer. The qualitative hCG blood test is about as accurate as a urine test.

How do you do a home pregnancy test?

There are many different types of home pregnancy tests, or HPTs. Most drugstores sell HPTs over-the-counter. They cost between $8 and $20 depending on the brand and how many tests come in the box.

Most popular HPTs work in a similar way. The majority tell the user to hold a stick in the urine stream. Others involve collecting urine in a cup and then dipping the stick into it. At least one brand tells the woman to collect urine in a cup and then put a few drops into a special container with a dropper. Testing the urine first thing in the morning may help boost accuracy.

Then the woman needs to wait a few minutes. Different brands instruct the woman to wait different amounts of time. Once the time has passed, the user should inspect the "result window." If a line or plus symbol appears, you are pregnant. It does not matter how faint the line is. A line, whether bold or faint, means the result is positive.

Most tests also have a "control indicator" in the result window. This line or symbol shows whether the test is working or not. If the control indicator does not appear, the test is not working properly. You should not rely on any results from a HPT that may be faulty.

Most brands tell users to repeat the test in a few days, no matter what the results. One negative result (especially soon after a missed period) does not always mean you're not pregnant. All HPTs come with written instructions. Most tests also have toll-free phone numbers to call in case of questions about use or results.

Which brand of pregnancy test is the most accurate?

In a 2004 study, researchers tested the accuracy of 18 HPTs sold in retail stores. They found that only one brand consistently detected the low levels of hCG usually present on the first day of the missed period. This was the First Response, Early Result Pregnancy Test. The other tests missed up to 85% of pregnancies on the first day of the missed period. Most tests accurately confirmed pregnancies one week after the missed period.

Some brands of tests can pick up lower levels of hCG than others. But limited research makes it impossible to say for sure which one is the best. Even so, two studies suggest that First Response, Early Result Pregnancy Test may be more sensitive than others. So for women who want test early, this is probably the best product.

How soon after a missed period can I take a home pregnancy test and get accurate results?

Many home pregnancy tests (HPTs) claim to be 99% accurate on the day you miss your period. But research suggests that most HPTs do not consistently spot pregnancy that early. And when they do, the results are often so faint they are misunderstood. If you can wait one week after your missed period, most home pregnancy tests will give you an accurate answer. Ask your doctor for a more sensitive test if you need to know earlier.

When a home pregnancy test will give an accurate result depends on many things:

- **How long it takes for the fertilized egg to implant in the uterus after ovulation:** Pregnancy tests look for the hormone human chorionic gonadotropin (hCG) that is only produced once the fertilized egg has implanted in the uterine wall. In most cases, this happens about six days after conception. But studies show that in up to 10 percent of women, the embryo doesn't implant until much later, after the first day of the missed period. So, home pregnancy tests will be accurate as soon as one day after a missed period for some women but not for others.

- **How you use them:** Be sure to follow the directions and check the expiration date.

- **When you use them:** The amount of hCG in a pregnant woman's urine increases with time. So, the earlier after a missed period you take a HPT, the harder it is to spot the hCG. If you wait one week after a missed period to test, you are more apt to have an accurate result. Also, testing your urine first thing in the morning may boost the accuracy.

- **Who uses them:** The amount of hCG in the urine at different points in early pregnancy is different for every woman. So, some women will have accurate results on the day of the missed period while others will need to wait longer.

- **The brand of test:** Some home pregnancy tests are more sensitive than others. So, some tests are better than others at spotting hCG early on.

I got a negative result on a home pregnancy test. Might I still be pregnant?

Yes. So, most HPTs suggest women take the test again in a few days or a week.

Every woman ovulates at different times in her menstrual cycle. Plus, embryos implant in the uterus at different times. So, the accuracy of HPT results varies from woman to woman. Other things can also affect the accuracy.

Sometimes women get false negative results (when the test says you are not pregnant and you are) when they test too early in the pregnancy. Other times, problems with the pregnancy can affect the amount of hCG in the urine.

If your HPT is negative, test yourself again in a few days or one week. If you keep getting a negative result but think you are pregnant, talk with your doctor right away.

Can anything interfere with home pregnancy test results?

Most medicines, over-the-counter and prescription, including birth control pills and antibiotics, should not affect the results of a home pregnancy test. Only medicines that have the pregnancy hormone hCG in them can give a false positive test result. A false positive is when a test says you are pregnant when you're not.

Sometimes medicines containing hCG are used to treat infertility (not being able to get pregnant). Alcohol and illegal drugs do not affect HPT results. But women who may become pregnant should not use these substances.

Chapter 47

Home-Use Tests for Gynecological Concerns

Chapter Contents

Section 47.1

Urine Test for Ovulation

"Home-Use Tests: Ovulation (Urine Test)," U.S. Food and Drug
Administration, Center for Devices and Radiological Health, February 2003.

What does this test do?

This is a home-use test kit to measure luteinizing hormone (LH) in
your urine. This helps detect the LH surge that happens in the middle
of your menstrual cycle, about 1–1½ days before ovulation. Some tests
also measure another hormone—estrone-3-glucuronide (E3G).

What is LH?

Luteinizing hormone (LH) is a hormone produced by your pituitary
gland. Your body always makes a small amount of LH, but just before you ovulate, you make much more LH. This test can detect this
LH surge, which usually happens 1–1½ days before you ovulate.

What is E3G?

E3G is produced when estrogen breaks down in your body. It accumulates in your urine around the time of ovulation and causes your
cervical mucus to become thin and slippery. Sperm may swim more
easily in your thin and slippery cervical mucus, increasing your
chances of getting pregnant.

What type of test is this?

This is a qualitative test—you find out whether or not you have
elevated LH or E3G levels, not if you will definitely become pregnant.

Why should you do this test?

You should do this test if you want to know when you expect to ovulate and be in the most fertile part of your menstrual cycle. This test
can be used to help you plan to become pregnant. You should not use

this test to help prevent pregnancy, because it is not reliable for that purpose.

How accurate is this test?

How well this test will predict your fertile period depends on how well you follow the instructions. These tests can detect LH and E3G reliably about nine times out of ten, but you must do the test carefully.

How do you do this test?

You add a few drops of your urine to the test, hold the tip of the test in your urine stream, or dip the test in a cup of your urine. You either read the test by looking for colored lines on the test or you put the test device into a monitor. You can get results in about five minutes. The details of what the color looks like, or how to use the monitor varies among the different brands.

Most kits come with multiple tests to allow you to take measurements over several days. This can help you find your most fertile period, the time during your cycle when you can expect to ovulate based on your hormone levels. Follow the instructions carefully to get good results. You will need to start your testing at the proper time during your cycle, otherwise the test will be unreliable, and you will not find your hormonal surges or your fertile period.

Is this test similar to the one my doctor uses?

The fertility tests your doctor uses are automated, and they may give more consistent results. Your doctor may use other tests that are not yet available for home use (that is, blood and urine laboratory tests) and information about your history to get a better view of your fertility status.

Where can you get more information about ovulation and ovulation tests?

- MEDLINEplus Health Information Medical Encyclopedia: LH Urine Test/Home Test (available online at http://www.nlm.nih.gov/medlineplus/ency/article/007062.htm)

- American Association for Clinical Chemistry Lab Tests Online: LH Test (available online at http://www.labtestsonline.org/understanding/analytes/lh/glance.html)

Section 47.2

Saliva Test for Ovulation

"Home-Use Tests: Ovulation (Saliva Test)," U.S. Food and Drug
Administration, Center for Devices and Radiological Health, February 2003.

What does this test do?

This is a home-use test kit to predict ovulation by looking at patterns formed by your saliva. When your estrogen increases near your time of ovulation, your dried saliva may form a fern-shaped pattern.

What type of test is this?

This is a qualitative test—you find out whether or not you may be near your ovulation time, not if you will definitely become pregnant.

Why should you do this test?

You should do this test if you want to know when you expect to ovulate and be in the most fertile part of your menstrual cycle. This test can be used to help you plan to become pregnant. You should not use this test to help prevent pregnancy, because it is not reliable for that purpose.

How accurate is this test?

This test may not work well for you. Some of the reasons include the following:

- Not all women fern.

- You may not be able to see the fern.

- Women who fern on some days of their fertile period, don't necessarily fern on all of their fertile days.

- Ferning may be disrupted by smoking, eating, drinking, brushing your teeth, how you put your saliva on the slide, and where you were when you did the test.

How do you do this test?

In this test, you get a small microscope with built-in or removable slides. You put some of your saliva on a glass slide, allow it to dry, and look at the pattern it makes. You will see dots and circles, a fern (full or partial), or a combination depending on where you are in your monthly cycle.

You will get your best results when you use the test within the five-day period around your expected ovulation. This period includes the two days before and the two days after your expected day of ovulation. The test is not perfect, though, and you might fern outside of this time period or when you are pregnant. Even some men will fern.

Is this test similar to the one my doctor uses?

The fertility tests your doctor uses are automated, and they may give more consistent results. Your doctor may use other tests that are not yet available for home use (that is, blood and urine laboratory tests) and information about your history to get a better view of your fertility status.

Does a positive test mean you are ovulating?

A positive test indicates that you may be near ovulation. It does not mean that you will definitely become pregnant.

Do negative test results mean that you are not ovulating?

No, there may be many reasons why you did not detect your time of ovulation. You should not use this test to help prevent pregnancy, because it is not reliable for that purpose.

Where can you get more information about ovulation and ovulation tests?

- MEDLINEplus Health Information Medical Encyclopedia: LH Urine Test/Home Test (available online at http://www.nlm.nih.gov/medlineplus/ency/article/007062.htm)

- American Association for Clinical Chemistry Lab Tests Online: LH Test (available online at http://www.labtestsonline.org/understanding/analytes/lh/glance.html)

Section 47.3

Testing Vaginal pH

"Home-Use Tests: Ovulation (Vaginal pH)," U.S. Food and Drug Administration, Center for Devices and Radiological Health, February 2003.

What does this test do?

This is a home-use test kit to measure the pH of your vaginal secretions. pH is a way to describe how acidic a substance is. It is given by a number on a scale of 1–14. The lower the number, the more acidic the substance.

What is pH?

pH is a way to describe how acidic a substance is. It is given by a number on a scale of 1–14. The lower the number, the more acidic the substance.

What type of test is this?

This is a quantitative test—you find out how acidic your vaginal secretions are.

Why should you do this test?

You should do this test to help evaluate if your vaginal symptoms (that is, itching, burning, unpleasant odor, or unusual discharge) are likely caused by an infection that needs medical treatment. The test is not intended for HIV, chlamydia, herpes, gonorrhea, syphilis, or group B streptococcus.

How accurate is this test?

Home vaginal pH tests showed good agreement with a doctor's diagnosis. However, just because you find changes in your vaginal pH, doesn't always mean that you have a vaginal infection. pH changes also do not help or differentiate one type of infection from another.

Your doctor diagnoses a vaginal infection by using a combination of: pH, microscopic examination of the vaginal discharge, amine odor, culture, wet preparation, and Gram stain.

Does a positive test mean you have a vaginal infection?

No, a positive test (elevated pH) could occur for other reasons. If you detect elevated pH, you should see your doctor for further testing and treatment. There are no over-the-counter medications for treatment of an elevated vaginal pH.

If test results are negative, can you be sure that you do not have a vaginal infection?

No, you may have an infection that does not show up in these tests. If you have no symptoms, your negative test could suggest the possibility of chemical, allergic, or other noninfectious irritation of the vagina. Or, a negative test could indicate the possibility of a yeast infection. You should see your doctor if you find changes in your vaginal pH or if you continue to have symptoms.

How do you do this test?

You hold a piece of pH paper against the wall of your vagina for a few seconds, then compare the color of the pH paper to the color on the chart provided with the test kit. The number on the chart for the color that best matches the color on the pH paper is the vaginal pH number.

Is the home test similar to your doctor's test?

Yes. The home vaginal pH tests are practically identical to the ones sold to doctors. But your doctor can provide a more thorough assessment of your vaginal status through your history, physical exam, and other laboratory tests than you can using a single pH test in your home.

Where can you get more information about vaginal pH and vaginal infection testing?

- MEDLINEplus Health Information: Vaginal Diseases (available online at http://www.nlm.nih.gov/medlineplus/vaginaldiseases .html)

Section 47.4

Testing for Menopause

"Home-Use Tests: Ovulation (Menopause)," U.S. Food and Drug Administration, Center for Devices and Radiological Health, February 2003.

What does this test do?

This is a home-use test kit to measure follicle stimulating hormone (FSH) in your urine. This may help indicate if you are in menopause or perimenopause.

What is menopause?

Menopause is the stage in your life when menstruation stops for at least 12 months. The time before this is called perimenopause and could last for several years. You may reach menopause in your early 40s or as late as your 60s.

What is FSH?

Follicle stimulating hormone (FSH) is a hormone produced by your pituitary gland. FSH levels increase temporarily each month to stimulate your ovaries to produce eggs. When you enter menopause and your ovaries stop working, your FSH levels also increase.

What type of test is this?

This is a qualitative test—you find out whether or not you have elevated FSH levels, not if you definitely are in menopause or perimenopause.

Why should you do this test?

You should use this test if you want to know if your symptoms, such as irregular periods, hot flashes, vaginal dryness, or sleep problems are part of menopause. While many women may have little or no trouble when going through the stages of menopause, others may have moderate to severe discomfort and may want treatment to alleviate their symptoms. This test may help you be better informed about your current condition when you see your doctor.

How accurate is this test?

These tests will accurately detect FSH about nine out of ten times. This test does not detect menopause or perimenopause. As you grow older, your FSH levels may rise and fall during your menstrual cycle. While your hormone levels are changing, your ovaries continue to release eggs and you can still become pregnant.

Your test will depend on whether you used your first morning urine, drank large amounts of water before the test, or use (or recently stopped using) oral or patch contraceptives, hormone replacement therapy, or estrogen supplements.

How do you do this test?

In this test, you put a few drops of your urine on a test device, put the end of the testing device in your urine stream, or dip the test device into a cup of urine. Chemicals in the test device react with FSH and produce a color. Read the instructions with the test you buy to learn exactly what to look for in this test.

Are the home menopause tests similar to the ones my doctor uses?

Some home menopause tests are identical to the one your doctor uses. However, doctors would not use this test by itself. Your doctor would use your medical history, physical exam, and other laboratory tests to get a more thorough assessment of your condition.

Does a positive test mean you are in menopause?

A positive test indicates that you may be in a stage of menopause. If you have a positive test, or if you have any symptoms of menopause, you should see your doctor. Do not stop taking contraceptives based on the results of these tests because they are not foolproof and you could become pregnant.

Do negative test results indicate that you are not in menopause?

If you have a negative test result, but you have symptoms of menopause, you may be in perimenopause or menopause. You should not assume that a negative test means you have not reached menopause, there could be other reasons for the negative result. You should always discuss your symptoms and your test results with your doctor. Do not use these tests to determine if you are fertile or can become pregnant. These tests will not give you a reliable answer on your ability to become pregnant.

Where can you get more information about menopause and menopause testing?

- MEDLINEplus Health Information: Menopause (available online at http://www.nlm.nih.gov/medlineplus/menopause.html)

Chapter 48

Home-Use Test for Human Immunodeficiency Virus

Privacy and confidentiality are main factors that lead people to choose home testing kits to find out if they are infected with human immunodeficiency virus (HIV), which causes AIDS.

It is important that consumers know there is only one product currently approved by U.S. Food and Drug Administration (FDA) and legally sold in the United States as a "home" testing system for HIV.

This product is a kit marketed as either "The Home Access HIV-1 Test System" or "The Home Access Express HIV-1 Test System." The kit is a home collection-test system that requires users to collect a blood specimen, and then mail it to a laboratory for professional testing. No test kits allow consumers to interpret the results at home.

Beware of False Claims

Numerous HIV home test systems that have not been approved by FDA are currently being marketed online and in newspapers and magazines.

Manufacturers of unapproved systems have falsely claimed that their products can detect antibodies to HIV in blood or saliva samples, and that they can provide results in the home in 15 minutes or less. Some have even claimed that their systems are approved by FDA or are manufactured in a facility that is registered with FDA.

"Vital Facts about HIV Home Test Kits," U.S. Food and Drug Administration (www.fda.gov), January 29, 2008.

FDA takes appropriate action against people or firms that sell unapproved and ineffective tests.

About the Approved Product

The FDA-approved Home Access System kits allow people to collect a blood sample. Using a personal identification number (PIN), they then mail the sample anonymously to a laboratory for testing. The PIN can then be used to obtain results.

The kits, manufactured by Illinois-based Home Access Health Corp., can be purchased at pharmacies, by mail order, or online. They only allow testing for the presence of antibodies of the virus known as HIV-1. They do not provide the ability to test for HIV-2, a less common cause of AIDS.

The Home Access System offers users pre- and post-test, anonymous and confidential counseling through both printed material and telephone interaction. It also provides the user with an interpretation of the test result.

Checking for Antibodies to HIV

Like most HIV tests, the approved Home Access testing system checks for the presence of antibodies to HIV that are produced once the virus enters the body. The rate at which individuals infected with HIV produce these antibodies differs.

There's a "window period" between the time someone is infected with HIV and the time the body produces enough antibodies to be detected through testing. During this time, an HIV-infected person will still get a negative test result.

According to FDA's Center for Biologics and Research (CBER), which regulates all HIV tests, detectable antibodies usually develop within two to eight weeks. The average is about 22 days.

Still, some people take longer to develop detectable antibodies. Most will develop antibodies within three months following infection. In very rare cases, it can take up to six months to develop detectable antibodies to HIV.

Rapid Tests: A Clinical Option

Consumers do have the option of taking a rapid test, some of which test for both HIV-1 and HIV-2. These tests are run where the sample is collected, and produce results within 20 minutes.

Because HIV testing requires interpretation and confirmation, rapid antibody tests are only approved and available in a professional health care setting, such as doctors' offices, clinics, and outreach testing sites.

According to the Centers for Disease Control and Prevention (CDC), there are tests that look for HIV's genetic material directly, but these are not in widespread use. Tests using saliva or urine are also available, although not for "at-home" use.

If you are unsure whether a certain type of HIV test is FDA-approved, look for the test on the agency's list of at www.fda.gov/cber/products/testkits.htm. You can also contact CBER by phone at (800) 835-4709, or e-mail at OCTMA@CBER.FDA.GOV.

Chapter 49

Home-Use Test for Hepatitis C

What does this test do?

This is a home-use collection kit to determine if you may have a hepatitis C infection now or had one in the past. You collect a blood sample and send it to a testing laboratory for analysis.

What is hepatitis C infection?

Hepatitis C infection is caused by the hepatitis C virus (HCV). Untreated, hepatitis C can cause liver disease.

What type of test is this?

This is a qualitative test—you find out whether or not you may have this infection, not how advanced your disease is.

Why should you do this test?

You should do this test if you think you may have been infected with HCV. If you are infected with HCV, you should take steps to avoid spreading the disease to others. At least eight out of ten people with acute hepatitis C develop chronic liver infection, and two to three out of 10 develop cirrhosis. A small number of people may also develop

---

"Home-Use Tests: Hepatitis C," U.S. Food and Drug Administration, Center for Devices and Radiological Health, February 2003.

liver cancer. Hepatitis C infection is the number one cause for liver transplantation in the US.

When should you do this test?

The Centers for Disease Control (CDC) recommend that you do this test if you any of the following characteristics apply to you:

- have ever injected illegal drugs
- received clotting factor concentrates produced before 1987
- were ever on long-term dialysis
- received a blood transfusion before July 1992
- received an organ transplant before July 1992
- are a health care, emergency medicine, or public safety worker who contacted HCV-positive blood through needlesticks, sharps, or mucosal exposure

How accurate is this test?

This test is about as accurate as the test your doctor uses, but you must carefully follow the directions about getting the sample and sending it the testing laboratory. Proper sample collection is important for obtaining accurate results.

Researchers found that about 90 of 100 home users were able to obtain acceptable samples to send to the laboratory. After the laboratory got these 90 samples, it could get results for about 81 of them. Of these 81 samples, the laboratory got correct results in 77 and incorrect results in four.

Does a positive test mean you have HCV?

If you have a positive test, you either are infected with HCV now or you have been infected with HCV in the past. You need to see your doctor to find out if you have an active infection and what therapy you should have. Some people who become infected with HCV develop antibodies and then are no longer infected.

If your test results are negative, can you be sure that you do not have HCV infection?

A negative test does not guarantee that you don't have HCV infection since it takes some time for you to develop antibodies after you are infected with this virus. If you think you were exposed to the virus and might be infected, you should see your doctor for a more accurate laboratory test.

How do you do this test?

The test kit comes with a small piece of filter paper, a lancet, and instructions for obtaining a blood sample and placing it on the filter paper. You first prick your finger with the lancet to get a drop of blood. Then, you put your drop of blood on a piece of filter paper and send it in a special container to the testing laboratory. You get the results of your test by phone from the laboratory.

The laboratory performs a preliminary (screening) test that separates the samples into three groups:

- Samples that are clearly positive

- Samples that might be positive

- Samples that are negative

All samples that "might be positive" receive a more specific (confirmatory) test to find those that are truly positive. All the "clearly positives" from the preliminary test and the "truly positives" from the more specific test are reported to you as positive.

You should note that a positive result does not mean that you are infected with HCV. If you receive a positive result from this test, you should see your doctor for further testing and information.

Where can you get more information about hepatitis C infection and HCV testing?

- MEDLINEplus Medical Encyclopedia: Hepatitis C (available online at http://www.nlm.nih.gov/medlineplus/ency/article/000284.htm)

- National Institutes of Health (NIH) Information on Hepatitis C (available online at http://www.labtestsonline.org/understanding/analytes/hepatitis_c/glance.html)

- Lab Tests Online: Hepatitis C Virus (available online at http://health.nih.gov/result.asp?disease_id=323&selectbox.x=10&selectbox .y=10)

Chapter 50

Home-Use Tests for Drugs of Abuse

Chapter Contents

Section 50.1

First Check 12 Drug Test

"Home-Use Tests Drugs of Abuse (First Check 12 Drug Test),"
Office of In Vitro Diagnostic Device Evaluation and Safety,
U.S. Food and Drug Administration, March 2006.

What does this test do?

The First Check 12 Drug Test indicates if one or more prescription or illegal drugs are present in urine. It is currently the only over the counter test available designed to detect prescription drugs that are being abused. The test detects the presence of 12 prescription and illegal drugs: marijuana, cocaine, opiates, methamphetamine, amphetamines, PCP, benzodiazepine, barbiturates, methadone, tricyclic antidepressants, ecstasy, and oxycodone.

This test is done in two steps. First, you do a quick at-home test. Second, if the test suggests that drugs may be present, you send the sample to a laboratory for additional testing.

What are prescription drugs of abuse?

Prescription drugs of abuse are medicines (for example, Oxycodone or Valium) that are obtained legally with a doctor's prescription but are being taken for a non-medical purpose. Non-medical purposes include taking the medication for longer than your doctor prescribed it for or for a purpose other than what the doctor prescribed it for. Medications are not drugs of abuse if they are taken according to your doctor's instructions.

What type of test is this?

This is a qualitative test—you find out if a particular drug may be in the urine, not how much is present.

Why should you do this test?

You should use this test when you think someone you care about might be abusing prescription or illegal drugs. If you are worried about a specific drug, make sure to check the label to confirm that this test is designed to detect the drug you are looking for.

How accurate is this test?

The at-home testing part of this test is fairly sensitive to the presence of drugs in the urine. This means that if drugs are present, you will usually get a preliminary (or presumptive) positive test result. If you get a preliminary positive result, you should send the urine sample to the laboratory for a second test.

It is very important to send the urine sample to the laboratory to confirm a positive at-home result because certain foods, food supplements, beverages, or medicines can affect the results of at-home tests. Laboratory tests are the most reliable way to confirm drugs of abuse.

Note that all amphetamine results should be considered carefully, even those from the laboratory. Some over-the-counter medications cannot be distinguished from illegally-abused amphetamines.

Many things can affect the accuracy of this test, including (but not limited to) the following factors:

- The way you did the test
- The way you stored the test or urine
- What the person ate or drank before taking the test
- Any other prescription or over-the-counter drugs the person may have taken before the test

Does a positive test mean that you found drugs of abuse?

No. Take no serious actions until you get the laboratory's result. Remember that many factors may cause a false positive result in the home test.

Remember that a positive test for a prescription drug does not mean that a person is abusing the drug, because there is no way for the test to indicate acceptable levels compared to abusive levels of prescribed drugs.

If the test results are negative, can you be sure that the person you tested did not abuse drugs?

No. There are several factors that can make the test results negative even though the person is abusing drugs. First, you may have tested for the wrong drugs. Or, you may not have tested the urine when it contained drugs. It takes time for drugs to appear in the urine after a person takes them, and they do not stay in the urine indefinitely; you may have collected the urine too late or too soon. It is also possible that the chemicals in the test went bad because they were stored incorrectly or they passed their expiration date.

If you get a negative test result, but still suspect that someone is abusing drugs, you can test again at a later time. Talk to your doctor if you need more help deciding what steps to take next.

How soon after a person takes drugs, will they show up in a drug test? And how long after a person takes drugs, will they continue to show up in a drug test?

The drug clearance rate tells how soon a person may have a positive test after taking a particular drug. It also tells how long the person may continue to test positive after the last time he or she took the drug. Clearance rates for common drugs of abuse are given in Table 50.1. These are only guidelines, however, and the times can vary significantly from these estimates based on how long the person has been taking the drug, the amount of drug they use, or the person's metabolism.

Table 50.1. Typical Drug Clearance Rates.

Drug	How soon after taking drug will there be a positive drug test?	How long after taking drug will there continue to be positive drug test?
Marijuana/Pot	1–3 hours	1–7 days
Crack (Cocaine)	2–6 hours	2–3 days
Heroin (Opiates)	2–6 hours	1–3 days
Speed/Uppers (Amphetamine, methamphetamine)	4–6 hours	2–3 days
Angel Dust/PCP	4–6 hours	7–14 days
Ecstasy	2–7 hours	2–4 days
Benzodiazepine	2–7 hours	1–4 days
Barbiturates	2–4 hours	1–3 weeks
Methadone	3–8 hours	1–3 days
Tricyclic Antidepressants	8–12 hours	2–7 days
Oxycodone	1–3 hours	1–2 days

How do you do the two-step test?

The kit contains a urine collection cup, a plastic lid containing 12 test strips, and an instruction booklet. It also includes a numbered sticker for confidential confirmation testing and packaging for sending samples to the laboratory for confirmation.

You collect a urine sample in the collection cup, and secure the lid onto the cup. The test strips in the lid contain chemicals that react with each possible drug and show a visible result for each drug they detect. Read and follow the directions carefully and exactly. If the test indicates the presence of one or more drugs, you should send the urine sample to the laboratory for confirmation.

Section 50.2

Home Collection Kit for Drug Testing

"Home-Use Test Kits - Drugs of Abuse (Collection Kit),"
Office of In Vitro Diagnostic Device Evaluation and Safety,
U.S. Food and Drug Administration, February 2003.

What does this test do?

This is a home collection kit for drugs of abuse. You collect a sample of urine, hair, saliva, or other human material and send it to a laboratory for analysis. The laboratory does a quick screening test for drugs, then, if the test suggests that one or more drugs may be present, it performs additional testing.

What are drugs of abuse?

Examples of drugs of abuse include marijuana, cocaine, opiates (including heroin), amphetamines (including Ecstasy or MDMA), and PCP (angel dust). Prescription drugs, such as codeine or other painkillers, also may be abused.

What type of test is this?

This is a qualitative test—you find out whether or not the person tested took drugs of abuse, not how much is present.

Why should you use this test?

You should use this test when you think someone you care about might be using drugs of abuse.

How accurate is this test?

Laboratories use a very reliable test, with very few errors, to determine whether or not your sample contains drugs of abuse.

Note that all amphetamine results should be considered carefully, even those from the laboratory. Some over-the-counter medications contain amphetamines that cannot be distinguished from illegally-abused amphetamines.

Many things can affect the accuracy of this test, including (but not limited to) the following factors:

- the way you did the test;
- the way you stored the test or urine;
- what the person ate or drank before taking the test; and
- any prescription or over-the-counter drugs the person may have taken before the test.

If the test results are negative, can you be sure that the person you tested did not take drugs?

No. You may not have taken a sample when it contained drugs. It takes time for drugs to appear in urine, hair, saliva, or other human materials, and they do not stay in the in the materials indefinitely; you may have gotten the sample too soon or too late.

If you get a negative test result, but still suspect that someone is abusing drugs, you can test again at a later time. Talk to your doctor if you need more help deciding what steps to take next.

How do you do this test?

You do not do the testing yourself. You simply collect a sample of urine, hair, saliva, or other human material and send it to a laboratory for analysis. The laboratory does a preliminary analysis to see if the sample might contain drugs of abuse. If the result is positive, they will do a more complete analysis of the sample and report the results to you. These collection kits contain the sample containers, instructions, and shipping containers. The price you pay for the kit usually pays for the analysis.

Section 50.3

Two-Step Test for Drugs of Abuse

"Home-Use Tests - Drugs of Abuse (Two-Step Test),"
Office of In Vitro Diagnostic Device Evaluation and Safety,
U.S. Food and Drug Administration, November 2007.

What does this test do?

This is a two-step test that shows if one or more drugs of abuse are present in urine. Step 1: do a quick home test. Step 2: if you get a presumptive positive (non-negative) test that suggests that one or more drugs may be present, send the sample to a laboratory for additional testing. The kit should have the sample container, the mailing materials and instructions for mailing the sample to the laboratory. The kit will have a toll-free customer service number if you have questions about the test. There are many different tests on the market. You must buy a test that checks for the drug or drugs you are looking for.

How do I know that FDA has cleared the test for marketing?

You can find information about each home drug test that FDA has cleared by searching FDA's database of in vitro devices (IVDs) (available online at http://www.accessdata.fda.gov/scripts/cdrh/cfdocs/cfIVD/Search.cfm).

To use this database, follow these instructions:

1. Enter a search term (test name, manufacturer name, test type) in the blank space.

2. For example if you select test type, enter the name of the drug you are testing (for example, amphetamines, or oxycodone, or methadone). If the drug test contains more than one drug, your search will pull up all drugs for the test kit you purchased.

3. Click on "Search."

4. Review the tests that match your search term.

5. Select any tests for additional information such as a summary of FDA's review of the product.

6. There is a "help" link with questions about searching this database available.

What are drugs of abuse?

Drugs of abuse can be illegal drugs (for example, marijuana, cocaine, heroin, methadone (fizzies), or PCP (angel dust)) or prescribed medications that are abused (for example, benzodiazepines, barbiturates or painkillers such as oxycodone or codeine).

What does the home drug test tell you?

This type of test can tell you whether or not a particular drug or drugs are in the urine, but not how much drug is present.

Why should you do this test?

You should use this test when you think someone you care about might be abusing drugs.

How reliable are these types of tests?

Home drug tests are fairly sensitive to the presence of drugs in the urine. This means that if drugs are present, you will usually get a presumptive positive (non-negative) test result. If this happens, you should send the urine sample to the laboratory for a second, more reliable test.

It is very important to send the urine sample to the laboratory, because home tests can give positive results when no drugs are present. Some tests are wrong more than 50% of the time because certain foods, food supplements, beverages, diet pills, or over-the-counter medicines can cause a reaction with the tests.

Laboratories use a more reliable test to show whether or not your sample contains drugs of abuse.

Note that all amphetamine results should be considered carefully, even those from the laboratory. Some over-the-counter medications contain amphetamines that cannot be distinguished from illegally-abused amphetamines.

Many things can affect the test, including (but not limited to) the following factors:

- The way you did the test
- The way you stored the test or urine
- Whether the urine was tampered with before you did the test
- What the person ate or drank before taking the test
- Prescription or over-the-counter drugs the person may have taken before the test

Does a positive (non-negative) test mean that you found drugs of abuse?

No. Take no action until you get the laboratory's result. Remember that many factors may cause a false positive result in the home test.

If the test results are negative, can you be sure that the person you tested did not take drugs?

No. There are several factors that can make the test results negative even though the person is using drugs.

- You may have tested for drugs that are not present in the urine.
- You may have gotten the urine too soon after drugs were taken or too late after they left the body.
- The urine sample may have been tampered with.
- The chemicals in the test may have gone bad.
- The test may have been stored improperly.

If you get a negative test result, but still suspect that someone is abusing drugs, you can test at a later time. Also, consider using a test that looks for other types of drugs. Talk to your doctor if you need help deciding what actions to take next.

How soon after a person takes drugs, will they show up in a drug test? And how long after a person takes drugs, will they continue to show up in a drug test?

The drug clearance rate tells how soon a person will have a positive test after taking a particular drug. It also tells how long the person will continue to test positive after the last time he or she took the drug. Clearance rates for common drugs of abuse are given in Table 50.1. These are guidelines and the times can vary depending on how long the person has been taking the drug, the amount of drug they took, or their metabolism.

How do you do the two-step test?

Step 1: Check the expiration date of the home test. Do not use the home test if it has expired. Carefully read the instructions before starting the test. Collect the urine sample and follow the directions exactly on how to perform the test and how to read the results of the test. The test cards, cassettes or strips contain chemicals that react with the drug and show some visible result such as a color change. Often a visible change such as the presence of a line for the test may mean the drug of abuse is not present.

Step 2: If you get a presumptive positive (non-negative) test that suggests that one or more drugs may be present, send the sample to a laboratory for additional testing. The kit should have the sample container, the mailing materials and instructions for mailing the sample to the laboratory.

Where can you get more information about drug abuse and drugs of abuse testing?

- MEDLINEplus Health Information: Drug Abuse (available online at http://www.nlm.nih.gov/medlineplus/drugabuse.html)

- National Institute on Drug Abuse, Understanding Drug Abuse and Addiction (available online at http://www.drugabuse.gov/Infofacts/understand.html)

- National Institute on Drug Abuse, Nationwide Trends (available online at http://www.drugabuse.gov/Infofacts/nationtrends.html)

Section 50.4

American Academy of Pediatrics Believes Adolescents Should Not Be Drug Tested without Their Knowledge and Consent

"Testing for Drugs of Abuse in Children and Adolescents: Addendum—Testing in Schools and at Home," an abstract reproduced with permission from *Pediatrics*, Volume 119, Page 627. © 2007 American Academy of Pediatrics.

Committee on Substance Abuse and Council on School Health

The American Academy of Pediatrics continues to believe that adolescents should not be drug tested without their knowledge and consent. Recent U.S. Supreme Court decisions and market forces have resulted in recommendations for drug testing of adolescents at school and products for parents to use to test adolescents at home. The American Academy of Pediatrics has strong reservations about testing adolescents at school or at home and believes that more research is needed on both safety and efficacy before school-based testing programs are implemented. The American Academy of Pediatrics also believes that more adolescent-specific substance abuse treatment resources are needed to ensure that testing leads to early rehabilitation rather than to punitive measures only.

Part Seven

Additional Help and Information

Chapter 51

Terms Related to Medical Tests

abdominal washings: Instillation of approximately 200 ml. of saline solution into the abdomen during laparotomy. After the solution is allowed to contact surfaces in the abdomen for about five minutes, it is aspirated and sent for cytologic examination. This procedure is used to determine whether tumor is present in the abdomen in the absence of ascites.[1]

accuracy: A measure of closeness of agreement between a test result and an accepted reference value. For example, if you have a standardized reference material at a known value (such as 180 mg/dl of cholesterol), accuracy measures how close the result of the test you are using will get to the known value. You may have a test that is very precise yet very inaccurate, which would be the case if your device measures 180 mg/dl of cholesterol reproducibly as 240 mg/dl.[2]

analyte: The part of the sample that the test is designed to find or measure. For example, a home pregnancy test measures human chorionic gonadotropin (hCG) in urine. The analyte is hCG.[2]

approved test: A test that has been approved by Food and Drug Association (FDA), based on the manufacturer's data showing that it is safe and effective for its intended use. For a new type of test, or for a

---

Terms marked [1] were excerpted from "Pathology," Surveillance, Epidemiology, and End Results (SEER), National Cancer Institute (www.cancer.gov), 2000; terms marked [2] were excerpted from "Glossary," Center for Devices and Radiological Health, U.S. Food and Drug Administration (FDA), 2005.

test that presents higher risk to the patient, the manufacturer performs studies to show that the test does what it claims to do and does not present any unreasonable risk. The manufacturer submits the results in a "premarket approval application" that FDA reviews. If FDA approves the application, the manufacturer can begin selling the test.[2]

bladder washings: Instillation of saline solution into the bladder during cystoscopy. After the solution is allowed to contact surfaces in the area for about five minutes, it is aspirated and sent for cytologic examination. This procedure is used to determine whether tumor is present in the absence of visible tumor.[1]

bone marrow biopsy: Also called bone marrow aspiration. Aspiration of bone marrow cells to determine involvement by tumor. This procedure is optional in low stage lymphoma cases. Bilateral bone marrow biopsies and aspirations should be done for higher stage and symptomatic lymphoma cases.[1]

bronchial washings: Bronchial brushings obtained through a bronchoscope.[1]

brushings: Also called: exfoliative cytology. Tumor is obtained by passing a small brush through an endoscopy tube and scraping cells from the lesion. This tissue is analyzed cytologically.[1]

cerebrospinal fluid (CSF) studies: Cytologic analysis of cerebrospinal fluid for detection of bacteria, fungi, and malignant cells, as well as protein and glucose values.[1]

cleared test: A test that has been cleared by FDA, based on the manufacturer's data showing that it is similar to other tests that are already being sold. For a test that is similar to others already on the market and that is considered to have low risk to the user, manufacturers submit information to show that the test performs similarly to the other tests. The manufacturer submits the results in a "premarket notification" that FDA reviews. If FDA determines that the test is substantially equivalent to another test, the manufacturer can begin selling the test.[2]

closed chest needle biopsy: Includes: skinny-needle biopsy of chest, fine needle aspiration (FNA). This procedure is performed by inserting a long needle through the surface of the chest to penetrate the lung cavity. Fluid suitable for cytologic analysis is drawn up into the needle, which is then withdrawn from the chest. Excludes: any procedure requiring incision into chest cavity.[1]

cytology: Aspiration (fine or skinny needle) of a cyst or tumor, cells, or fluid from a mass or lymph node; also pleural effusion or ascites; procedures include endoscopic brushings or washings of ulcerated areas, Pap smears; cytology of vaginal, cervical, endometrial, and/or abdominal fluid.[1]

cytology reports: Cytologic examination of urinary sediment for malignant cells; fine needle aspiration of a cyst or tumor (detects 70% of bladder cancers); also pleural effusion (thoracentesis) or ascites (paracentesis).[1]

dilatation and curettage (D&C): Dilation of the cervix and scraping or aspirating the contents for cytologic examination. Key words/ possible involvement: tumor, lesion, mass, neoplastic tissue, atypical epithelium, friable tissue. Other words/no involvement: if there is no reference to abnormality in the cervix.[1]

endometrial or pelvic washings: Instillation of saline solution into a body cavity to evaluate for occult tumor. After the solution is allowed to contact surfaces in the area for about five minutes, it is aspirated and sent for cytologic examination.[1]

exempt test: A test that is considered to have such low risk to the patient that FDA does not require manufacturers to submit any premarket approval application or notification.[2]

false negative: A test result that incorrectly says the analyte, disease, or condition is not present when it actually is present. False negatives can be due to human error, test error, or substances in the sample that interfere with the test. For example, a woman who is pregnant receives a test result saying that she is not pregnant.[2]

false positive: A test result that incorrectly says the analyte, disease, or condition is present when it is actually not present. False positives can be due to human error, test error, or substances in the sample that interfere with the test. For example, a woman who is not pregnant woman receives a test result saying she is pregnant.[2]

fractional curettage: Separate scraping of material from the endocervix and walls of uterine corpus in a set order to determine which site may be the source of the malignancy. This is the preferred diagnostic procedure for endometrial cancer. Key words/possible involvement: tumor, lesion, mass, chunky material, neoplastic tissue, abnormal tissue, gray, necrotic, or friable tissue. Other words/no involvement: if there is no reference to abnormality in the endometrium or endocervix.[1]

indications for use: a description of why a patient would use a certain test.[2]

intended use: A description of what the manufacturer intended to measure with a certain test.[2]

in vitro diagnostic test: A medical test that analyzes body samples, such as blood, urine, stool, or saliva, for specific components or analytes.[2]

label: Written material and instructions that accompany the medical test. Labeling includes the writing on the outside of the box as well as instructions packaged with the test.[2]

needle biopsy and aspiration: Includes: skinny-needle biopsy, fine needle aspiration (FNA). This procedure is performed by inserting a needle through the surface into the questionable mass. Fluid suitable for cytologic analysis is drawn up into the needle, which is then withdrawn from the mass.[1]

omentectomy: Surgical removal of the omentum, the fatty covering in the anterior abdomen, usually performed in the presence of ovarian cancer. The omentum can then be examined for nonpalpable metastases. This may be either a partial or complete omentectomy.[1]

over-the-counter (OTC): Products that can be purchased and used by anyone at home. These do not require a doctor's prescription. If manufacturers intend to sell their test kits over-the-counter, they must demonstrate that untrained users can perform the test and get results.[2]

package insert: Information about the test and/or instructions that come inside the box or package.[2]

Pap smear: Aspiration, scraping, or brushing of the cervix for cytologic evaluation. Pap smear is not a reliable method for ruling out endometrial cancer when used by itself.[1]

paracentesis: Removal of fluid from abdomen for cytologic analysis by inserting a long-needle syringe into the abdominal cavity.[1]

pelvic lymphadenectomy: A procedure during which the lymph nodes of the pelvis are removed for evaluation. Also called: staging lymphadenectomy, pelvic lymph node dissection. May also be performed via a laparoscope.[1]

peritoneal/pelvic washings: Instillation of saline solution into a body cavity to evaluate for occult tumor. After the solution is allowed to contact surfaces in the area for about five minutes, it is aspirated and sent for cytologic examination.[1]

qualitative test: Tests that give results in terms of negative or positive. For example, pregnancy tests, ovulation tests, and drugs of abuse detection tests indicate whether or not the person has the condition.[2]

quantitative test: Tests that give results in terms of numbers. For example, glucose meters indicate how much glucose is present in the sample.[2]

screening test: An initial or preliminary test. Screening tests do not tell you if you definitely have a disease or condition. Rather, positive results indicate that you may need additional tests or a doctor's evaluation to see if you have a particular disease or condition.[2]

splenectomy: Surgical removal of the spleen. Splenectomy may occur as part of a full staging laparotomy or occasionally as a separate procedure.[1]

sputum cytology: A specimen of lung secretions obtained by deep cough for cytologic examination.[1]

thoracentesis: Removal of part of an abnormal collection of fluid from the pleural cavity for cytologic analysis by inserting a long needle-syringe instrument into the pleural cavity. Also called: chest tapping, paracentesis thoracic, paracentesis pulmonis.[1]

transrectal/transperineal needle biopsy: Includes: standard needle biopsy, core biopsy, skinny-needle biopsy, fine needle aspiration (FNA). Sometimes called a sextant biopsy because needle biopsies are taken from all regions of the prostate. Excludes: any procedure requiring incision or transurethral approach. This procedure is performed by inserting a needle through the perineum (external) or via the rectum through the rectal wall to penetrate areas of nodularity or induration of the prostate. Fluid or tissue suitable for cytologic analysis is drawn up into the needle, which is withdrawn from the prostate. Multiple random needle biopsies may be performed to determine if tumor is multifocal.[1]

urine cytology: Cytologic examination of urinary sediment for malignant cells; fine needle aspiration of a cyst or tumor (detects 70% of bladder cancers).[1]

washings: Instillation of approximately 200 ml. of saline solution into the abdomen or pelvis during laparotomy. After the solution is allowed to contact surfaces in the area for about five minutes, it is aspirated and sent for cytologic examination. This procedure is used to determine whether tumor is present in the abdomen in the absence of ascites.[1]

Chapter 52

Online Health Screening Tools

Addictions

Alcoholism
Addicted.com
Website: http://www.addicted.com/addiction-resources/self-tests/
alcohol-addiction-alcoholism-quiz

Drug Addiction
Addicted.com
Website: http://www.addicted.com/addiction-resources/self-tests/
drug-addiction-quiz

Food Addiction
Addicted.com
Website: http://www.addicted.com/addiction-resources/self-tests/
food-addiction-quiz

Tobacco Dependence
Addicted.com
Website: http://www.addicted.com/addiction-resources/self-tests/
tobacco-addiction-quiz

This list of online health and health risk assessment tools was compiled from many sources deemed accurate. They are not intended to be used as a substitute for appropriate care from a qualified health care provider. Inclusion does not constitute endorsement and there is no implication associated with omission. All website addresses were verified in May 2008.

Allergy

Allergy Assessment Screen
Health A to Z
Website: http://www.healthatoz.com/healthatoz/Atoz/tl/rq/
allergy_1.jsp

Auditory

Equal Loudness Contours and Audiometry
The University of New South Wales
School of Physics
Website: http://www.phys.unsw.edu.au/jw/hearing.html

Five Minute Hearing Test
New ENT
Website: http://www.newent.com/pateducathearingfivetest.htm

Autism

The AQ Test
Autism Research Centre
Website: http://www.wired.com/wired/archive/9.12/aqtest.html

Milestone Checklist
Centers for Disease Control and Prevention
Website: http://www.cdc.gov/ncbddd/autism/actearly/interactive/
index.html

Cancer Risk

Am I at Risk for Developing Bladder Cancer?
Health A to Z
Website: http://www.healthatoz.com/healthatoz/Atoz/tl/rq/
bladder_1.jsp

Are You at High Risk for Skin Cancer?
Health A to Z
Website: http://www.healthatoz.com/healthatoz/Atoz/tl/rq/
skincancer_1.jsp

Bowel Cancer Risk
Better Health
Website: http://www.betterhealth.vic.gov.au/bhcv2/bhcarticles.nsf/
pages/Quiz_what_are_the_risk_factors_of_bowel_cancer?Open

Breast Cancer Risk Calculator
National Breast and Ovarian Cancer Centre
Website: http://www.nbcc.org.au/risk/yourrisk.html

Colon Cancer Risk Assessment Screen
Health A to Z
Website: http://www.healthatoz.com/healthatoz/Atoz/tl/rq/colon_1.jsp

Prostate Cancer Risk Calculator
National Cancer Institute
Website: http://www.compass.fhcrc.org/edrnnci/bin/calculator/
main.asp?t=prostate&sub=disclaimer&v=prostate&m=&x
=Prostate%20Cancer

Risk Assessment Screen for Cancer of the Uterus
Health A to Z
Website: http://www.healthatoz.com/healthatoz/Atoz/tl/rq/uterus_1.jsp

Cholesterol Levels

LDL Cholesterol Goal Calculator
Medical College of Wisconsin
Website: http://www.intmed.mcw.edu/clincalc/chol.html

Depression

Confidential Depression-Screening Test
Mental Health America
Website: http://www.depression-screening.org/screeningtest/
screeningtestMain.htm

Online Depression Screening Test
NYU School of Medicine
Department of Psychiatry
Website: http://www.med.nyu.edu/psych/screens/depres.html

Online Screening for Anxiety
NYU School of Medicine
Department of Psychiatry
Website: http://www.med.nyu.edu/psych/screens/anxiety.html

Diabetes and Kidney Disease Risk

Could You Be at Risk for Diabetes?
Health A to Z
Website: http://www.healthatoz.com/healthatoz/Atoz/tl/rq/
diabetes_1.jsp

Diabetes Risk Test
American Diabetes Association
Website: http://www.diabetes.org/risk-test.jsp

Diabetes Risk Test
My Dr.
Website: http://www.mydr.com.au/tools/diabetes-quiz.asp

GRF Calculator
DaVita
Website: http://www.davita.com/gfr-calculator/noflash

Heart Attack and Heart Disease Risk

Coronary Heart Disease Risk Calculator
Medical College of Wisconsin
Website: http://www.intmed.mcw.edu/clincalc/heartrisk.html

Heart Disease Risk Calculator
University of Maryland Heart Center
Website: http://www.healthcalculators.org/calculators/
heart_disease_risk.asp

Risk Assessment Screen for Coronary Heart Disease
Health A to Z
Website: http://www.healthatoz.com/healthatoz/Atoz/tl/rq/
coronary_1.jsp

Risk Assessment Tool for Estimating You 10-year Risk of Having a Heart Attack
National Cholesterol Education Program
Website: http://hp2010.nhlbihin.net/atpiii/calculator.asp?usertype =pub

Pregnancy Due Date

Pregnancy Calculator
Medical College of Wisconsin
Website: http://www.intmed.mcw.edu/clincalc/pregnancy.html

Pregnancy Due Date Calculator
Pathways to Women's Sexual Health
Website: http://www.pathways-womens-sexual-health.com/ pregnancy-due-date.html

Sexual Health

Free HIV Test
AIDSGame.com
Website: http://www.aidsgame.com/quick_hiv_test.aspx

HIV/AIDS Risk Assessment Screening
Health A to Z
Website: http://www.healthatoz.com/healthatoz/Atoz/tl/rq/aids _1.jsp

Online Sexual Disorders Screening for Men
NYU School of Medicine
Department of Psychiatry
Website: http://www.med.nyu.edu/psych/screens/disorder_male .html

Online Sexual Disorders Screening for Women
NYU School of Medicine
Department of Psychiatry
Website: http://www.med.nyu.edu/psych/screens/ disorder_women.html

Sleep Disorder

Sleep Disorders
Provena Mercy Medical Center
Website: http://www.provena.org/mercy/body.cfm?id=161&oTopID=0

Take a Sleep Test
Sleepnet.com
Website: http://www.sleepnet.com/sleeptest.html

Stress

How Stressed Are You?
Health A to Z
Website: http://www.healthatoz.com/healthatoz/Atoz/tl/rq/stress.jsp

Online Stress Test
Suicide and Mental Health Association International
Website: http://suicideandmentalhealthassociationinternational
.org/stresstest.html

Stress Test
Lessons 4 Life
Website: http://www.lessons4living.com/stress_test.htm

Visual Tests

Color Vision Testing Made Easy
Color Vision Testing
Website: http://colorvisiontesting.com/online%20test.htm

Distance Vision Test for Adults
Prevent Blindness America
Website: http://www.preventblindness.org/eye_tests/
Adult_distance_test.html

Ishihara Color Blindness Test
Archimedes' Laboratory
Website: http://www.archimedes-lab.org/colorblindnesstest.html

Near Vision Test for Adults
Prevent Blindness America
Website: http://www.preventblindness.org/eye_tests/near_vision
_test.html

Weight Risk

Adult BMI Calculator
Center for Disease Control and Prevention
Website: http://www.cdc.gov/nccdphp/dnpa/bmi/adult_BMI/english
_bmi_calculator/bmi_calculator.htm

Aim for a Healthy Weight
National Heart Lung and Blood Institute
Website: http://www.nhlbi.nih.gov/health/public/heart/obesity/lose
_wt/risk.htm

Body Surface Area, Body Mass Index
Medical College of Wisconsin
Website: http://www.intmed.mcw.edu/clincalc/body.html

Is Your Child at Risk for Being Overweight?
Health A to Z
Website: http://www.healthatoz.com/healthatoz/Atoz/tl/rq/
obesity_1.jsp

Chapter 53

Resources for More Information about Medical Tests

Medical Testing: General Information

Agency for Healthcare Research and Quality
P.O. Box 8547
Silver Springs, MD 20907-8547
Toll-Free: 800-358-9295
Phone: 301-427-1364
Website: http://www.ahrq.gov
E-mail: info@ahrq.gov

American Academy of Family Physicians
11400 Tomahawk Creek Pkwy.
Leawood, KS 66211-2672
Toll-Free: 800-274-2237
Phone: 913-906-6000
Website: http://www.aafp.org
E-mail: contactcenter@aafp.org

American Academy of Pediatrics
141 Northwest Point Blvd.
Elk Grove Village, IL 60007-1098
Phone: 847-434-4000
Fax: 847-434-8000
Website: http://www.aap.org
E-mail: kidsdocs@aap.org

American Association for Clinical Chemistry
Lab Tests Online
1850 K St., NW, Suite 625
Washington, DC 20006
Website: http://
www.labtestsonline.org
E-mail:
2labtestsonline@aacc.org
Website: http://
www.labtestsonline.org

Resources listed in this chapter were compiled from many sources deemed accurate. Inclusion does not constitute endorsement and there is no implication associated with omission. Contact information was verified in May 2008.

American College of Physicians
American Society of Internal Medicine
190 N. Independence Mall W.
Philadelphia, PA 19106-1572
Toll-Free (customer service):
800-523-1546, ext. 2600
Phone: 215-351-2600
Website: http://
www.acponline.org

American College of Radiology
CT Accreditation Department
1891 Preston White Dr.
Reston, VA 20191-4397
Toll-Free: 800-347-7748
Phone: 703-648-8900
Fax: 703-264-2093
Website: http://www.acr.org
E-mail: info@acr.org

American Society for Clinical Laboratory Science
6701 Democracy Boulevard
Suite 300
Bethesda, MD 20817
Phone: 301-657-2768
Fax: 301-657-2909
Website: http://www.ascls.org
E-mail: ascls@ascls.org

American Society of Radiologic Technologists
15000 Central Ave. SE
Albuquerque, NM 87123-3909
Toll-Free: 800-444-2778
Phone: 505-298-4500
Fax: 505-298-5063
Website: http://www.asrt.org
E-mail: customerinfo@asrt.org

Centers for Disease Control and Prevention
1600 Clifton Rd., N.E.
Atlanta, GA 30333
Toll-Free: 800-CDC INFO
Phone: 404-639-3311
Website: http://www.cdc.gov

Cleveland Clinic
9500 Euclid Avenue
Cleveland, OH 44195
Toll Free: 800-223-2273
Phone: 216-444-2200
TTY: 216-444-0261
Website: http://
www.clevelandclinic.org

Frederick Memorial Healthcare System
Frederick Memorial Hospital
400 West Seventh St.
Frederick, MD 21701
Phone: 240-566-3300
Website: http://www.fmh.org

Health-Care-Information.org
Website: http://
www.health-care-information.org

Health Resources and Services Administration (HRSA) Information Center
U.S. Department of Health and Human Services
Parklawn Building
5600 Fishers Lane
Rockville, MD 20857
Toll-Free: 888-275-4772
Website: http://
www.ask.hrsa.gov
E-mail: ask@arsa.gov

Healthline
Website: http://
www.healthline.com

Medicine Net
Website: http://
www.medicinenet.com

Nemours Foundation
1600 Rockland Road
Wilmington, DE 19803
Phone: 302-651-4000
Website: http://
www.kidshealth.org
E-mail: info@kidshealth.org

Radiological Society of North America, Inc.
820 Jorie Blvd.
Oak Brook, IL 60523-2251
Toll-Free: 800-381-6660
Phone: 630-571-2670
Fax: 630-571-7837
Website: http://www.rsna.org or
http://www.radiologyinfo.org

U.S. Department of Health and Human Services
Public Health Service
200 Independence Avenue, S.W.
Washington, DC 20201
Toll-Free: 877-696-6775
Phone: 202-619-0257
Website: http://www.hhs.gov

U.S. Food and Drug Administration
Office of Consumer Affairs
5600 Fishers Lane
Rockville, MD 20857-0001
Toll-Free: 888-463-6332
Phone: 301-827-4420
Website: http://www.fda.gov

WebMD
111 8th Ave, 7th Floor
New York, NY 10011
Phone: 212-624-3700
Website: http://www.webmd.com

Disorder-Specific Testing

American Academy of Allergy, Asthma, and Immunology
555 East Wells St.
Milwaukee, WI 53202
Toll-Free: 800-822-2762
Phone: 414-272-6071
Website: http://www.aaaai.org
E-mail: info@aaaai.org

American College of Cardiology
Heart House
2400 N Street NW
Washington DC, 20037
Phone: 202-375-6000
Fax: 202-375-7000
Website: http://www.acc.org
E-mail: resource@aac.org

American College of Gastroenterology
6400 Goldsboro, Suite 450
Bethesda, MD 20817
Phone: 301-263-9000
Fax: 301-263-9025
Website: http://www.acg.gi.org

American Heart Association
7272 Greenville Ave.
Dallas, TX 75231
Toll-Free: 800-AHA-USA-1
(242-8721)
Website: http://
www.americanheart.org

American Pregnancy Association
1425 Greenway Drive
Suite 440
Irving, TX 75038
Phone: 972-550-0140
Fax: 972-550-0800
Website: http://
www.americanpregnancy.org
E-mail: Questions
@AmericanPregnancy.org

American Stroke Association
7272 Greenville Ave.
Dallas, TX 75231
Toll-Free: 888-478-7653
Website:
www.strokeassociation.org

Imaginis Corporation
P.O. Box 8398
Greenville, SC 29604
Phone: 864-335-1139
Website: http://
www.imaginis.com
E-mail:
learnmore@imaginis.com

Juvenile Diabetes Research Foundation International
120 Wall St.
New York, NY 10005-4001
Toll-Free: 800-533-CURE (2873)
Phone: 212-785-9500
Website: http://www.jdrf.org
E-mail: info@jdrf.org

March of Dimes
1275 Mamaroneck Avenue
White Plains, NY 10605
Toll-Free: 888-MODIMES
(663-4637)
Phone: 914-428-7100
Fax: 914-428-8203
Website: http://
www.marchofdimes.com
E-mail:
askus@marchofdimes.com

National Cancer Institute
6116 Executive Boulevard,
Room 3036A
Bethesda, MD 20892-8322
Toll-Free: 800-4-CANCER
(422-6237)
TTY Toll-Free: 800-332-8615
Website: http://www.cancer.gov
E-mail:
cancergovstaff@mail.nih.gov

National Diabetes Information Clearinghouse
1 Information Way
Bethesda, MD 20892-3560
Toll-Free: 800-860-8747
Phone: 301-654-3327
Fax: 301-907-8906
Website: http://
diabetes.niddk.nih.gov
E-mail: ndic@info.niddk.nih.gov

National Digestive Diseases Information Clearinghouse
2 Information Way
Bethesda, MD 20892-3570
Toll-Free: 800-891-5389
Phone: 301-654-3810
Fax: 301-907-8906
Website: http://
digestive.niddk.nih.gov
E-mail:
nddic@info.niddk.nih.gov

National Dissemination Center for Children with Disabilities (NICHCY)
U.S. Department of Education
Office of Special Education Programs
P.O. Box 1492
Washington, DC 20013
Toll-Free: 800-695-0285 (Voice/TTY)
Phone: 202-884-8200 (Voice/TTY)
Fax: 202-884-8441
Website: http://www.nichcy.org
E-mail: nichcy@aed.org

National Heart, Lung, and Blood Institute
Information Center
P.O. Box 30105
Bethesda, MD 20824-0105
Phone: 301-592-8573
TTY: 240-629-3255
Fax: 301-592-8563
Website: http://
www.nhlbi.nih.gov
E-mail: nhlbiinfo@nhlbi.nih.gov

National Institute of Mental Health
6001 Executive Boulevard
Bethesda, MD 20892-9663
Phone: 301-443-4513
Fax: 301-443-4279
TTY: 301-443-8431
Website: http://
www.nimh.nih.gov
E-mail: nimhinfo@nih.gov

National Jewish Medical and Research Center
1400 Jackson Street
Denver, CO 80206
Phone: 303-388-4461
Website: http://
www.nationaljewish.org

National Kidney and Urologic Diseases Information Clearinghouse
3 Information Way
Bethesda, MD 20892-3580
Toll-Free: 800-891-5390
Phone: 301-654-4415
Website: http://
kidney.niddk.nih.gov/index.htm
E-mail:
nkudic@info.niddk.nih.gov

Mental Health America
2000 N. Beauregard St., 6th Floor
Alexandria, VA 22311
Toll-Free: 800-969-6642
Phone: 703-684-7722
TTY: 800-433-5959
Fax: 703-684-5968
Website: http://
www.mentalhealthamerica.net

National Women's Health Information Center

Office on Women's Health
200 Independence Ave., S.W.,
Room 712E
Washington, DC 20201
Toll-Free: 800-994-9662
Toll-Free TDD: 888-220-5446
Phone: 202-690-7650
Fax: 202-205-2631
Website: http://
www.4woman.gov

RESOLVE

The National Infertility
Association
8405 Greensboro Drive
Suite 800
McLean, VA 22102-5105
Phone: 703-556-7172
Fax: 703-506-3266
Website: http://www.resolve.org
E-mail: info@resolve.org

Society of American Gastrointestinal Endoscopic Surgeons (SAGES)

11300 W. Olympic Blvd.
Suite 600
Los Angeles, CA 90064
Phone: 310-437-0544
Fax: 310-437-0585
Website: http://www.sages.org
E-mail: sagesweb@sages.org

WISEWOMAN

Division for Heart Disease and
Stroke Prevention
National Center for Chronic
Disease Prevention and Health
Promotion
Centers for Disease Control and
Prevention
4770 Buford Highway, NE
MS/K–77
Atlanta, GA 30341–3717
Phone: 800-CDC-INFO
(800-232-4636 Choose Option #1)
Website: http://www.cdc.gov/
wisewoman
E-mail: cdcinfo@cdc.gov

Index

Index

Page numbers followed by 'n' indicate a footnote. Page numbers in *italics* indicate a table or illustration.

American Society of
Echocardiography, heart
ultrasound publication 340n
American Society of Radiologic
Technologists (ASRT)
contact information 598
publications
barium enema 309n
magnetic resonance
imaging 376n
myelograms 317n
x-rays 284n
American Speech-Language-Hearing
Association, hearing test
publication 139n
American Stroke Association,
contact information 600
American Thyroid Association,
thyroid function tests
publication 77n
amino acid metabolism
disorders 6–7
aminotransaminases,
hepatitis C 128
amniocentesis, described 92–94
Amsler grid *160*, 161
analyte, defined 583
anemia
described 179
prenatal tests 83, 85
anencephaly, prenatal tests 84
antibody, defined 124
antibody tests
hepatitis C 129–31
HIV testing 119
pediatric HIV/AIDS 114
thyroid function 78–80
antigen, defined 124
antigen-presenting cells 180
approved test, defined 583–84
argininosuccinic acidemia 7
arterial blood gas test 504, 506, 510
arterial duplex 352–53
arterial pressures/waveforms 353
"Arthrograms" (University of
Washington Medical Center) 315n
arthrograms, overview 315–16
ASCLS *see* American Society for
Clinical Laboratory Science

ascorbic acid, diabetes testing 68
aspartate aminotransferase (AST),
liver function tests 192–93
ASRT *see* American Society of
Radiologic Technologists
atherosclerosis, C-reactive
protein 54–57
athletes, twelve-step
screening 57–60
audiograms, described 143–46
audiologic evaluation,
described 139–40
auditory evoked potentials,
described 147
autism, online health
screening tools 590
axons, nerve conduction
velocities 430

B

bacterial vaginosis (BV),
described 110
"Bacterial Vaginosis"
(NIAID) 110n
bad cholesterol
see low-density lipoprotein
balance system assessment,
described 148
barium enema, described 34,
309–11
"Barium Enema Examination"
(ASRT) 309n
barium sulfate
described 296–97
upper/lower GI series 307–8
"Basic Blood Tests"
(Nemours Foundation) 185n
basophils
complete blood count 188
described 179
B cells, described 181
Bernstein, David 128n
beta-ketothiolase deficiency 6
beta thalassemia, prenatal tests 83
bicarbonate, blood tests 186
bilirubin, described 129, 193–94
biological marker, described 40

home testing kits
  cholesterol levels 527–29
  diabetes management 535–44
  fecal occult blood 531–33
  hepatitis C 565–67
  HIV infection 561–63
  HIV testing 121
  menopause 558–60
  overview 516–25
  ovulation 552–55
  pregnancy 547–50
  prothrombin 545–46
  substance abuse 570–79
  vaginal pH 556–57
"Home-Use Test Kits - Drugs of
  Abuse (Collection Kit)" (FDA)
  573n
"Home-Use Tests: Cholesterol"
  (FDA) 527n
"Home-Use Tests Drugs of Abuse
  (First Check 12 Drug Test)"
  (FDA) 570n
"Home Use Tests - Drugs of Abuse
  (Two-Step Test)" (FDA) 575n
"Home-Use Tests: Fecal Occult
  Blood" (FDA) 531n
"Home-Use Tests: Glucose"
  (FDA) 535n
"Home-Use Tests: Hepatitis C"
  (FDA) 565n
"Home-Use Tests: Ovulation
  (Menopause)" (FDA) 558n
"Home-Use Tests: Ovulation
  (Saliva Test)" (FDA) 554n
"Home-Use Tests: Ovulation
  (Urine Test)" (FDA) 552n
"Home-Use Tests: Ovulation
  (Vaginal pH)" (FDA) 556n
"Home-Use Tests: Prothrombin
  Time" (FDA) 545n
homocystinuria 7
hormone tests, fertility testing
  100
HPV *see* human papillomavirus
HRSA *see* Health Resources and
  Services Administration
HRT-II *see* Heidelberg retinal
  tomography
HSG *see* hysterosalpingogram

human papillomavirus (HPV)
  described 32, 114
  oral cancer 40
"Human Papillomavirus and
  Genital Warts" (NIAID) 110n
Huntington disease, prenatal
  tests 83
hyperthyroidism *78*
hypo-osmotic swelling test 102
hypothyroidism 4, *78*
hysterosalpingogram (HSG)
  described 100
  overview 312–14
"Hysterosalpingogram (HSG)"
  (American Society for
  Reproductive Medicine) 312n
hysteroscopy 100–101

I

IDEA *see* Individuals with
  Disabilities Education Act
imaging tests *see* computed axial
  tomography scan; contrast
  radiography; magnetic resonance
  imaging; mammograms; nuclear
  imaging tests; ultrasound; x-rays
Imaginis Corporation
  breast biopsy publication 203n
  contact information 600
immunizations, pediatric
  recommendations 12–15
immunohistochemistry,
  described 224
impaired fasting glucose,
  described 63
impaired glucose tolerance,
  described 63
"The Importance of Laboratory
  Test Results in Hepatitis B
  Infection" (Bernstein) 128n
"The Importance of Regular Eye
  Exams" (American Optometric
  Association) 150n
incisional biopsy
  described 198
  skin tissue 227
indications for use, defined 586

Health Reference Series

COMPLETE CATALOG

List price $87 per volume. **School and library price $78 per volume.**

Adolescent Health Sourcebook, 2nd Edition

Basic Consumer Health Information about the Physical, Mental, and Emotional Growth and Development of Adolescents, Including Medical Care, Nutritional and Physical Activity Requirements, Puberty, Sexual Activity, Acne, Tanning, Body Piercing, Common Physical Illnesses and Disorders, Eating Disorders, Attention Deficit Hyperactivity Disorder, Depression, Bullying, Hazing, and Adolescent Injuries Related to Sports, Driving, and Work

Along with Substance Abuse Information about Nicotine, Alcohol, and Drug Use, a Glossary, and Directory of Additional Resources

Edited by Joyce Brennfleck Shannon. 683 pages. 2006. 978-0-7808-0943-7.

"It is written in clear, nontechnical language aimed at general readers. . . . Recommended for public libraries, community colleges, and other agencies serving health care consumers."
— *American Reference Books Annual, 2003*

"Recommended for school and public libraries. Parents and professionals dealing with teens will appreciate the easy-to-follow format and the clearly written text. This could become a 'must have' for every high school teacher." — *E-Streams, Jan '03*

"A good starting point for information related to common medical, mental, and emotional concerns of adolescents." — *School Library Journal, Nov '02*

"This book provides accurate information in an easy to access format. It addresses topics that parents and caregivers might not be aware of and provides practical, useable information."
— *Doody's Health Sciences Book Review Journal, Sep-Oct '02*

"Recommended reference source."
— *Booklist, American Library Association, Sep '02*

AIDS Sourcebook, 3rd Edition

Basic Consumer Health Information about Acquired Immune Deficiency Syndrome (AIDS) and Human Immunodeficiency Virus (HIV) Infection, Including Facts about Transmission, Prevention, Diagnosis, Treatment, Opportunistic Infections, and Other Complications, with a Section for Women and Children, Including Details about Associated Gynecological Concerns, Pregnancy, and Pediatric Care

Along with Updated Statistical Information, Reports on Current Research Initiatives, a Glossary, and Directories of Internet, Hotline, and Other Resources

Edited by Dawn D. Matthews. 664 pages. 2003. 978-0-7808-0631-3.

"The 3rd edition of the *AIDS Sourcebook*, part of Omnigraphics' *Health Reference Series*, is a welcome update. . . . This resource is highly recommended for academic and public libraries."
— *American Reference Books Annual, 2004*

"Excellent sourcebook. This continues to be a highly recommended book. There is no other book that provides as much information as this book provides."
— *AIDS Book Review Journal, Dec-Jan '00*

"Recommended reference source."
— *Booklist, American Library Association, Dec '99*

Alcoholism Sourcebook, 2nd Edition

Basic Consumer Health Information about Alcohol Use, Abuse, and Dependence, Featuring Facts about the Physical, Mental, and Social Health Effects of Alcohol Addiction, Including Alcoholic Liver Disease, Pancreatic Disease, Cardiovascular Disease, Neurological Disorders, and the Effects of Drinking during Pregnancy

Along with Information about Alcohol Treatment, Medications, and Recovery Programs, in Addition to Tips for Reducing the Prevalence of Underage Drinking, Statistics about Alcohol Use, a Glossary of Related Terms, and Directories of Resources for More Help and Information

Edited by Amy L. Sutton. 653 pages. 2006. 978-0-7808-0942-0.

"This title is one of the few reference works on alcoholism for general readers. For some readers this will be a welcome complement to the many self-help books on the market. Recommended for collections serving general readers and consumer health collections."
— *E-Streams, Mar '01*

"This book is an excellent choice for public and academic libraries."
— *American Reference Books Annual, 2001*

"Recommended reference source."
— *Booklist, American Library Association, Dec '00*

"Presents a wealth of information on alcohol use and abuse and its effects on the body and mind, treatment, and prevention." — *SciTech Book News, Dec '00*

"Important new health guide which packs in the latest consumer information about the problems of alcoholism." — *Reviewer's Bookwatch, Nov '00*

SEE ALSO Drug Abuse Sourcebook

Allergies Sourcebook, 3rd Edition

Basic Consumer Health Information about Allergic Disorders, Such as Anaphylaxis, Hives, Eczema, Rhinitis, Sinusitis, and Conjunctivitis, and Their Triggers, Including Pollen, Mold, Dust Mites, Animal Dander, Insects, Chemicals, Food, Food Additives, and Medications;

Along with Advice about the Diagnosis and Treatment of Allergy Symptoms, a Glossary of Related Terms, a Directory of Resources for Help and Information, and Suggestions for Additional Reading

Edited by Amy L. Sutton. 598 pages. 2007. 978-0-7808-0950-5.

"This book brings a great deal of useful material together. . . . This is an excellent addition to public and consumer health library collections."
— *American Reference Books Annual, 2003*

"This second edition would be useful to laypersons with little or advanced knowledge of the subject matter. This book would also serve as a resource for nursing and other health care professions students. It would be useful in public, academic, and hospital libraries with consumer health collections." — *E-Streams, Jul '02*

Alternative Medicine Sourcebook

SEE Complementary & Alternative Medicine Sourcebook

Alzheimer's Disease Sourcebook, 3rd Edition

Basic Consumer Health Information about Alzheimer's Disease, Other Dementias, and Related Disorders, Including Multi-Infarct Dementia, AIDS Dementia Complex, Dementia with Lewy Bodies, Huntington's Disease, Wernicke-Korsakoff Syndrome (Alcohol-Related Dementia), Delirium, and Confusional States

Along with Information for People Newly Diagnosed with Alzheimer's Disease and Caregivers, Reports Detailing Current Research Efforts in Prevention, Diagnosis, and Treatment, Facts about Long-Term Care Issues, and Listings of Sources for Additional Information

Edited by Karen Bellenir. 645 pages. 2003. 978-0-7808-0666-5.

"This very informative and valuable tool will be a great addition to any library serving consumers, students and health care workers."
— *American Reference Books Annual, 2004*

"This is a valuable resource for people affected by dementias such as Alzheimer's. It is easy to navigate and includes important information and resources."
— *Doody's Review Service, Feb '04*

"Recommended reference source."
— *Booklist, American Library Association, Oct '99*

SEE ALSO *Brain Disorders Sourcebook*

Arthritis Sourcebook, 2nd Edition

Basic Consumer Health Information about Osteoarthritis, Rheumatoid Arthritis, Other Rheumatic Disorders, Infectious Forms of Arthritis, and Diseases with Symptoms Linked to Arthritis, Featuring Facts about Diagnosis, Pain Management, and Surgical Therapies

Along with Coping Strategies, Research Updates, a Glossary, and Resources for Additional Help and Information

Edited by Amy L. Sutton. 593 pages. 2004. 978-0-7808-0667-2.

"This easy-to-read volume is recommended for consumer health collections within public or academic libraries." — *E-Streams, May '05*

"As expected, this updated edition continues the excellent reputation of this series in providing sound, usable health information. . . . Highly recommended."
— *American Reference Books Annual, 2005*

"Excellent reference." — *The Bookwatch, Jan '05*

Asthma Sourcebook, 2nd Edition

Basic Consumer Health Information about the Causes, Symptoms, Diagnosis, and Treatment of Asthma in Infants, Children, Teenagers, and Adults, Including Facts about Different Types of Asthma, Common Co-Occurring Conditions, Asthma Management Plans, Triggers, Medications, and Medication Delivery Devices

Along with Asthma Statistics, Research Updates, a Glossary, a Directory of Asthma-Related Resources, and More

Edited by Karen Bellenir. 609 pages. 2006. 978-0-7808-0866-9.

"A worthwhile reference acquisition for public libraries and academic medical libraries whose readers desire a quick introduction to the wide range of asthma information." — *Choice, Association of College & Research Libraries, Jun '01*

"Recommended reference source."
— *Booklist, American Library Association, Feb '01*

"Highly recommended." — *The Bookwatch, Jan '01*

"There is much good information for patients and their families who deal with asthma daily."
— *American Medical Writers Association Journal, Winter '01*

"This informative text is recommended for consumer health collections in public, secondary school, and community college libraries and the libraries of universities with a large undergraduate population."
— *American Reference Books Annual, 2001*

Attention Deficit Disorder Sourcebook

Basic Consumer Health Information about Attention Deficit/Hyperactivity Disorder in Children and Adults,

Including Facts about Causes, Symptoms, Diagnostic Criteria, and Treatment Options Such as Medications, Behavior Therapy, Coaching, and Homeopathy

Along with Reports on Current Research Initiatives, Legal Issues, and Government Regulations, and Featuring a Glossary of Related Terms, Internet Resources, and a List of Additional Reading Material

Edited by Dawn D. Matthews. 470 pages. 2002. 978-0-7808-0624-5.

"Recommended reference source."
— Booklist, American Library Association, Jan '03

"This book is recommended for all school libraries and the reference or consumer health sections of public libraries." — American Reference Books Annual, 2003

Back & Neck Sourcebook, 2nd Edition

Basic Consumer Health Information about Spinal Pain, Spinal Cord Injuries, and Related Disorders, Such as Degenerative Disk Disease, Osteoarthritis, Scoliosis, Sciatica, Spina Bifida, and Spinal Stenosis, and Featuring Facts about Maintaining Spinal Health, Self-Care, Pain Management, Rehabilitative Care, Chiropractic Care, Spinal Surgeries, and Complementary Therapies

Along with Suggestions for Preventing Back and Neck Pain, a Glossary of Related Terms, and a Directory of Resources

Edited by Amy L. Sutton. 633 pages. 2004. 978-0-7808-0738-9.

"Recommended . . . an easy to use, comprehensive medical reference book." — E-Streams, Sep '05

"The strength of this work is its basic, easy-to-read format. Recommended." — Reference and User Services Quarterly, American Library Association, Winter '97

Blood & Circulatory Disorders Sourcebook, 2nd Edition

Basic Consumer Health Information about the Blood and Circulatory System and Related Disorders, Such as Anemia and Other Hemoglobin Diseases, Cancer of the Blood and Associated Bone Marrow Disorders, Clotting and Bleeding Problems, and Conditions That Affect the Veins, Blood Vessels, and Arteries, Including Facts about the Donation and Transplantation of Bone Marrow, Stem Cells, and Blood and Tips for Keeping the Blood and Circulatory System Healthy

Along with a Glossary of Related Terms and Resources for Additional Help and Information

Edited by Amy L. Sutton. 659 pages. 2005. 978-0-7808-0746-4.

"Highly recommended pick for basic consumer health reference holdings at all levels."
— The Bookwatch, Aug '05

"Recommended reference source."
— Booklist, American Library Association, Feb '99

"An important reference sourcebook written in simple language for everyday, non-technical users. "
— Reviewer's Bookwatch, Jan '99

Brain Disorders Sourcebook, 2nd Edition

Basic Consumer Health Information about Acquired and Traumatic Brain Injuries, Infections of the Brain, Epilepsy and Seizure Disorders, Cerebral Palsy, and Degenerative Neurological Disorders, Including Amyotrophic Lateral Sclerosis (ALS), Dementias, Multiple Sclerosis, and More

Along with Information on the Brain's Structure and Function, Treatment and Rehabilitation Options, Reports on Current Research Initiatives, a Glossary of Terms Related to Brain Disorders and Injuries, and a Directory of Sources for Further Help and Information

Edited by Sandra J. Judd. 625 pages. 2005. 978-0-7808-0744-0.

"Highly recommended pick for basic consumer health reference holdings at all levels."
— The Bookwatch, Aug '05

"Belongs on the shelves of any library with a consumer health collection." — E-Streams, Mar '00

"Recommended reference source."
— Booklist, American Library Association, Oct '99

SEE ALSO Alzheimer's Disease Sourcebook

Breast Cancer Sourcebook, 2nd Edition

Basic Consumer Health Information about Breast Cancer, Including Facts about Risk Factors, Prevention, Screening and Diagnostic Methods, Treatment Options, Complementary and Alternative Therapies, Post-Treatment Concerns, Clinical Trials, Special Risk Populations, and New Developments in Breast Cancer Research

Along with Breast Cancer Statistics, a Glossary of Related Terms, and a Directory of Resources for Additional Help and Information

Edited by Sandra J. Judd. 595 pages. 2004. 978-0-7808-0668-9.

"This book will be an excellent addition to public, community college, medical, and academic libraries."
— American Reference Books Annual, 2006

"It would be a useful reference book in a library or on loan to women in a support group."
— Cancer Forum, Mar '03

"Recommended reference source."
— Booklist, American Library Association, Jan '02

"This reference source is highly recommended. It is quite informative, comprehensive and detailed in nature, and yet it offers practical advice in easy-to-read language. It could be thought of as the 'bible' of breast cancer for the consumer." — *E-Streams, Jan '02*

"From the pros and cons of different screening methods and results to treatment options, *Breast Cancer Sourcebook* provides the latest information on the subject." — *Library Bookwatch, Dec '01*

"This thoroughgoing, very readable reference covers all aspects of breast health and cancer. . . . Readers will find much to consider here. Recommended for all public and patient health collections." — *Library Journal, Sep '01*

SEE ALSO *Cancer Sourcebook for Women, Women's Health Concerns Sourcebook*

Breastfeeding Sourcebook

Basic Consumer Health Information about the Benefits of Breastmilk, Preparing to Breastfeed, Breastfeeding as a Baby Grows, Nutrition, and More, Including Information on Special Situations and Concerns Such as Mastitis, Illness, Medications, Allergies, Multiple Births, Prematurity, Special Needs, and Adoption

Along with a Glossary and Resources for Additional Help and Information

Edited by Jenni Lynn Colson. 388 pages. 2002. 978-0-7808-0332-9.

"Particularly useful is the information about professional lactation services and chapters on breastfeeding when returning to work. . . . *Breastfeeding Sourcebook* will be useful for public libraries, consumer health libraries, and technical schools offering nurse assistant training, especially in areas where Internet access is problematic." — *American Reference Books Annual, 2003*

SEE ALSO *Pregnancy & Birth Sourcebook*

Burns Sourcebook

Basic Consumer Health Information about Various Types of Burns and Scalds, Including Flame, Heat, Cold, Electrical, Chemical, and Sun Burns

Along with Information on Short-Term and Long-Term Treatments, Tissue Reconstruction, Plastic Surgery, Prevention Suggestions, and First Aid

Edited by Allan R. Cook. 604 pages. 1999. 978-0-7808-0204-9.

"This is an exceptional addition to the series and is highly recommended for all consumer health collections, hospital libraries, and academic medical centers." — *E-Streams, Mar '00*

"This key reference guide is an invaluable addition to all health care and public libraries in confronting this ongoing health issue." — *American Reference Books Annual, 2000*

"Recommended reference source." — *Booklist, American Library Association, Dec '99*

SEE ALSO *Dermatological Disorders Sourcebook*

Cancer Sourcebook, 5th Edition

Basic Consumer Health Information about Major Forms and Stages of Cancer, Featuring Facts about Head and Neck Cancers, Lung Cancers, Gastrointestinal Cancers, Genitourinary Cancers, Lymphomas, Blood Cell Cancers, Endocrine Cancers, Skin Cancers, Bone Cancers, Metastatic Cancers, and More

Along with Facts about Cancer Treatments, Cancer Risks and Prevention, a Glossary of Related Terms, Statistical Data, and a Directory of Resources for Additional Information

Edited by Karen Bellenir. 1,133 pages. 2007. 978-0-7808-0947-5.

"With cancer being the second leading cause of death for Americans, a prodigious work such as this one, which locates centrally so much cancer-related information, is clearly an asset to this nation's citizens and others." — *Journal of the National Medical Association, 2004*

"This title is recommended for health sciences and public libraries with consumer health collections." — *E-Streams, Feb '01*

". . . can be effectively used by cancer patients and their families who are looking for answers in a language they can understand. Public and hospital libraries should have it on their shelves." — *American Reference Books Annual, 2001*

"Recommended reference source." — *Booklist, American Library Association, Dec '00*

SEE ALSO *Breast Cancer Sourcebook, Cancer Sourcebook for Women, Pediatric Cancer Sourcebook, Prostate Cancer Sourcebook*

Cancer Sourcebook for Women, 3rd Edition

Basic Consumer Health Information about Leading Causes of Cancer in Women, Featuring Facts about Gynecologic Cancers and Related Concerns, Such as Breast Cancer, Cervical Cancer, Endometrial Cancer, Uterine Sarcoma, Vaginal Cancer, Vulvar Cancer, and Common Non-Cancerous Gynecologic Conditions, in Addition to Facts about Lung Cancer, Colorectal Cancer, and Thyroid Cancer in Women

Along with Information about Cancer Risk Factors, Screening and Prevention, Treatment Options, and Tips on Coping with Life after Cancer Treatment, a Glossary of Cancer Terms, and a Directory of Resources for Additional Help and Information

Edited by Amy L. Sutton. 715 pages. 2006. 978-0-7808-0867-6.

"An excellent addition to collections in public, consumer health, and women's health libraries." — *American Reference Books Annual, 2003*

"Overall, the information is excellent, and complex topics are clearly explained. As a reference book for the consumer it is a valuable resource to assist them to make informed decisions about cancer and its treatments." — *Cancer Forum, Nov '02*

"Highly recommended for academic and medical reference collections." —*Library Bookwatch, Sep '02*

"This is a highly recommended book for any public or consumer library, being reader friendly and containing accurate and helpful information." —*E-Streams, Aug '02*

"Recommended reference source." —*Booklist, American Library Association, Jul '02*

SEE ALSO *Breast Cancer Sourcebook, Women's Health Concerns Sourcebook*

Cancer Survivorship Sourcebook

Basic Consumer Health Information about the Physical, Educational, Emotional, Social, and Financial Needs of Cancer Patients from Diagnosis, through Cancer Treatment, and Beyond, Including Facts about Researching Specific Types of Cancer and Learning about Clinical Trials and Treatment Options, and Featuring Tips for Coping with the Side Effects of Cancer Treatments and Adjusting to Life after Cancer Treatment Concludes

Along with Suggestions for Caregivers, Friends, and Family Members of Cancer Patients, a Glossary of Cancer Care Terms, and Directories of Related Resources

Edited by Karen Bellenir. 6561 pages. 2007. 978-0-7808-0985-7.

Cardiovascular Diseases & Disorders Sourcebook, 3rd Edition

Basic Consumer Health Information about Heart and Vascular Diseases and Disorders, Such as Angina, Heart Attacks, Arrhythmias, Cardiomyopathy, Valve Disease, Atherosclerosis, and Aneurysms, with Information about Managing Cardiovascular Risk Factors and Maintaining Heart Health, Medications and Procedures Used to Treat Cardiovascular Disorders, and Concerns of Special Significance to Women

Along with Reports on Current Research Initiatives, a Glossary of Related Medical Terms, and a Directory of Sources for Further Help and Information

Edited by Sandra J. Judd. 713 pages. 2005. 978-0-7808-0739-6.

"This updated sourcebook is still the best first stop for comprehensive introductory information on cardiovascular diseases." —*American Reference Books Annual, 2006*

"Recommended for public libraries and libraries supporting health care professionals." —*E-Streams, Sep '05*

"This should be a standard health library reference." —*The Bookwatch, Jun '05*

"Recommended reference source." —*Booklist, American Library Association, Dec '00*

"... comprehensive format provides an extensive overview on this subject." —*Choice, Association of College & Research Libraries*

Caregiving Sourcebook

Basic Consumer Health Information for Caregivers, Including a Profile of Caregivers, Caregiving Responsibilities and Concerns, Tips for Specific Conditions, Care Environments, and the Effects of Caregiving

Along with Facts about Legal Issues, Financial Information, and Future Planning, a Glossary, and a Listing of Additional Resources

Edited by Joyce Brennfleck Shannon. 600 pages. 2001. 978-0-7808-0331-2.

"Essential for most collections." —*Library Journal, Apr 1, 2002*

"An ideal addition to the reference collection of any public library. Health sciences information professionals may also want to acquire the *Caregiving Sourcebook* for their hospital or academic library for use as a ready reference tool by health care workers interested in aging and caregiving." —*E-Streams, Jan '02*

"Recommended reference source." —*Booklist, American Library Association, Oct '01*

Child Abuse Sourcebook

Basic Consumer Health Information about the Physical, Sexual, and Emotional Abuse of Children, with Additional Facts about Neglect, Munchausen Syndrome by Proxy (MSBP), Shaken Baby Syndrome, and Controversial Issues Related to Child Abuse, Such as Withholding Medical Care, Corporal Punishment, and Child Maltreatment in Youth Sports, and Featuring Facts about Child Protective Services, Foster Care, Adoption, Parenting Challenges, and Other Abuse Prevention Efforts

Along with a Glossary of Related Terms and Resources for Additional Help and Information

Edited by Dawn D. Matthews. 620 pages. 2004. 978-0-7808-0705-1.

"A valuable and highly recommended resource for school, academic and public libraries whether used on its own or as a starting point for more in-depth research." —*E-Streams, Apr '05*

"Every week the news brings cases of child abuse or neglect, so it is useful to have a source that supplies so much helpful information. . . . Recommended. Public and academic libraries, and child welfare offices." —*Choice, Association of College & Research Libraries, Mar '05*

"Packed with insights on all kinds of issues, from foster care and adoption to parenting and abuse prevention." —*The Bookwatch, Nov '04*

SEE ALSO: *Domestic Violence Sourcebook*

Childhood Diseases & Disorders Sourcebook

Basic Consumer Health Information about Medical Problems Often Encountered in Pre-Adolescent Children, Including Respiratory Tract Ailments, Ear Infections, Sore Throats, Disorders of the Skin and Scalp, Digestive and Genitourinary Diseases, Infectious Diseases, Inflammatory Disorders, Chronic Physical and Developmental Disorders, Allergies, and More

Along with Information about Diagnostic Tests, Common Childhood Surgeries, and Frequently Used Medications, with a Glossary of Important Terms and Resource Directory

Edited by Chad T. Kimball. 662 pages. 2003. 978-0-7808-0458-6.

"This is an excellent book for new parents and should be included in all health care and public libraries."
—*American Reference Books Annual, 2004*

SEE ALSO: Healthy Children Sourcebook

■

Colds, Flu & Other Common Ailments Sourcebook

Basic Consumer Health Information about Common Ailments and Injuries, Including Colds, Coughs, the Flu, Sinus Problems, Headaches, Fever, Nausea and Vomiting, Menstrual Cramps, Diarrhea, Constipation, Hemorrhoids, Back Pain, Dandruff, Dry and Itchy Skin, Cuts, Scrapes, Sprains, Bruises, and More

Along with Information about Prevention, Self-Care, Choosing a Doctor, Over-the-Counter Medications, Folk Remedies, and Alternative Therapies, and Including a Glossary of Important Terms and a Directory of Resources for Further Help and Information

Edited by Chad T. Kimball. 638 pages. 2001. 978-0-7808-0435-7.

"A good starting point for research on common illnesses. It will be a useful addition to public and consumer health library collections."
—*American Reference Books Annual, 2002*

"Will prove valuable to any library seeking to maintain a current, comprehensive reference collection of health resources. . . . Excellent reference."
—*The Bookwatch, Aug '01*

"Recommended reference source."
—*Booklist, American Library Association, Jul '01*

■

Communication Disorders Sourcebook

Basic Information about Deafness and Hearing Loss, Speech and Language Disorders, Voice Disorders, Balance and Vestibular Disorders, and Disorders of Smell, Taste, and Touch

Edited by Linda M. Ross. 533 pages. 1996. 978-0-7808-0077-9.

"This is skillfully edited and is a welcome resource for the layperson. It should be found in every public and medical library." —*Booklist Health Sciences Supplement, American Library Association, Oct '97*

■

Complementary & Alternative Medicine Sourcebook, 3rd Edition

Basic Consumer Health Information about Complementary and Alternative Medical Therapies, Including Acupuncture, Ayurveda, Traditional Chinese Medicine, Herbal Medicine, Homeopathy, Naturopathy, Biofeedback, Hypnotherapy, Yoga, Art Therapy, Aromatherapy, Clinical Nutrition, Vitamin and Mineral Supplements, Chiropractic, Massage, Reflexology, Crystal Therapy, Therapeutic Touch, and More

Along with Facts about Alternative and Complementary Treatments for Specific Conditions Such as Cancer, Diabetes, Osteoarthritis, Chronic Pain, Menopause, Gastrointestinal Disorders, Headaches, and Mental Illness, a Glossary, and a Resource List for Additional Help and Information

Edited by Sandra J. Judd. 657 pages. 2006. 978-0-7808-0864-5.

"Recommended for public, high school, and academic libraries that have consumer health collections. Hospital libraries that also serve the public will find this to be a useful resource." —*E-Streams, Feb '03*

"Recommended reference source."
—*Booklist, American Library Association, Jan '03*

"An important alternate health reference."
—*MBR Bookwatch, Oct '02*

"A great addition to the reference collection of every type of library." —*American Reference Books Annual, 2000*

■

Congenital Disorders Sourcebook, 2nd Edition

Basic Consumer Health Information about Nonhereditary Birth Defects and Disorders Related to Prematurity, Gestational Injuries, Congenital Infections, and Birth Complications, Including Heart Defects, Hydrocephalus, Spina Bifida, Cleft Lip and Palate, Cerebral Palsy, and More

Along with Facts about the Prevention of Birth Defects, Fetal Surgery and Other Treatment Options, Research Initiatives, a Glossary of Related Terms, and Resources for Additional Information and Support

Edited by Sandra J. Judd. 647 pages. 2006. 978-0-7808-0945-1.

"Recommended reference source."
—*Booklist, American Library Association, Oct '97*

SEE ALSO Pregnancy & Birth Sourcebook

■

Contagious Diseases Sourcebook

Basic Consumer Health Information about Infectious Diseases Spread by Person-to-Person Contact through

Direct Touch, Airborne Transmission, Sexual Contact, or Contact with Blood or Other Body Fluids, Including Hepatitis, Herpes, Influenza, Lice, Measles, Mumps, Pinworm, Ringworm, Severe Acute Respiratory Syndrome (SARS), Streptococcal Infections, Tuberculosis, and Others

Along with Facts about Disease Transmission, Antimicrobial Resistance, and Vaccines, with a Glossary and Directories of Resources for More Information

Edited by Karen Bellenir. 643 pages. 2004. 978-0-7808-0736-5.

"This easy-to-read volume is recommended for consumer health collections within public or academic libraries." —E-Streams, May '05

"This informative book is highly recommended for public libraries, consumer health collections, and secondary schools and undergraduate libraries." —American Reference Books Annual, 2005

"Excellent reference." —The Bookwatch, Jan '05

■

Death & Dying Sourcebook, 2nd Edition

Basic Consumer Health Information about End-of-Life Care and Related Perspectives and Ethical Issues, Including End-of-Life Symptoms and Treatments, Pain Management, Quality-of-Life Concerns, the Use of Life Support, Patients' Rights and Privacy Issues, Advance Directives, Physician-Assisted Suicide, Caregiving, Organ and Tissue Donation, Autopsies, Funeral Arrangements, and Grief

Along with Statistical Data, Information about the Leading Causes of Death, a Glossary, and Directories of Support Groups and Other Resources

Edited by Joyce Brennfleck Shannon. 653 pages. 2006. 978-0-7808-0871-3.

"Public libraries, medical libraries, and academic libraries will all find this sourcebook a useful addition to their collections." —American Reference Books Annual, 2001

"An extremely useful resource for those concerned with death and dying in the United States." —Respiratory Care, Nov '00

"Recommended reference source." —Booklist, American Library Association, Aug '00

"This book is a definite must for all those involved in end-of-life care." —Doody's Review Service, 2000

■

Dental Care & Oral Health Sourcebook, 2nd Edition

Basic Consumer Health Information about Dental Care, Including Oral Hygiene, Dental Visits, Pain Management, Cavities, Crowns, Bridges, Dental Implants, and Fillings, and Other Oral Health Concerns, Such as Gum Disease, Bad Breath, Dry Mouth, Genetic and Developmental Abnormalities, Oral Cancers, Orthodontics, and Temporomandibular Disorders

Along with Updates on Current Research in Oral Health, a Glossary, a Directory of Dental and Oral Health Organizations, and Resources for People with Dental and Oral Health Disorders

Edited by Amy L. Sutton. 609 pages. 2003. 978-0-7808-0634-4.

"This book could serve as a turning point in the battle to educate consumers in issues concerning oral health." —American Reference Books Annual, 2004

"Unique source which will fill a gap in dental sources for patients and the lay public. A valuable reference tool even in a library with thousands of books on dentistry. Comprehensive, clear, inexpensive, and easy to read and use. It fills an enormous gap in the health care literature." —Reference & User Services Quarterly, American Library Association, Summer '98

"Recommended reference source." —Booklist, American Library Association, Dec '97

■

Depression Sourcebook

Basic Consumer Health Information about Unipolar Depression, Bipolar Disorder, Postpartum Depression, Seasonal Affective Disorder, and Other Types of Depression in Children, Adolescents, Women, Men, the Elderly, and Other Selected Populations

Along with Facts about Causes, Risk Factors, Diagnostic Criteria, Treatment Options, Coping Strategies, Suicide Prevention, a Glossary, and a Directory of Sources for Additional Help and Information

Edited by Karen Bellenir. 602 pages. 2002. 978-0-7808-0611-5.

"Depression Sourcebook is of a very high standard. Its purpose, which is to serve as a reference source to the lay reader, is very well served." —Journal of the National Medical Association, 2004

"Invaluable reference for public and school library collections alike." —Library Bookwatch, Apr '03

"Recommended for purchase." —American Reference Books Annual, 2003

■

Dermatological Disorders Sourcebook, 2nd Edition

Basic Consumer Health Information about Conditions and Disorders Affecting the Skin, Hair, and Nails, Such as Acne, Rosacea, Rashes, Dermatitis, Pigmentation Disorders, Birthmarks, Skin Cancer, Skin Injuries, Psoriasis, Scleroderma, and Hair Loss, Including Facts about Medications and Treatments for Dermatological Disorders and Tips for Maintaining Healthy Skin, Hair, and Nails

Along with Information about How Aging Affects the Skin, a Glossary of Related Terms, and a Directory of Resources for Additional Help and Information

Edited by Amy L. Sutton. 645 pages. 2005. 978-0-7808-0795-2.

"... comprehensive, easily read reference book."
—Doody's Health Sciences Book Reviews, Oct '97

SEE ALSO *Burns Sourcebook*

■

Diabetes Sourcebook, 3rd Edition

Basic Consumer Health Information about Type 1 Diabetes (Insulin-Dependent or Juvenile-Onset Diabetes), Type 2 Diabetes (Noninsulin-Dependent or Adult-Onset Diabetes), Gestational Diabetes, Impaired Glucose Tolerance (IGT), and Related Complications, Such as Amputation, Eye Disease, Gum Disease, Nerve Damage, and End-Stage Renal Disease, Including Facts about Insulin, Oral Diabetes Medications, Blood Sugar Testing, and the Role of Exercise and Nutrition in the Control of Diabetes

Along with a Glossary and Resources for Further Help and Information

Edited by Dawn D. Matthews. 622 pages. 2003. 978-0-7808-0629-0.

"This edition is even more helpful than earlier versions. . . . It is a truly valuable tool for anyone seeking readable and authoritative information on diabetes."
— American Reference Books Annual, 2004

"An invaluable reference." *— Library Journal, May '00*

Selected as one of the 250 "Best Health Sciences Books of 1999." *— Doody's Rating Service, Mar-Apr '00*

"Provides useful information for the general public."
— Healthlines, University of Michigan Health Management Research Center, Sep/Oct '99

"... provides reliable mainstream medical information ... belongs on the shelves of any library with a consumer health collection." *— E-Streams, Sep '99*

"Recommended reference source."
— Booklist, American Library Association, Feb '99

■

Diet & Nutrition Sourcebook, 3rd Edition

Basic Consumer Health Information about Dietary Guidelines and the Food Guidance System, Recommended Daily Nutrient Intakes, Serving Proportions, Weight Control, Vitamins and Supplements, Nutrition Issues for Different Life Stages and Lifestyles, and the Needs of People with Specific Medical Concerns, Including Cancer, Celiac Disease, Diabetes, Eating Disorders, Food Allergies, and Cardiovascular Disease

Along with Facts about Federal Nutrition Support Programs, a Glossary of Nutrition and Dietary Terms, and Directories of Additional Resources for More Information about Nutrition

Edited by Joyce Brennfleck Shannon. 633 pages. 2006. 978-0-7808-0800-3.

"This book is an excellent source of basic diet and nutrition information." *— Booklist Health Sciences Supplement, American Library Association, Dec '00*

"This reference document should be in any public library, but it would be a very good guide for beginning students in the health sciences. If the other books in this publisher's series are as good as this, they should all be in the health sciences collections."
— American Reference Books Annual, 2000

"This book is an excellent general nutrition reference for consumers who desire to take an active role in their health care for prevention. Consumers of all ages who select this book can feel confident they are receiving current and accurate information." *— Journal of Nutrition for the Elderly, Vol. 19, No. 4, 2000*

SEE ALSO *Digestive Diseases & Disorders Sourcebook, Eating Disorders Sourcebook, Gastrointestinal Diseases & Disorders Sourcebook, Vegetarian Sourcebook*

■

Digestive Diseases & Disorders Sourcebook

Basic Consumer Health Information about Diseases and Disorders that Impact the Upper and Lower Digestive System, Including Celiac Disease, Constipation, Crohn's Disease, Cyclic Vomiting Syndrome, Diarrhea, Diverticulosis and Diverticulitis, Gallstones, Heartburn, Hemorrhoids, Hernias, Indigestion (Dyspepsia), Irritable Bowel Syndrome, Lactose Intolerance, Ulcers, and More

Along with Information about Medications and Other Treatments, Tips for Maintaining a Healthy Digestive Tract, a Glossary, and Directory of Digestive Diseases Organizations

Edited by Karen Bellenir. 335 pages. 2000. 978-0-7808-0327-5.

"This title would be an excellent addition to all public or patient-research libraries."
— American Reference Books Annual, 2001

"This title is recommended for public, hospital, and health sciences libraries with consumer health collections." *— E-Streams, Jul-Aug '00*

"Recommended reference source."
— Booklist, American Library Association, May '00

SEE ALSO *Eating Disorders Sourcebook, Gastrointestinal Diseases & Disorders Sourcebook*

■

Disabilities Sourcebook

Basic Consumer Health Information about Physical and Psychiatric Disabilities, Including Descriptions of Major Causes of Disability, Assistive and Adaptive Aids, Workplace Issues, and Accessibility Concerns

Along with Information about the Americans with Disabilities Act, a Glossary, and Resources for Additional Help and Information

Edited by Dawn D. Matthews. 616 pages. 2000. 978-0-7808-0389-3.

"It is a must for libraries with a consumer health section." *— American Reference Books Annual, 2002*

"A much needed addition to the Omnigraphics *Health Reference Series*. A current reference work to provide people with disabilities, their families, caregivers or those who work with them, a broad range of information in one volume, has not been available until now. . . . It is recommended for all public and academic library reference collections."   —*E-Streams, May '01*

"An excellent source book in easy-to-read format covering many current topics; highly recommended for all libraries."   —*Choice, Association of College & Research Libraries, Jan '01*

"Recommended reference source."
  —*Booklist, American Library Association, Jul '00*

■

Domestic Violence Sourcebook, 2nd Edition

Basic Consumer Health Information about the Causes and Consequences of Abusive Relationships, Including Physical Violence, Sexual Assault, Battery, Stalking, and Emotional Abuse, and Facts about the Effects of Violence on Women, Men, Young Adults, and the Elderly, with Reports about Domestic Violence in Selected Populations, and Featuring Facts about Medical Care, Victim Assistance and Protection, Prevention Strategies, Mental Health Services, and Legal Issues

Along with a Glossary of Related Terms and Resources for Additional Help and Information

Edited by Dawn D. Matthews. 628 pages. 2004. 978-0-7808-0669-6.

"Educators, clergy, medical professionals, police, and victims and their families will benefit from this realistic and easy-to-understand resource."
  —*American Reference Books Annual, 2005*

"Recommended for all collections supporting consumer health information. It should also be considered for any collection needing general, readable information on domestic violence."   —*E-Streams, Jan '05*

"This sourcebook complements other books in its field, providing a one-stop resource . . . Recommended."
  —*Choice, Association of College & Research Libraries, Jan '05*

"Interested lay persons should find the book extremely beneficial. . . . A copy of *Domestic Violence and Child Abuse Sourcebook* should be in every public library in the United States."
  —*Social Science & Medicine, No. 56, 2003*

"This is important information. The Web has many resources but this sourcebook fills an important societal need. I am not aware of any other resources of this type."   —*Doody's Review Service, Sep '01*

"Recommended reference source."
  —*Booklist, American Library Association, Apr '01*

"Important pick for college-level health reference libraries."   —*The Bookwatch, Mar '01*

"Because this problem is so widespread and because this book includes a lot of issues within one volume, this work is recommended for all public libraries."
  —*American Reference Books Annual, 2001*

SEE ALSO Child Abuse Sourcebook

■

Drug Abuse Sourcebook, 2nd Edition

Basic Consumer Health Information about Illicit Substances of Abuse and the Misuse of Prescription and Over-the-Counter Medications, Including Depressants, Hallucinogens, Inhalants, Marijuana, Stimulants, and Anabolic Steroids

Along with Facts about Related Health Risks, Treatment Programs, Prevention Programs, a Glossary of Abuse and Addiction Terms, a Glossary of Drug-Related Street Terms, and a Directory of Resources for More Information

Edited by Catherine Ginther. 607 pages. 2004. 978-0-7808-0740-2.

"Commendable for organizing useful, normally scattered government and association-produced data into a logical sequence."
  —*American Reference Books Annual, 2006*

"This easy-to-read volume is recommended for consumer health collections within public or academic libraries."   —*E-Streams, Sep '05*

"An excellent library reference."
  —*The Bookwatch, May '05*

"Containing a wealth of information, this book will be useful to the college student just beginning to explore the topic of substance abuse. This resource belongs in libraries that serve a lower-division undergraduate or community college clientele as well as the general public."   —*Choice, Association of College & Research Libraries, Jun '01*

"Recommended reference source."
  —*Booklist, American Library Association, Feb '01*

SEE ALSO Alcoholism Sourcebook

■

Ear, Nose & Throat Disorders Sourcebook, 2nd Edition

Basic Consumer Health Information about Disorders of the Ears, Hearing Loss, Vestibular Disorders, Nasal and Sinus Problems, Throat and Vocal Cord Disorders, and Otolaryngologic Cancers, Including Facts about Ear Infections and Injuries, Genetic and Congenital Deafness, Sensorineural Hearing Disorders, Tinnitus, Vertigo, Ménière Disease, Rhinitis, Sinusitis, Snoring, Sore Throats, Hoarseness, and More

Along with Reports on Current Research Initiatives, a Glossary of Related Medical Terms, and a Directory of Sources for Further Help and Information

Edited by Sandra J. Judd. 659 pages. 2006. 978-0-7808-0872-0.

"Overall, this sourcebook is helpful for the consumer seeking information on ENT issues. It is recommended for public libraries."
—*American Reference Books Annual, 1999*

"Recommended reference source."
—*Booklist, American Library Association, Dec '98*

Eating Disorders Sourcebook, 2nd Edition

Basic Consumer Health Information about Anorexia Nervosa, Bulimia Nervosa, Binge Eating, Compulsive Exercise, Female Athlete Triad, and Other Eating Disorders, Including Facts about Body Image and Other Cultural and Age-Related Risk Factors, Prevention Efforts, Adverse Health Effects, Treatment Options, and the Recovery Process

Along with Guidelines for Healthy Weight Control, a Glossary, and Directories of Additional Resources

Edited by Joyce Brennfleck Shannon. 585 pages. 2007. 978-0-7808-0948-2.

"Recommended for health science libraries that are open to the public, as well as hospital libraries. This book is a good resource for the consumer who is concerned about eating disorders." — *E-Streams, Mar '02*

"This volume is another convenient collection of excerpted articles. Recommended for school and public library patrons; lower-division undergraduates; and two-year technical program students."
—*Choice, Association of College & Research Libraries, Jan '02*

"Recommended reference source."
— *Booklist, American Library Association, Oct '01*

SEE ALSO *Diet & Nutrition Sourcebook, Digestive Diseases & Disorders Sourcebook, Gastrointestinal Diseases & Disorders Sourcebook*

Emergency Medical Services Sourcebook

Basic Consumer Health Information about Preventing, Preparing for, and Managing Emergency Situations, When and Who to Call for Help, What to Expect in the Emergency Room, the Emergency Medical Team, Patient Issues, and Current Topics in Emergency Medicine

Along with Statistical Data, a Glossary, and Sources of Additional Help and Information

Edited by Jenni Lynn Colson. 494 pages. 2002. 978-0-7808-0420-3.

"Handy and convenient for home, public, school, and college libraries. Recommended."
— *Choice, Association of College & Research Libraries, Apr '03*

"This reference can provide the consumer with answers to most questions about emergency care in the United States, or it will direct them to a resource where the answer can be found."
—*American Reference Books Annual, 2003*

"Recommended reference source."
— *Booklist, American Library Association, Feb '03*

Endocrine & Metabolic Disorders Sourcebook

Basic Information for the Layperson about Pancreatic and Insulin-Related Disorders Such as Pancreatitis, Diabetes, and Hypoglycemia; Adrenal Gland Disorders Such as Cushing's Syndrome, Addison's Disease, and Congenital Adrenal Hyperplasia; Pituitary Gland Disorders Such as Growth Hormone Deficiency, Acromegaly, and Pituitary Tumors; Thyroid Disorders Such as Hypothyroidism, Graves' Disease, Hashimoto's Disease, and Goiter; Hyperparathyroidism; and Other Diseases and Syndromes of Hormone Imbalance or Metabolic Dysfunction

Along with Reports on Current Research Initiatives

Edited by Linda M. Shin. 574 pages. 1998. 978-0-7808-0207-0.

"Omnigraphics has produced another needed resource for health information consumers."
—*American Reference Books Annual, 2000*

"Recommended reference source."
— *Booklist, American Library Association, Dec '98*

Environmental Health Sourcebook, 2nd Edition

Basic Consumer Health Information about the Environment and Its Effect on Human Health, Including the Effects of Air Pollution, Water Pollution, Hazardous Chemicals, Food Hazards, Radiation Hazards, Biological Agents, Household Hazards, Such as Radon, Asbestos, Carbon Monoxide, and Mold, and Information about Associated Diseases and Disorders, Including Cancer, Allergies, Respiratory Problems, and Skin Disorders

Along with Information about Environmental Concerns for Specific Populations, a Glossary of Related Terms, and Resources for Further Help and Information

Edited by Dawn D. Matthews. 673 pages. 2003. 978-0-7808-0632-0.

"This recently updated edition continues the level of quality and the reputation of the numerous other volumes in Omnigraphics' *Health Reference Series*."
— *American Reference Books Annual, 2004*

"An excellent updated edition."
— *The Bookwatch, Oct '03*

"Recommended reference source."
— *Booklist, American Library Association, Sep '98*

"This book will be a useful addition to anyone's library." — *Choice Health Sciences Supplement, Association of College & Research Libraries, May '98*

". . . a good survey of numerous environmentally induced physical disorders . . . a useful addition to anyone's library."
— *Doody's Health Sciences Book Reviews, Jan '98*

Ethnic Diseases Sourcebook

Basic Consumer Health Information for Ethnic and Racial Minority Groups in the United States, Including General Health Indicators and Behaviors, Ethnic Diseases, Genetic Testing, the Impact of Chronic Diseases, Women's Health, Mental Health Issues, and Preventive Health Care Services

Along with a Glossary and a Listing of Additional Resources

Edited by Joyce Brennfleck Shannon. 664 pages. 2001. 978-0-7808-0336-7.

"Recommended for health sciences libraries where public health programs are a priority."
— E-Streams, Jan '02

"Not many books have been written on this topic to date, and the *Ethnic Diseases Sourcebook* is a strong addition to the list. It will be an important introductory resource for health consumers, students, health care personnel, and social scientists. It is recommended for public, academic, and large hospital libraries."
— American Reference Books Annual, 2002

"Recommended reference source."
— Booklist, American Library Association, Oct '01

"Will prove valuable to any library seeking to maintain a current, comprehensive reference collection of health resources. . . . An excellent source of health information about genetic disorders which affect particular ethnic and racial minorities in the U.S."
— The Bookwatch, Aug '01

Eye Care Sourcebook, 2nd Edition

Basic Consumer Health Information about Eye Care and Eye Disorders, Including Facts about the Diagnosis, Prevention, and Treatment of Common Refractive Problems Such as Myopia, Hyperopia, Astigmatism, and Presbyopia, and Eye Diseases, Including Glaucoma, Cataract, Age-Related Macular Degeneration, and Diabetic Retinopathy

Along with a Section on Vision Correction and Refractive Surgeries, Including LASIK and LASEK, a Glossary, and Directories of Resources for Additional Help and Information

Edited by Amy L. Sutton. 543 pages. 2003. 978-0-7808-0635-1.

". . . a solid reference tool for eye care and a valuable addition to a collection."
— American Reference Books Annual, 2004

Family Planning Sourcebook

Basic Consumer Health Information about Planning for Pregnancy and Contraception, Including Traditional Methods, Barrier Methods, Hormonal Methods, Permanent Methods, Future Methods, Emergency Contraception, and Birth Control Choices for Women at Each Stage of Life

Along with Statistics, a Glossary, and Sources of Additional Information

Edited by Amy Marcaccio Keyzer. 520 pages. 2001. 978-0-7808-0379-4.

"Recommended for public, health, and undergraduate libraries as part of the circulating collection."
— E-Streams, Mar '02

"Information is presented in an unbiased, readable manner, and the sourcebook will certainly be a necessary addition to those public and high school libraries where Internet access is restricted or otherwise problematic." — American Reference Books Annual, 2002

"Recommended reference source."
— Booklist, American Library Association, Oct '01

"Will prove valuable to any library seeking to maintain a current, comprehensive reference collection of health resources. . . . Excellent reference."
— The Bookwatch, Aug '01

SEE ALSO Pregnancy & Birth Sourcebook

Fitness & Exercise Sourcebook, 3rd Edition

Basic Consumer Health Information about the Physical and Mental Benefits of Fitness, Including Cardiorespiratory Endurance, Muscular Strength, Muscular Endurance, and Flexibility, with Facts about Sports Nutrition and Exercise-Related Injuries and Tips about Physical Activity and Exercises for People of All Ages and for People with Health Concerns

Along with Advice on Selecting and Using Exercise Equipment, Maintaining Exercise Motivation, a Glossary of Related Terms, and a Directory of Resources for More Help and Information

Edited by Amy L. Sutton. 663 pages. 2007. 978-0-7808-0946-8.

"This work is recommended for all general reference collections."
— American Reference Books Annual, 2002

"Highly recommended for public, consumer, and school grades fourth through college." — E-Streams, Nov '01

"Recommended reference source."
— Booklist, American Library Association, Oct '01

"The information appears quite comprehensive and is considered reliable. . . . This second edition is a welcomed addition to the series."
— Doody's Review Service, Sep '01

Food Safety Sourcebook

Basic Consumer Health Information about the Safe Handling of Meat, Poultry, Seafood, Eggs, Fruit Juices, and Other Food Items, and Facts about Pesticides, Drinking Water, Food Safety Overseas, and the Onset, Duration, and Symptoms of Foodborne Illnesses, Including Types of Pathogenic Bacteria, Parasitic Protozoa, Worms, Viruses, and Natural Toxins

Along with the Role of the Consumer, the Food Handler, and the Government in Food Safety; a Glossary, and Resources for Additional Help and Information

Edited by Dawn D. Matthews. 339 pages. 1999. 978-0-7808-0326-8.

"This book is recommended for public libraries and universities with home economic and food science programs."
—E-Streams, Nov '00

"Recommended reference source."
—Booklist, American Library Association, May '00

"This book takes the complex issues of food safety and foodborne pathogens and presents them in an easily understood manner. [It does] an excellent job of covering a large and often confusing topic."
—American Reference Books Annual, 2000

■

Forensic Medicine Sourcebook

Basic Consumer Information for the Layperson about Forensic Medicine, Including Crime Scene Investigation, Evidence Collection and Analysis, Expert Testimony, Computer-Aided Criminal Identification, Digital Imaging in the Courtroom, DNA Profiling, Accident Reconstruction, Autopsies, Ballistics, Drugs and Explosives Detection, Latent Fingerprints, Product Tampering, and Questioned Document Examination

Along with Statistical Data, a Glossary of Forensics Terminology, and Listings of Sources for Further Help and Information

Edited by Annemarie S. Muth. 574 pages. 1999. 978-0-7808-0232-2.

"Given the expected widespread interest in its content and its easy to read style, this book is recommended for most public and all college and university libraries."
—E-Streams, Feb '01

"Recommended for public libraries."
—Reference & User Services Quarterly, American Library Association, Spring 2000

"Recommended reference source."
—Booklist, American Library Association, Feb '00

"A wealth of information, useful statistics, references are up-to-date and extremely complete. This wonderful collection of data will help students who are interested in a career in any type of forensic science. It is a great resource for attorneys who need information about types of expert witnesses needed in a particular case. It also offers useful information for fiction and nonfiction writers whose work involves a crime. A fascinating compilation. All levels."
—Choice, Association of College & Research Libraries, Jan '00

"There are several items that make this book attractive to consumers who are seeking certain forensic data. . . . This is a useful current source for those seeking general forensic medical answers."
—American Reference Books Annual, 2000

Gastrointestinal Diseases & Disorders Sourcebook, 2nd Edition

Basic Consumer Health Information about the Upper and Lower Gastrointestinal (GI) Tract, Including the Esophagus, Stomach, Intestines, Rectum, Liver, and Pancreas, with Facts about Gastroesophageal Reflux Disease, Gastritis, Hernias, Ulcers, Celiac Disease, Diverticulitis, Irritable Bowel Syndrome, Hemorrhoids, Gastrointestinal Cancers, and Other Diseases and Disorders Related to the Digestive Process

Along with Information about Commonly Used Diagnostic and Surgical Procedures, Statistics, Reports on Current Research Initiatives and Clinical Trials, a Glossary, and Resources for Additional Help and Information

Edited by Sandra J. Judd. 681 pages. 2006. 978-0-7808-0798-3.

". . . very readable form. The successful editorial work that brought this material together into a useful and understandable reference makes accessible to all readers information that can help them more effectively understand and obtain help for digestive tract problems."
—Choice, Association of College & Research Libraries, Feb '97

SEE ALSO Diet & Nutrition Sourcebook, Digestive Diseases & Disorders Sourcebook, Eating Disorders Sourcebook

■

Genetic Disorders Sourcebook, 3rd Edition

Basic Consumer Health Information about Hereditary Diseases and Disorders, Including Facts about the Human Genome, Genetic Inheritance Patterns, Disorders Associated with Specific Genes, Such as Sickle Cell Disease, Hemophilia, and Cystic Fibrosis, Chromosome Disorders, Such as Down Syndrome, Fragile X Syndrome, and Turner Syndrome, and Complex Diseases and Disorders Resulting from the Interaction of Environmental and Genetic Factors, Such as Allergies, Cancer, and Obesity

Along with Facts about Genetic Testing, Suggestions for Parents of Children with Special Needs, Reports on Current Research Initiatives, a Glossary of Genetic Terminology, and Resources for Additional Help and Information

Edited by Karen Bellenir. 777 pages. 2004. 978-0-7808-0742-6.

"This text is recommended for any library with an interest in providing consumer health resources."
—E-Streams, Aug '05

"This is a valuable resource for anyone wishing to have an understandable description of any of the topics or disorders included. The editor succeeds in making complex genetic issues understandable."
—Doody's Book Review Service, May '05

"A good acquisition for public libraries."
—American Reference Books Annual, 2005

■

Head Trauma Sourcebook

Basic Information for the Layperson about Open-Head and Closed-Head Injuries, Treatment Advances, Recovery, and Rehabilitation

Along with Reports on Current Research Initiatives

Edited by Karen Bellenir. 414 pages. 1997. 978-0-7808-0208-7.

Headache Sourcebook

Basic Consumer Health Information about Migraine, Tension, Cluster, Rebound and Other Types of Headaches, with Facts about the Cause and Prevention of Headaches, the Effects of Stress and the Environment, Headaches during Pregnancy and Menopause, and Childhood Headaches

Along with a Glossary and Other Resources for Additional Help and Information

Edited by Dawn D. Matthews. 362 pages. 2002. 978-0-7808-0337-4.

■

Healthy Aging Sourcebook

Basic Consumer Health Information about Maintaining Health through the Aging Process, Including Advice on Nutrition, Exercise, and Sleep, Help in Making Decisions about Midlife Issues and Retirement, and Guidance Concerning Practical and Informed Choices in Health Consumerism

Along with Data Concerning the Theories of Aging, Different Experiences in Aging by Minority Groups, and Facts about Aging Now and Aging in the Future; and Featuring a Glossary, a Guide to Consumer Help, Additional Suggested Reading, and Practical Resource Directory

Edited by Jenifer Swanson. 536 pages. 1999. 978-0-7808-0390-9.

SEE ALSO *Physical & Mental Issues in Aging Sourcebook*

■

Healthy Children Sourcebook

Basic Consumer Health Information about the Physical and Mental Development of Children between the Ages of 3 and 12, Including Routine Health Care, Preventative Health Services, Safety and First Aid,

Healthy Sleep, Dental Care, Nutrition, and Fitness, and Featuring Parenting Tips on Such Topics as Bedwetting, Choosing Day Care, Monitoring TV and Other Media, and Establishing a Foundation for Substance Abuse Prevention

Along with a Glossary of Commonly Used Pediatric Terms and Resources for Additional Help and Information

Edited by Chad T. Kimball. 647 pages. 2003. 978-0-7808-0247-6.

SEE ALSO *Childhood Diseases & Disorders Sourcebook*

■

Healthy Heart Sourcebook for Women

Basic Consumer Health Information about Cardiac Issues Specific to Women, Including Facts about Major Risk Factors and Prevention, Treatment and Control Strategies, and Important Dietary Issues

Along with a Special Section Regarding the Pros and Cons of Hormone Replacement Therapy and Its Impact on Heart Health, and Additional Help, Including Recipes, a Glossary, and a Directory of Resources

Edited by Dawn D. Matthews. 336 pages. 2000. 978-0-7808-0329-9.

SEE ALSO *Cardiovascular Diseases & Disorders Sourcebook, Women's Health Concerns Sourcebook*

■

Hepatitis Sourcebook

Basic Consumer Health Information about Hepatitis A, Hepatitis B, Hepatitis C, and Other Forms of Hepatitis, Including Autoimmune Hepatitis, Alcoholic Hepatitis, Nonalcoholic Steatohepatitis, and Toxic Hepatitis, with

Facts about Risk Factors, Screening Methods, Diagnostic Tests, and Treatment Options

Along with Information on Liver Health, Tips for People Living with Chronic Hepatitis, Reports on Current Research Initiatives, a Glossary of Terms Related to Hepatitis, and a Directory of Sources for Further Help and Information

Edited by Sandra J. Judd. 597 pages. 2005. 978-0-7808-0749-5.

"Highly recommended."
— American Reference Books Annual, 2006

Household Safety Sourcebook

Basic Consumer Health Information about Household Safety, Including Information about Poisons, Chemicals, Fire, and Water Hazards in the Home

Along with Advice about the Safe Use of Home Maintenance Equipment, Choosing Toys and Nursery Furniture, Holiday and Recreation Safety, a Glossary, and Resources for Further Help and Information

Edited by Dawn D. Matthews. 606 pages. 2002. 978-0-7808-0338-1.

"This work will be useful in public libraries with large consumer health and wellness departments."
— American Reference Books Annual, 2003

"As a sourcebook on household safety this book meets its mark. It is encyclopedic in scope and covers a wide range of safety issues that are commonly seen in the home."
— E-Streams, Jul '02

Hypertension Sourcebook

Basic Consumer Health Information about the Causes, Diagnosis, and Treatment of High Blood Pressure, with Facts about Consequences, Complications, and Co-Occurring Disorders, Such as Coronary Heart Disease, Diabetes, Stroke, Kidney Disease, and Hypertensive Retinopathy, and Issues in Blood Pressure Control, Including Dietary Choices, Stress Management, and Medications

Along with Reports on Current Research Initiatives and Clinical Trials, a Glossary, and Resources for Additional Help and Information

Edited by Dawn D. Matthews and Karen Bellenir. 613 pages. 2004. 978-0-7808-0674-0.

"Academic, public, and medical libraries will want to add the *Hypertension Sourcebook* to their collections."
— E-Streams, Aug '05

"The strength of this source is the wide range of information given about hypertension."
— American Reference Books Annual, 2005

Immune System Disorders Sourcebook, 2nd Edition

Basic Consumer Health Information about Disorders of the Immune System, Including Immune System Function and Response, Diagnosis of Immune Disorders, Information about Inherited Immune Disease, Acquired Immune Disease, and Autoimmune Diseases, Including Primary Immune Deficiency, Acquired Immunodeficiency Syndrome (AIDS), Lupus, Multiple Sclerosis, Type 1 Diabetes, Rheumatoid Arthritis, and Graves' Disease

Along with Treatments, Tips for Coping with Immune Disorders, a Glossary, and a Directory of Additional Resources.

Edited by Joyce Brennfleck Shannon. 671 pages. 2005. 978-0-7808-0748-8.

"Highly recommended for academic and public libraries." — American Reference Books Annual, 2006

"The updated second edition is a 'must' for any consumer health library seeking a solid resource covering the treatments, symptoms, and options for immune disorder sufferers. . . . An excellent guide."
— MBR Bookwatch, Jan '06

Infant & Toddler Health Sourcebook

Basic Consumer Health Information about the Physical and Mental Development of Newborns, Infants, and Toddlers, Including Neonatal Concerns, Nutrition Recommendations, Immunization Schedules, Common Pediatric Disorders, Assessments and Milestones, Safety Tips, and Advice for Parents and Other Caregivers

Along with a Glossary of Terms and Resource Listings for Additional Help

Edited by Jenifer Swanson. 585 pages. 2000. 978-0-7808-0246-9.

"As a reference for the general public, this would be useful in any library." — E-Streams, May '01

"Recommended reference source."
— Booklist, American Library Association, Feb '01

"This is a good source for general use."
— American Reference Books Annual, 2001

Infectious Diseases Sourcebook

Basic Consumer Health Information about Non-Contagious Bacterial, Viral, Prion, Fungal, and Parasitic Diseases Spread by Food and Water, Insects and Animals, or Environmental Contact, Including Botulism, E. Coli, Encephalitis, Legionnaires' Disease, Lyme Disease, Malaria, Plague, Rabies, Salmonella, Tetanus, and Others, and Facts about Newly Emerging Diseases, Such as Hantavirus, Mad Cow Disease, Monkeypox, and West Nile Virus

Along with Information about Preventing Disease Transmission, the Threat of Bioterrorism, and Current Research Initiatives, with a Glossary and Directory of Resources for More Information

Edited by Karen Bellenir. 634 pages. 2004. 978-0-7808-0675-7.

"This reference continues the excellent tradition of the *Health Reference Series* in consolidating a wealth of information on a selected topic into a format that is easy to use and accessible to the general public."
— *American Reference Books Annual, 2005*

"Recommended for public and academic libraries."
— *E-Streams, Jan '05*

■

Injury & Trauma Sourcebook

Basic Consumer Health Information about the Impact of Injury, the Diagnosis and Treatment of Common and Traumatic Injuries, Emergency Care, and Specific Injuries Related to Home, Community, Workplace, Transportation, and Recreation

Along with Guidelines for Injury Prevention, a Glossary, and a Directory of Additional Resources

Edited by Joyce Brennfleck Shannon. 696 pages. 2002. 978-0-7808-0421-0.

"This publication is the most comprehensive work of its kind about injury and trauma."
— *American Reference Books Annual, 2003*

"This sourcebook provides concise, easily readable, basic health information about injuries. . . . This book is well organized and an easy to use reference resource suitable for hospital, health sciences and public libraries with consumer health collections."
— *E-Streams, Nov '02*

"Practitioners should be aware of guides such as this in order to facilitate their use by patients and their families."
— *Doody's Health Sciences Book Review Journal, Sep-Oct '02*

"Recommended reference source."
— *Booklist, American Library Association, Sep '02*

"Highly recommended for academic and medical reference collections." — *Library Bookwatch, Sep '02*

■

Kidney & Urinary Tract Diseases & Disorders Sourcebook

SEE *Urinary Tract & Kidney Diseases & Disorders Sourcebook*

■

Learning Disabilities Sourcebook, 2nd Edition

Basic Consumer Health Information about Learning Disabilities, Including Dyslexia, Developmental Speech and Language Disabilities, Non-Verbal Learning Disorders, Developmental Arithmetic Disorder, Developmental Writing Disorder, and Other Conditions That Impede Learning Such as Attention Deficit/Hyperactivity Disorder, Brain Injury, Hearing Impairment, Klinefelter Syndrome, Dyspraxia, and Tourette's Syndrome

Along with Facts about Educational Issues and Assistive Technology, Coping Strategies, a Glossary of Related Terms, and Resources for Further Help and Information

Edited by Dawn D. Matthews. 621 pages. 2003. 978-0-7808-0626-9.

"The second edition of Learning Disabilities Sourcebook far surpasses the earlier edition in that it is more focused on information that will be useful as a consumer health resource."
— *American Reference Books Annual, 2004*

"Teachers as well as consumers will find this an essential guide to understanding various syndromes and their latest treatments. [An] invaluable reference for public and school library collections alike."
— *Library Bookwatch, Apr '03*

Named "Outstanding Reference Book of 1999."
— *New York Public Library, Feb '00*

"An excellent candidate for inclusion in a public library reference section. It's a great source of information. Teachers will also find the book useful. Definitely worth reading."
— *Journal of Adolescent & Adult Literacy, Feb 2000*

"Readable . . . provides a solid base of information regarding successful techniques used with individuals who have learning disabilities, as well as practical suggestions for educators and family members. Clear language, concise descriptions, and pertinent information for contacting multiple resources add to the strength of this book as a useful tool." — *Choice, Association of College & Research Libraries, Feb '99*

"Recommended reference source."
— *Booklist, American Library Association, Sep '98*

"A useful resource for libraries and for those who don't have the time to identify and locate the individual publications." — *Disability Resources Monthly, Sep '98*

■

Leukemia Sourcebook

Basic Consumer Health Information about Adult and Childhood Leukemias, Including Acute Lymphocytic Leukemia (ALL), Chronic Lymphocytic Leukemia (CLL), Acute Myelogenous Leukemia (AML), Chronic Myelogenous Leukemia (CML), and Hairy Cell Leukemia, and Treatments Such as Chemotherapy, Radiation Therapy, Peripheral Blood Stem Cell and Marrow Transplantation, and Immunotherapy

Along with Tips for Life During and After Treatment, a Glossary, and Directories of Additional Resources

Edited by Joyce Brennfleck Shannon. 587 pages. 2003. 978-0-7808-0627-6.

"Unlike other medical books for the layperson, . . . the language does not talk down to the reader. . . . This volume is highly recommended for all libraries."
— *American Reference Books Annual, 2004*

". . . a fine title which ranges from diagnosis to alternative treatments, staging, and tips for life during and after diagnosis." — *The Bookwatch, Dec '03*

643

Liver Disorders Sourcebook

Basic Consumer Health Information about the Liver and How It Works; Liver Diseases, Including Cancer, Cirrhosis, Hepatitis, and Toxic and Drug Related Diseases; Tips for Maintaining a Healthy Liver; Laboratory Tests, Radiology Tests, and Facts about Liver Transplantation

Along with a Section on Support Groups, a Glossary, and Resource Listings

Edited by Joyce Brennfleck Shannon. 591 pages. 2000. 978-0-7808-0383-1.

"A valuable resource."
—*American Reference Books Annual, 2001*

"This title is recommended for health sciences and public libraries with consumer health collections."
—*E-Streams, Oct '00*

"Recommended reference source."
—*Booklist, American Library Association, Jun '00*

Lung Disorders Sourcebook

Basic Consumer Health Information about Emphysema, Pneumonia, Tuberculosis, Asthma, Cystic Fibrosis, and Other Lung Disorders, Including Facts about Diagnostic Procedures, Treatment Strategies, Disease Prevention Efforts, and Such Risk Factors as Smoking, Air Pollution, and Exposure to Asbestos, Radon, and Other Agents

Along with a Glossary and Resources for Additional Help and Information

Edited by Dawn D. Matthews. 678 pages. 2002. 978-0-7808-0339-8.

"This title is a great addition for public and school libraries because it provides concise health information on the lungs."
—*American Reference Books Annual, 2003*

"Highly recommended for academic and medical reference collections."   —*Library Bookwatch, Sep '02*

SEE ALSO *Respiratory Diseases & Disorders Sourcebook*

Medical Tests Sourcebook, 2nd Edition

Basic Consumer Health Information about Medical Tests, Including Age-Specific Health Tests, Important Health Screenings and Exams, Home-Use Tests, Blood and Specimen Tests, Electrical Tests, Scope Tests, Genetic Testing, and Imaging Tests, Such as X-Rays, Ultrasound, Computed Tomography, Magnetic Resonance Imaging, Angiography, and Nuclear Medicine

Along with a Glossary and Directory of Additional Resources

Edited by Joyce Brennfleck Shannon. 654 pages. 2004. 978-0-7808-0670-2.

"Recommended for hospital and health sciences

libraries with consumer health collections."
—*E-Streams, Mar '00*

"This is an overall excellent reference with a wealth of general knowledge that may aid those who are reluctant to get vital tests performed."
—*Today's Librarian, Jan '00*

"A valuable reference guide."
—*American Reference Books Annual, 2000*

Men's Health Concerns Sourcebook, 2nd Edition

Basic Consumer Health Information about the Medical and Mental Concerns of Men, Including Theories about the Shorter Male Lifespan, the Leading Causes of Death and Disability, Physical Concerns of Special Significance to Men, Reproductive and Sexual Concerns, Sexually Transmitted Diseases, Men's Mental and Emotional Health, and Lifestyle Choices That Affect Wellness, Such as Nutrition, Fitness, and Substance Use

Along with a Glossary of Related Terms and a Directory of Organizational Resources in Men's Health

Edited by Robert Aquinas McNally. 644 pages. 2004. 978-0-7808-0671-9.

"A very accessible reference for non-specialist general readers and consumers."   —*The Bookwatch, Jun '04*

"This comprehensive resource and the series are highly recommended."
—*American Reference Books Annual, 2000*

"Recommended reference source."
—*Booklist, American Library Association, Dec '98*

Mental Health Disorders Sourcebook, 3rd Edition

Basic Consumer Health Information about Mental and Emotional Health and Mental Illness, Including Facts about Depression, Bipolar Disorder, and Other Mood Disorders, Phobias, Post-Traumatic Stress Disorder (PTSD), Obsessive-Compulsive Disorder, and Other Anxiety Disorders, Impulse Control Disorders, Eating Disorders, Personality Disorders, and Psychotic Disorders, Including Schizophrenia and Dissociative Disorders

Along with Statistical Information, a Special Section Concerning Mental Health Issues in Children and Adolescents, a Glossary, and Directories of Resources for Additional Help and Information

Edited by Karen Bellenir. 661 pages. 2005. 978-0-7808-0747-1.

"Recommended for public libraries and academic libraries with an undergraduate program in psychology."
—*American Reference Books Annual, 2006*

"Recommended reference source."
—*Booklist, American Library Association, Jun '00*

Mental Retardation Sourcebook

Basic Consumer Health Information about Mental Retardation and Its Causes, Including Down Syndrome, Fetal Alcohol Syndrome, Fragile X Syndrome, Genetic Conditions, Injury, and Environmental Sources

Along with Preventive Strategies, Parenting Issues, Educational Implications, Health Care Needs, Employment and Economic Matters, Legal Issues, a Glossary, and a Resource Listing for Additional Help and Information

Edited by Joyce Brennfleck Shannon. 642 pages. 2000. 978-0-7808-0377-0.

"Public libraries will find the book useful for reference and as a beginning research point for students, parents, and caregivers."
— *American Reference Books Annual, 2001*

"The strength of this work is that it compiles many basic fact sheets and addresses for further information in one volume. It is intended and suitable for the general public. This sourcebook is relevant to any collection providing health information to the general public."
— *E-Streams, Nov '00*

"From preventing retardation to parenting and family challenges, this covers health, social and legal issues and will prove an invaluable overview."
— *Reviewer's Bookwatch, Jul '00*

Movement Disorders Sourcebook

Basic Consumer Health Information about Neurological Movement Disorders, Including Essential Tremor, Parkinson's Disease, Dystonia, Cerebral Palsy, Huntington's Disease, Myasthenia Gravis, Multiple Sclerosis, and Other Early-Onset and Adult-Onset Movement Disorders, Their Symptoms and Causes, Diagnostic Tests, and Treatments

Along with Mobility and Assistive Technology Information, a Glossary, and a Directory of Additional Resources

Edited by Joyce Brennfleck Shannon. 655 pages. 2003. 978-0-7808-0628-3.

"... a good resource for consumers and recommended for public, community college and undergraduate libraries." — *American Reference Books Annual, 2004*

Muscular Dystrophy Sourcebook

Basic Consumer Health Information about Congenital, Childhood-Onset, and Adult-Onset Forms of Muscular Dystrophy, Such as Duchenne, Becker, Emery-Dreifuss, Distal, Limb-Girdle, Facioscapulohumeral (FSHD), Myotonic, and Ophthalmoplegic Muscular Dystrophies, Including Facts about Diagnostic Tests, Medical and Physical Therapies, Management of Co-Occurring Conditions, and Parenting Guidelines

Along with Practical Tips for Home Care, a Glossary, and Directories of Additional Resources

Edited by Joyce Brennfleck Shannon. 577 pages. 2004. 978-0-7808-0676-4.

"This book is highly recommended for public and academic libraries as well as health care offices that support the information needs of patients and their families."
— *E-Streams, Apr '05*

"Excellent reference." — *The Bookwatch, Jan '05*

Obesity Sourcebook

Basic Consumer Health Information about Diseases and Other Problems Associated with Obesity, and Including Facts about Risk Factors, Prevention Issues, and Management Approaches

Along with Statistical and Demographic Data, Information about Special Populations, Research Updates, a Glossary, and Source Listings for Further Help and Information

Edited by Wilma Caldwell and Chad T. Kimball. 376 pages. 2001. 978-0-7808-0333-6.

"The book synthesizes the reliable medical literature on obesity into one easy-to-read and useful resource for the general public."
— *American Reference Books Annual, 2002*

"This is a very useful resource book for the lay public."
— *Doody's Review Service, Nov '01*

"Well suited for the health reference collection of a public library or an academic health science library that serves the general population." — *E-Streams, Sep '01*

"Recommended reference source."
— *Booklist, American Library Association, Apr '01*

"Recommended pick both for specialty health library collections and any general consumer health reference collection." — *The Bookwatch, Apr '01*

Oral Health Sourcebook

SEE *Dental Care & Oral Health Sourcebook*

Osteoporosis Sourcebook

Basic Consumer Health Information about Primary and Secondary Osteoporosis and Juvenile Osteoporosis and Related Conditions, Including Fibrous Dysplasia, Gaucher Disease, Hyperthyroidism, Hypophosphatasia, Myeloma, Osteopetrosis, Osteogenesis Imperfecta, and Paget's Disease

Along with Information about Risk Factors, Treatments, Traditional and Non-Traditional Pain Management, a Glossary of Related Terms, and a Directory of Resources

Edited by Allan R. Cook. 584 pages. 2001. 978-0-7808-0239-1.

"This would be a book to be kept in a staff or patient library. The targeted audience is the layperson, but the therapist who needs a quick bit of information on a particular topic will also find the book useful."
— *Physical Therapy, Jan '02*

"This resource is recommended as a great reference source for public, health, and academic libraries, and is another triumph for the editors of Omnigraphics."
— *American Reference Books Annual, 2002*

"Recommended for all public libraries and general health collections, especially those supporting patient education or consumer health programs."
— *E-Streams, Nov '01*

"Will prove valuable to any library seeking to maintain a current, comprehensive reference collection of health resources. . . . From prevention to treatment and associated conditions, this provides an excellent survey."
— *The Bookwatch, Aug '01*

"Recommended reference source."
— *Booklist, American Library Association, Jul '01*

SEE ALSO *Healthy Aging Sourcebook, Physical & Mental Issues in Aging Sourcebook, Women's Health Concerns Sourcebook*

■

Pain Sourcebook, 2nd Edition

Basic Consumer Health Information about Specific Forms of Acute and Chronic Pain, Including Muscle and Skeletal Pain, Nerve Pain, Cancer Pain, and Disorders Characterized by Pain, Such as Fibromyalgia, Shingles, Angina, Arthritis, and Headaches

Along with Information about Pain Medications and Management Techniques, Complementary and Alternative Pain Relief Options, Tips for People Living with Chronic Pain, a Glossary, and a Directory of Sources for Further Information

Edited by Karen Bellenir. 670 pages. 2002. 978-0-7808-0612-2.

"A source of valuable information. . . . This book offers help to nonmedical people who need information about pain and pain management. It is also an excellent reference for those who participate in patient education."
— *Doody's Review Service, Sep '02*

"Highly recommended for academic and medical reference collections." — *Library Bookwatch, Sep '02*

"The text is readable, easily understood, and well indexed. This excellent volume belongs in all patient education libraries, consumer health sections of public libraries, and many personal collections."
— *American Reference Books Annual, 1999*

"The information is basic in terms of scholarship and is appropriate for general readers. Written in journalistic style . . . intended for non-professionals. Quite thorough in its coverage of different pain conditions and summarizes the latest clinical information regarding pain treatment." — *Choice, Association of College and Research Libraries, Jun '98*

"Recommended reference source."
— *Booklist, American Library Association, Mar '98*

■

Pediatric Cancer Sourcebook

Basic Consumer Health Information about Leukemias, Brain Tumors, Sarcomas, Lymphomas, and Other Cancers in Infants, Children, and Adolescents, Including Descriptions of Cancers, Treatments, and Coping Strategies

Along with Suggestions for Parents, Caregivers, and Concerned Relatives, a Glossary of Cancer Terms, and Resource Listings

Edited by Edward J. Prucha. 587 pages. 1999. 978-0-7808-0245-2.

"An excellent source of information. Recommended for public, hospital, and health science libraries with consumer health collections." — *E-Streams, Jun '00*

"Recommended reference source."
— *Booklist, American Library Association, Feb '00*

"A valuable addition to all libraries specializing in health services and many public libraries."
— *American Reference Books Annual, 2000*

SEE ALSO *Childhood Diseases & Disorders Sourcebook, Healthy Children Sourcebook*

■

Physical & Mental Issues in Aging Sourcebook

Basic Consumer Health Information on Physical and Mental Disorders Associated with the Aging Process, Including Concerns about Cardiovascular Disease, Pulmonary Disease, Oral Health, Digestive Disorders, Musculoskeletal and Skin Disorders, Metabolic Changes, Sexual and Reproductive Issues, and Changes in Vision, Hearing, and Other Senses

Along with Data about Longevity and Causes of Death, Information on Acute and Chronic Pain, Descriptions of Mental Concerns, a Glossary of Terms, and Resource Listings for Additional Help

Edited by Jenifer Swanson. 660 pages. 1999. 978-0-7808-0233-9.

"This is a treasure of health information for the layperson." — *Choice Health Sciences Supplement, Association of College & Research Libraries, May '00*

"Recommended for public libraries."
— *American Reference Books Annual, 2000*

"Recommended reference source."
— *Booklist, American Library Association, Oct '99*

SEE ALSO *Healthy Aging Sourcebook*

■

Podiatry Sourcebook, 2nd Edition

Basic Consumer Health Information about Disorders, Diseases, Deformities, and Injuries that Affect the Foot and Ankle, Including Sprains, Corns, Calluses, Bunions, Plantar Warts, Plantar Fasciitis, Neuromas, Clubfoot, Flat Feet, Achilles Tendonitis, and Much More

Along with Information about Selecting a Foot Care Specialist, Foot Fitness, Shoes and Socks, Diagnostic Tests and Corrective Procedures, Financial Assistance for Corrective Devices, a Glossary of Related Terms, and a Directory of Resources for Additional Help and Information

Edited by Ivy L. Alexander. 543 pages. 2007. 978-0-7808-0944-4.

"Recommended reference source."
— *Booklist, American Library Association, Feb '02*

"There is a lot of information presented here on a topic that is usually only covered sparingly in most larger comprehensive medical encyclopedias."
— *American Reference Books Annual, 2002*

∎

Pregnancy & Birth Sourcebook, 2nd Edition

Basic Consumer Health Information about Conception and Pregnancy, Including Facts about Fertility, Infertility, Pregnancy Symptoms and Complications, Fetal Growth and Development, Labor, Delivery, and the Postpartum Period, as Well as Information about Maintaining Health and Wellness during Pregnancy and Caring for a Newborn

Along with Information about Public Health Assistance for Low-Income Pregnant Women, a Glossary, and Directories of Agencies and Organizations Providing Help and Support

Edited by Amy L. Sutton. 626 pages. 2004. 978-0-7808-0672-6.

"Will appeal to public and school reference collections strong in medicine and women's health. . . . Deserves a spot on any medical reference shelf."
— *The Bookwatch, Jul '04*

"A well-organized handbook. Recommended."
— *Choice, Association of College & Research Libraries, Apr '98*

"Recommended reference source."
— *Booklist, American Library Association, Mar '98*

"Recommended for public libraries."
— *American Reference Books Annual, 1998*

SEE ALSO *Breastfeeding Sourcebook, Congenital Disorders Sourcebook, Family Planning Sourcebook*

∎

Prostate & Urological Disorders Sourcebook

Basic Consumer Health Information about Urogenital and Sexual Disorders in Men, Including Prostate and Other Andrological Cancers, Prostatitis, Benign Prostatic Hyperplasia, Testicular and Penile Trauma, Cryptorchidism, Peyronie Disease, Erectile Dysfunction, and Male Factor Infertility, and Facts about Commonly Used Tests and Procedures, Such as Prostatectomy, Vasectomy, Vasectomy Reversal, Penile Implants, and Semen Analysis

Along with a Glossary of Andrological Terms and a Directory of Resources for Additional Information

Edited by Karen Bellenir. 631 pages. 2005. 978-0-7808-0797-6.

Prostate Cancer Sourcebook

Basic Consumer Health Information about Prostate Cancer, Including Information about the Associated Risk Factors, Detection, Diagnosis, and Treatment of Prostate Cancer

Along with Information on Non-Malignant Prostate Conditions, and Featuring a Section Listing Support and Treatment Centers and a Glossary of Related Terms

Edited by Dawn D. Matthews. 358 pages. 2001. 978-0-7808-0324-4.

"Recommended reference source."
— *Booklist, American Library Association, Jan '02*

"A valuable resource for health care consumers seeking information on the subject. . . . All text is written in a clear, easy-to-understand language that avoids technical jargon. Any library that collects consumer health resources would strengthen their collection with the addition of the *Prostate Cancer Sourcebook*."
— *American Reference Books Annual, 2002*

SEE ALSO *Men's Health Concerns Sourcebook*

∎

Reconstructive & Cosmetic Surgery Sourcebook

Basic Consumer Health Information on Cosmetic and Reconstructive Plastic Surgery, Including Statistical Information about Different Surgical Procedures, Things to Consider Prior to Surgery, Plastic Surgery Techniques and Tools, Emotional and Psychological Considerations, and Procedure-Specific Information

Along with a Glossary of Terms and a Listing of Resources for Additional Help and Information

Edited by M. Lisa Weatherford. 374 pages. 2001. 978-0-7808-0214-8.

"An excellent reference that addresses cosmetic and medically necessary reconstructive surgeries. . . . The style of the prose is calm and reassuring, discussing the many positive outcomes now available due to advances in surgical techniques."
— *American Reference Books Annual, 2002*

"Recommended for health science libraries that are open to the public, as well as hospital libraries that are open to the patients. This book is a good resource for the consumer interested in plastic surgery."
— *E-Streams, Dec '01*

"Recommended reference source."
— *Booklist, American Library Association, Jul '01*

∎

Rehabilitation Sourcebook

Basic Consumer Health Information about Rehabilitation for People Recovering from Heart Surgery, Spinal Cord Injury, Stroke, Orthopedic Impairments, Amputation, Pulmonary Impairments, Traumatic Injury, and More, Including Physical Therapy, Occupational Therapy, Speech/Language Therapy, Massage Therapy, Dance Therapy, Art Therapy, and Recreational Therapy

Along with Information on Assistive and Adaptive Devices, a Glossary, and Resources for Additional Help and Information

Edited by Dawn D. Matthews. 531 pages. 1999. 978-0-7808-0236-0.

"This is an excellent resource for public library reference and health collections."
— American Reference Books Annual, 2001

"Recommended reference source."
— Booklist, American Library Association, May '00

■

Respiratory Diseases & Disorders Sourcebook

Basic Information about Respiratory Diseases and Disorders, Including Asthma, Cystic Fibrosis, Pneumonia, the Common Cold, Influenza, and Others, Featuring Facts about the Respiratory System, Statistical and Demographic Data, Treatments, Self-Help Management Suggestions, and Current Research Initiatives

Edited by Allan R. Cook and Peter D. Dresser. 771 pages. 1995. 978-0-7808-0037-3.

"Designed for the layperson and for patients and their families coping with respiratory illness. . . . an extensive array of information on diagnosis, treatment, management, and prevention of respiratory illnesses for the general reader." — Choice, Association of College & Research Libraries, Jun '96

"A highly recommended text for all collections. It is a comforting reminder of the power of knowledge that good books carry between their covers."
— Academic Library Book Review, Spring '96

"A comprehensive collection of authoritative information presented in a nontechnical, humanitarian style for patients, families, and caregivers."
— Association of Operating Room Nurses, Sep/Oct '95

SEE ALSO *Lung Disorders Sourcebook*

■

Sexually Transmitted Diseases Sourcebook, 3rd Edition

Basic Consumer Health Information about Chlamydial Infections, Gonorrhea, Hepatitis, Herpes, HIV/AIDS, Human Papillomavirus, Pubic Lice, Scabies, Syphilis, Trichomoniasis, Vaginal Infections, and Other Sexually Transmitted Diseases, Including Facts about Risk Factors, Symptoms, Diagnosis, Treatment, and the Prevention of Sexually Transmitted Infections

Along with Updates on Current Research Initiatives, a Glossary of Related Terms, and Resources for Additional Help and Information

Edited by Amy L. Sutton. 629 pages. 2006. 978-0-7808-0824-9.

"Recommended for consumer health collections in public libraries, and secondary school and community college libraries."
— American Reference Books Annual, 2002

"Every school and public library should have a copy of this comprehensive and user-friendly reference book."
— Choice, Association of College & Research Libraries, Sep '01

"This is a highly recommended book. This is an especially important book for all school and public libraries."
— AIDS Book Review Journal, Jul-Aug '01

"Recommended reference source."
— Booklist, American Library Association, Apr '01

■

Sleep Disorders Sourcebook, 2nd Edition

Basic Consumer Health Information about Sleep and Sleep Disorders, Including Insomnia, Sleep Apnea, Restless Legs Syndrome, Narcolepsy, Parasomnias, and Other Health Problems That Affect Sleep, Plus Facts about Diagnostic Procedures, Treatment Strategies, Sleep Medications, and Tips for Improving Sleep Quality

Along with a Glossary of Related Terms and Resources for Additional Help and Information

Edited by Amy L. Sutton. 567 pages. 2005. 978-0-7808-0743-3.

"This book will be useful for just about everybody, especially the 40 million Americans with sleep disorders."
— American Reference Books Annual, 2006

"Recommended for public libraries and libraries supporting health care professionals." — E-Streams, Sep '05

". . . key medical library acquisition."
— The Bookwatch, Jun '05

■

Smoking Concerns Sourcebook

Basic Consumer Health Information about Nicotine Addiction and Smoking Cessation, Featuring Facts about the Health Effects of Tobacco Use, Including Lung and Other Cancers, Heart Disease, Stroke, and Respiratory Disorders, Such as Emphysema and Chronic Bronchitis

Along with Information about Smoking Prevention Programs, Suggestions for Achieving and Maintaining a Smoke-Free Lifestyle, Statistics about Tobacco Use, Reports on Current Research Initiatives, a Glossary of Related Terms, and Directories of Resources for Additional Help and Information

Edited by Karen Bellenir. 621 pages. 2004. 978-0-7808-0323-7.

"Provides everything needed for the student or general reader seeking practical details on the effects of tobacco use." — The Bookwatch, Mar '05

"Public libraries and consumer health care libraries will find this work useful."
— American Reference Books Annual, 2005

Sports Injuries Sourcebook, 3rd Edition

Basic Consumer Health Information about Sprains and Strains, Fractures, Growth Plate Injuries, Overtraining Injuries, and Injuries to the Head, Face, Shoulders, Elbows, Hands, Spinal Column, Knees, Ankles, and Feet, and with Facts about Heat-Related Illness, Steroids and Sport Supplements, Protective Equipment, Diagnostic Procedures, Treatment Options, and Rehabilitation

Along with a Glossary of Related Terms and a Directory of Resources for Additional Help and Information

Edited by Sandra J. Judd. 651 pages. 2007. 978-0-7808-0949-9.

"This is an excellent reference for consumers and it is recommended for public, community college, and undergraduate libraries."
— *American Reference Books Annual, 2003*

"Recommended reference source."
— *Booklist, American Library Association, Feb '03*

■

Stress-Related Disorders Sourcebook

Basic Consumer Health Information about Stress and Stress-Related Disorders, Including Stress Origins and Signals, Environmental Stress at Work and Home, Mental and Emotional Stress Associated with Depression, Post-Traumatic Stress Disorder, Panic Disorder, Suicide, and the Physical Effects of Stress on the Cardiovascular, Immune, and Nervous Systems

Along with Stress Management Techniques, a Glossary, and a Listing of Additional Resources

Edited by Joyce Brennfleck Shannon. 610 pages. 2002. 978-0-7808-0560-6.

"Well written for a general readership, the *Stress-Related Disorders Sourcebook* is a useful addition to the health reference literature."
— *American Reference Books Annual, 2003*

"I am impressed by the amount of information. It offers a thorough overview of the causes and consequences of stress for the layperson. . . . A well-done and thorough reference guide for professionals and nonprofessionals alike."
— *Doody's Review Service, Dec '02*

■

Stroke Sourcebook

Basic Consumer Health Information about Stroke, Including Ischemic, Hemorrhagic, Transient Ischemic Attack (TIA), and Pediatric Stroke, Stroke Triggers and Risks, Diagnostic Tests, Treatments, and Rehabilitation Information

Along with Stroke Prevention Guidelines, Legal and Financial Information, a Glossary, and a Directory of Additional Resources

Edited by Joyce Brennfleck Shannon. 606 pages. 2003. 978-0-7808-0630-6.

"This volume is highly recommended and should be in every medical, hospital, and public library."
— *American Reference Books Annual, 2004*

"Highly recommended for the amount and variety of topics and information covered." — *Choice, Nov '03*

■

Surgery Sourcebook

Basic Consumer Health Information about Inpatient and Outpatient Surgeries, Including Cardiac, Vascular, Orthopedic, Ocular, Reconstructive, Cosmetic, Gynecologic, and Ear, Nose, and Throat Procedures and More

Along with Information about Operating Room Policies and Instruments, Laser Surgery Techniques, Hospital Errors, Statistical Data, a Glossary, and Listings of Sources for Further Help and Information

Edited by Annemarie S. Muth and Karen Bellenir. 596 pages. 2002. 978-0-7808-0380-0.

"Large public libraries and medical libraries would benefit from this material in their reference collections."
— *American Reference Books Annual, 2004*

"Invaluable reference for public and school library collections alike." — *Library Bookwatch, Apr '03*

■

Thyroid Disorders Sourcebook

Basic Consumer Health Information about Disorders of the Thyroid and Parathyroid Glands, Including Hypothyroidism, Hyperthyroidism, Graves Disease, Hashimoto Thyroiditis, Thyroid Cancer, and Parathyroid Disorders, Featuring Facts about Symptoms, Risk Factors, Tests, and Treatments

Along with Information about the Effects of Thyroid Imbalance on Other Body Systems, Environmental Factors That Affect the Thyroid Gland, a Glossary, and a Directory of Additional Resources

Edited by Joyce Brennfleck Shannon. 599 pages. 2005. 978-0-7808-0745-7.

"Recommended for consumer health collections."
— *American Reference Books Annual, 2006*

"Highly recommended pick for basic consumer health reference holdings at all levels."
— *The Bookwatch, Aug '05*

■

Transplantation Sourcebook

Basic Consumer Health Information about Organ and Tissue Transplantation, Including Physical and Financial Preparations, Procedures and Issues Relating to Specific Solid Organ and Tissue Transplants, Rehabilitation, Pediatric Transplant Information, the Future of Transplantation, and Organ and Tissue Donation

Along with a Glossary and Listings of Additional Resources

Edited by Joyce Brennfleck Shannon. 628 pages. 2002. 978-0-7808-0322-0.

"Along with these advances [in transplantation technology] have come a number of daunting questions for potential transplant patients, their families, and their health care providers. This reference text is the best single tool to address many of these questions. . . . It will be a much-needed addition to the reference collections in health care, academic, and large public libraries."
— *American Reference Books Annual, 2003*

"Recommended for libraries with an interest in offering consumer health information." — *E-Streams, Jul '02*

"This is a unique and valuable resource for patients facing transplantation and their families."
— *Doody's Review Service, Jun '02*

■

Traveler's Health Sourcebook

Basic Consumer Health Information for Travelers, Including Physical and Medical Preparations, Transportation Health and Safety, Essential Information about Food and Water, Sun Exposure, Insect and Snake Bites, Camping and Wilderness Medicine, and Travel with Physical or Medical Disabilities

Along with International Travel Tips, Vaccination Recommendations, Geographical Health Issues, Disease Risks, a Glossary, and a Listing of Additional Resources

Edited by Joyce Brennfleck Shannon. 613 pages. 2000. 978-0-7808-0384-8.

"Recommended reference source."
— *Booklist, American Library Association, Feb '01*

"This book is recommended for any public library, any travel collection, and especially any collection for the physically disabled."
— *American Reference Books Annual, 2001*

SEE ALSO Worldwide Health Sourcebook

■

Urinary Tract & Kidney Diseases & Disorders Sourcebook, 2nd Edition

Basic Consumer Health Information about the Urinary System, Including the Bladder, Urethra, Ureters, and Kidneys, with Facts about Urinary Tract Infections, Incontinence, Congenital Disorders, Kidney Stones, Cancers of the Urinary Tract and Kidneys, Kidney Failure, Dialysis, and Kidney Transplantation

Along with Statistical and Demographic Information, Reports on Current Research in Kidney and Urologic Health, a Summary of Commonly Used Diagnostic Tests, a Glossary of Related Terms, and a Directory of Resources for Additional Help and Information

Edited by Ivy L. Alexander. 649 pages. 2005. 978-0-7808-0750-1.

"A good choice for a consumer health information library or for a medical library needing information to refer to their patients."
— *American Reference Books Annual, 2006*

Vegetarian Sourcebook

Basic Consumer Health Information about Vegetarian Diets, Lifestyle, and Philosophy, Including Definitions of Vegetarianism and Veganism, Tips about Adopting Vegetarianism, Creating a Vegetarian Pantry, and Meeting Nutritional Needs of Vegetarians, with Facts Regarding Vegetarianism's Effect on Pregnant and Lactating Women, Children, Athletes, and Senior Citizens

Along with a Glossary of Commonly Used Vegetarian Terms and Resources for Additional Help and Information

Edited by Chad T. Kimball. 360 pages. 2002. 978-0-7808-0439-5.

"Organizes into one concise volume the answers to the most common questions concerning vegetarian diets and lifestyles. This title is recommended for public and secondary school libraries." — *E-Streams, Apr '03*

"Invaluable reference for public and school library collections alike." — *Library Bookwatch, Apr '03*

"The articles in this volume are easy to read and come from authoritative sources. The book does not necessarily support the vegetarian diet but instead provides the pros and cons of this important decision. The Vegetarian Sourcebook is recommended for public libraries and consumer health libraries."
— *American Reference Books Annual, 2003*

SEE ALSO Diet & Nutrition Sourcebook

■

Women's Health Concerns Sourcebook, 2nd Edition

Basic Consumer Health Information about the Medical and Mental Concerns of Women, Including Maintaining Health and Wellness, Gynecological Concerns, Breast Health, Sexuality and Reproductive Issues, Menopause, Cancer in Women, Leading Causes of Death and Disability among Women, Physical Concerns of Special Significance to Women, and Women's Mental and Emotional Health

Along with a Glossary of Related Terms and Directories of Resources for Additional Help and Information

Edited by Amy L. Sutton. 746 pages. 2004. 978-0-7808-0673-3.

"This is a useful reference book, which makes the reader knowledgeable about several issues that concern women's health. It is recommended for public libraries and home library collections." — *E-Streams, May '05*

"A useful addition to public and consumer health library collections."
— *American Reference Books Annual, 2005*

"A highly recommended title."
— *The Bookwatch, May '04*

"Handy compilation. There is an impressive range of diseases, devices, disorders, procedures, and other physical and emotional issues covered . . . well organized, illustrated, and indexed." — *Choice, Association of College & Research Libraries, Jan '98*

SEE ALSO *Breast Cancer Sourcebook, Cancer Sourcebook for Women, Healthy Heart Sourcebook for Women, Osteoporosis Sourcebook*

■

Workplace Health & Safety Sourcebook

Basic Consumer Health Information about Workplace Health and Safety, Including the Effect of Workplace Hazards on the Lungs, Skin, Heart, Ears, Eyes, Brain, Reproductive Organs, Musculoskeletal System, and Other Organs and Body Parts

Along with Information about Occupational Cancer, Personal Protective Equipment, Toxic and Hazardous Chemicals, Child Labor, Stress, and Workplace Violence

Edited by Chad T. Kimball. 626 pages. 2000. 978-0-7808-0231-5.

"As a reference for the general public, this would be useful in any library." —*E-Streams, Jun '01*

"Provides helpful information for primary care physicians and other caregivers interested in occupational medicine. . . . General readers; professionals."
—*Choice, Association of College & Research Libraries, May '01*

"Recommended reference source."
—*Booklist, American Library Association, Feb '01*

"Highly recommended." —*The Bookwatch, Jan '01*

■

Worldwide Health Sourcebook

Basic Information about Global Health Issues, Including Malnutrition, Reproductive Health, Disease Dispersion and Prevention, Emerging Diseases, Risky Health Behaviors, and the Leading Causes of Death

Along with Global Health Concerns for Children, Women, and the Elderly, Mental Health Issues, Research and Technology Advancements, and Economic, Environmental, and Political Health Implications, a Glossary, and a Resource Listing for Additional Help and Information

Edited by Joyce Brennfleck Shannon. 614 pages. 2001. 978-0-7808-0330-5.

"Named an Outstanding Academic Title."
—*Choice, Association of College & Research Libraries, Jan '02*

"Yet another handy but also unique compilation in the extensive *Health Reference Series*, this is a useful work because many of the international publications reprinted or excerpted are not readily available. Highly recommended." —*Choice, Association of College & Research Libraries, Nov '01*

"Recommended reference source."
—*Booklist, American Library Association, Oct '01*

SEE ALSO *Traveler's Health Sourcebook*

Teen Health Series
Helping Young Adults Understand, Manage, and Avoid Serious Illness

List price $65 per volume. **School and library price $58 per volume.**

Alcohol Information for Teens
Health Tips about Alcohol and Alcoholism

Including Facts about Underage Drinking, Preventing Teen Alcohol Use, Alcohol's Effects on the Brain and the Body, Alcohol Abuse Treatment, Help for Children of Alcoholics, and More

Edited by Joyce Brennfleck Shannon. 370 pages. 2005. 978-0-7808-0741-9.

"Boxed facts and tips add visual interest to the well-researched and clearly written text."
— *Curriculum Connection, Apr '06*

Allergy Information for Teens
Health Tips about Allergic Reactions Such as Anaphylaxis, Respiratory Problems, and Rashes

Including Facts about Identifying and Managing Allergies to Food, Pollen, Mold, Animals, Chemicals, Drugs, and Other Substances

Edited by Karen Bellenir. 410 pages. 2006. 978-0-7808-0799-0.

Asthma Information for Teens
Health Tips about Managing Asthma and Related Concerns

Including Facts about Asthma Causes, Triggers, Symptoms, Diagnosis, and Treatment

Edited by Karen Bellenir. 386 pages. 2005. 978-0-7808-0770-9.

"Highly recommended for medical libraries, public school libraries, and public libraries."
— *American Reference Books Annual, 2006*

"It is so clearly written and well organized that even hesitant readers will be able to find the facts they need, whether for reports or personal information. . . . A succinct but complete resource."
— *School Library Journal, Sep '05*

Body Information for Teens
Health Tips about Maintaining Well-Being for a Lifetime

Including Facts about the Development and Functioning of the Body's Systems, Organs, and Structures and the Health Impact of Lifestyle Choices

Edited by Sandra Augustyn Lawton. 458 pages. 2007. 978-0-7808-0443-2.

Cancer Information for Teens
Health Tips about Cancer Awareness, Prevention, Diagnosis, and Treatment

Including Facts about Frequently Occurring Cancers, Cancer Risk Factors, and Coping Strategies for Teens Fighting Cancer or Dealing with Cancer in Friends or Family Members

Edited by Wilma R. Caldwell. 428 pages. 2004. 978-0-7808-0678-8.

"Recommended for school libraries, or consumer libraries that see a lot of use by teens."
— *E-Streams, May '05*

"A valuable educational tool."
— *American Reference Books Annual, 2005*

"Young adults and their parents alike will find this new addition to the *Teen Health Series* an important reference to cancer in teens."
— *Children's Bookwatch, Feb '05*

Complementary and Alternative Medicine Information for Teens
Health Tips about Non-Traditional and Non-Western Medical Practices

Including Information about Acupuncture, Chiropractic Medicine, Dietary and Herbal Supplements, Hypnosis, Massage Therapy, Prayer and Spirituality, Reflexology, Yoga, and More

Edited by Sandra Augustyn Lawton. 405 pages. 2006. 978-0-7808-0966-6.

Diabetes Information for Teens
Health Tips about Managing Diabetes and Preventing Related Complications

Including Information about Insulin, Glucose Control, Healthy Eating, Physical Activity, and Learning to Live with Diabetes

Edited by Sandra Augustyn Lawton. 410 pages. 2006. 978-0-7808-0811-9.

Diet Information for Teens, 2nd Edition

Health Tips about Diet and Nutrition

Including Facts about Dietary Guidelines, Food Groups, Nutrients, Healthy Meals, Snacks, Weight Control, Medical Concerns Related to Diet, and More

Edited by Karen Bellenir. 432 pages. 2006. 978-0-7808-0820-1.

"Full of helpful insights and facts throughout the book. ... An excellent resource to be placed in public libraries or even in personal collections."
— *American Reference Books Annual, 2002*

"Recommended for middle and high school libraries and media centers as well as academic libraries that educate future teachers of teenagers. It is also a suitable addition to health science libraries that serve patrons who are interested in teen health promotion and education." — *E-Streams, Oct '01*

"This comprehensive book would be beneficial to collections that need information about nutrition, dietary guidelines, meal planning, and weight control. ... This reference is so easy to use that its purchase is recommended." — *The Book Report, Sep-Oct '01*

"This book is written in an easy to understand format describing issues that many teens face every day, and then provides thoughtful explanations so that teens can make informed decisions. This is an interesting book that provides important facts and information for today's teens." — *Doody's Health Sciences Book Review Journal, Jul-Aug '01*

"A comprehensive compendium of diet and nutrition. The information is presented in a straightforward, plain-spoken manner. This title will be useful to those working on reports on a variety of topics, as well as to general readers concerned about their dietary health."
— *School Library Journal, Jun '01*

Drug Information for Teens, 2nd Edition

Health Tips about the Physical and Mental Effects of Substance Abuse

Including Information about Marijuana, Inhalants, Club Drugs, Stimulants, Hallucinogens, Opiates, Prescription and Over-the-Counter Drugs, Herbal Products, Tobacco, Alcohol, and More

Edited by Sandra Augustyn Lawton. 468 pages. 2006. 978-0-7808-0862-1.

"A clearly written resource for general readers and researchers alike." — *School Library Journal*

"This book is well-balanced. ... a must for public and school libraries."
— *VOYA: Voice of Youth Advocates, Dec '03*

"The chapters are quick to make a connection to their teenage reading audience. The prose is straightforward and the book lends itself to spot reading. It should be useful both for practical information and for research, and it is suitable for public and school libraries."
— *American Reference Books Annual, 2003*

"Recommended reference source."
— *Booklist, American Library Association, Feb '03*

"This is an excellent resource for teens and their parents. Education about drugs and substances is key to discouraging teen drug abuse and this book provides this much needed information in a way that is interesting and factual." — *Doody's Review Service, Dec '02*

Eating Disorders Information for Teens

Health Tips about Anorexia, Bulimia, Binge Eating, and Other Eating Disorders

Including Information on the Causes, Prevention, and Treatment of Eating Disorders, and Such Other Issues as Maintaining Healthy Eating and Exercise Habits

Edited by Sandra Augustyn Lawton. 337 pages. 2005. 978-0-7808-0783-9.

"An excellent resource for teens and those who work with them."
— *VOYA: Voice of Youth Advocates, Apr '06*

"A welcome addition to high school and undergraduate libraries." — *American Reference Books Annual, 2006*

"This book covers the topic in a lucid manner but delves deeper into every aspect of an eating disorder. A solid addition for any nonfiction or reference collection." — *School Library Journal, Dec '05*

Fitness Information for Teens

Health Tips about Exercise, Physical Well-Being, and Health Maintenance

Including Facts about Aerobic and Anaerobic Conditioning, Stretching, Body Shape and Body Image, Sports Training, Nutrition, and Activities for Non-Athletes

Edited by Karen Bellenir. 425 pages. 2004. 978-0-7808-0679-5.

"Another excellent offering from Omnigraphics in their *Teen Health Series.* ... This book will be a great addition to any public, junior high, senior high, or secondary school library."
— *American Reference Books Annual, 2005*

Learning Disabilities Information for Teens

Health Tips about Academic Skills Disorders and Other Disabilities That Affect Learning

Including Information about Common Signs of Learning Disabilities, School Issues, Learning to Live with a Learning Disability, and Other Related Issues

Edited by Sandra Augustyn Lawton. 337 pages. 2005. 978-0-7808-0796-9.

"This book provides a wealth of information for any reader interested in the signs, causes, and consequences

of learning disabilities, as well as related legal rights and educational interventions. . . . Public and academic libraries should want this title for both students and general readers."
— *American Reference Books Annual, 2006*

Mental Health Information for Teens, 2nd Edition
Health Tips about Mental Wellness and Mental Illness

Including Facts about Mental and Emotional Health, Depression and Other Mood Disorders, Anxiety Disorders, Behavior Disorders, Self-Injury, Psychosis, Schizophrenia, and More

Edited by Karen Bellenir. 400 pages. 2006. 978-0-7808-0863-8.

"In both language and approach, this user-friendly entry in the *Teen Health Series* is on target for teens needing information on mental health concerns."
— *Booklist, American Library Association, Jan '02*

"Readers will find the material accessible and informative, with the shaded notes, facts, and embedded glossary insets adding appropriately to the already interesting and succinct presentation."
— *School Library Journal, Jan '02*

"This title is highly recommended for any library that serves adolescents and parents/caregivers of adolescents." — *E-Streams, Jan '02*

"Recommended for high school libraries and young adult collections in public libraries. Both health professionals and teenagers will find this book useful."
— *American Reference Books Annual, 2002*

"This is a nice book written to enlighten the society, primarily teenagers, about common teen mental health issues. It is highly recommended to teachers and parents as well as adolescents."
— *Doody's Review Service, Dec '01*

Sexual Health Information for Teens
Health Tips about Sexual Development, Human Reproduction, and Sexually Transmitted Diseases

Including Facts about Puberty, Reproductive Health, Chlamydia, Human Papillomavirus, Pelvic Inflammatory Disease, Herpes, AIDS, Contraception, Pregnancy, and More

Edited by Deborah A. Stanley. 391 pages. 2003. 978-0-7808-0445-6.

"This work should be included in all high school libraries and many larger public libraries. . . . highly recommended."
— *American Reference Books Annual, 2004*

"*Sexual Health* approaches its subject with appropriate seriousness and offers easily accessible advice and information." — *School Library Journal, Feb '04*

Skin Health Information for Teens
Health Tips about Dermatological Concerns and Skin Cancer Risks

Including Facts about Acne, Warts, Hives, and Other Conditions and Lifestyle Choices, Such as Tanning, Tattooing, and Piercing, That Affect the Skin, Nails, Scalp, and Hair

Edited by Robert Aquinas McNally. 429 pages. 2003. 978-0-7808-0446-3.

"This volume, as with others in the series, will be a useful addition to school and public library collections." — *American Reference Books Annual, 2004*

"There is no doubt that this reference tool is valuable."
— *VOYA: Voice of Youth Advocates, Feb '04*

"This volume serves as a one-stop source and should be a necessity for any health collection."
— *Library Media Connection*

Sports Injuries Information for Teens
Health Tips about Sports Injuries and Injury Protection

Including Facts about Specific Injuries, Emergency Treatment, Rehabilitation, Sports Safety, Competition Stress, Fitness, Sports Nutrition, Steroid Risks, and More

Edited by Joyce Brennfleck Shannon. 405 pages. 2003. 978-0-7808-0447-0.

"This work will be useful in the young adult collections of public libraries as well as high school libraries."
— *American Reference Books Annual, 2004*

Suicide Information for Teens
Health Tips about Suicide Causes and Prevention

Including Facts about Depression, Risk Factors, Getting Help, Survivor Support, and More

Edited by Joyce Brennfleck Shannon. 368 pages. 2005. 978-0-7808-0737-2.

Tobacco Information for Teens
Health Tips about the Hazards of Using Cigarettes, Smokeless Tobacco, and Other Nicotine Products

Including Facts about Nicotine Addiction, Immediate and Long-Term Health Effects of Tobacco Use, Related Cancers, Smoking Cessation, Tobacco Use Prevention, and Tobacco Use Statistics

Edited by Karen Bellenir. 440 pages. 2007. 978-0-7808-0976-5.

UMDNJ-SMITH LIBRARY

30 12th Avenue

Newark, NJ 07103

Health Reference Series